T0248897

Immunology Handbook

Immunology Handbook

Edited by **Jim Wang**

FOSTER
ACADEMICS

New Jersey

Published by Foster Academics,
61 Van Reypen Street,
Jersey City, NJ 07306, USA
www.fosteracademics.com

Immunology Handbook
Edited by Jim Wang

International Standard Book Number: 978-1-63242-240-8 (Hardback)

Printed in the United States of America.

Contents

Preface

I am honored to present to you this unique book which encompasses the most up-to-date data in the field. I was extremely pleased to get this opportunity of editing the work of experts from across the globe. I have also written papers in this field and researched the various aspects revolving around the progress of the discipline. I have tried to unify my knowledge along with that of stalwarts from every corner of the world, to produce a text which not only benefits the readers but also facilitates the growth of the field.

This book provides information on immunology, which is a branch of biomedical sciences to study the immune system physiology in both diseased and healthy states. Some aspects of autoimmunity enable us to understand that it is not always related to pathology. For example, autoimmune reactions are effective in clearing off the unwanted, excess or aged tissues from the body. Also, autoimmunity occurs after the exposure the non-self-antigen which is structurally similar to the self, assisted by the stimulatory molecules such as cytokines. Therefore, it can be said that there's a minor difference between immunity and auto-immunity. The question of how physiologic immunity changes to pathologic autoimmunity continue to interest researchers. Answer to such questions can be found by understanding physiology of the immune system. This book covers various topics organized under two sections: Nutrition & Immunology and Parasite Immunology. The contributors of this book have carefully selected topics which would be of reader's interests.

Finally, I would like to thank all the contributing authors for their valuable time and contributions. This book would not have been possible without their efforts. I would also like to thank my friends and family for their constant support.

Editor

Section 1

Nutrition and Immunology

Innate Immune Responses in the Geriatric Population

Nathalie Compté and Stanislas Goriely
Institute for Medical Immunology,
Université Libre de Bruxelles
Belgium

1. Introduction

Demographic evolution represents a challenge for public health. Global population, especially in the developed countries is aging. The proportion of the population above 60 years has increased from 8% in 1950 to 10% in 2000 and is expected to reach 21% by 2050. Older people suffer from more frequent and more severe community-acquired and nosocomial infections than younger people. The clinical presentation is often atypical making diagnostic more difficult. "Latent" intracellular pathogens such as viruses (Herpesviridae) or Mycobacteriae are more prone to reactivate while opportunistic infections (such as Candida) manifest at increased rates (Ongradi & Kovesdi, 2010). Older individuals suffer from reactivation of mycobacterium tuberculosis that counts for 15 percent of all geriatric pulmonary infections. There is also an age-related decline in the magnitude of the responses to vaccination. Low-level chronic inflammation, a process referred to as "inflamm-aging", is commonly observed in older people. It results in both decreased immunity to exogenous antigens and increased autoreactivity. It is well documented that a significant fraction of older people are positive for low affinity autoantibodies without clinical significance. Rheumatoid factors are present in up to 5% of young healthy individuals, a proportion that increases up to five times in older persons. Similarly, the prevalence of antinuclear antibodies is higher in healthy individuals over 70 years of age compared to healthy young adults (Grolleau-Julius et al., 2010). Furthermore, older persons are more susceptible to develop cancer, probably because of accumulation of cell damages and reduced "immunosurveillance"(Malaguarnera et al., 2010; Fulop et al., 2010).

There is clear evidence of an age-related decline in effectiveness of the immune system in humans; it is common to most if not all vertebrates and to some invertebrates. For example, drosophilae display pro-inflammatory status with increasing age and have reduced capacity to produce antimicrobial peptides in response to infection. There is also substantial body of evidence reporting immunosenescence in wild birds (decline of T- and B-cell functions and altered innate immune responses) and mice (thymic atrophy and reduced recent thymic emigrants) (Shanley et al., 2009). Immunosenescence is characterized by the deleterious "filling" of the immunological space with memory and effector cells as a consequence of exposure to a variety of antigens. The continuous attrition caused by clinical and subclinical infections as well as the continuous exposure to other types of antigens (food, allergens) is likely to be responsible for the chronic activation of the immune system and inflammation. Immunosenescence process along with morbidity and mortality will be accelerated in those subjects who are exposed to an extra-burden of antigenic load. The phenomenology of HIV+ patients after several years of infection shows striking similarities (regarding T cell subset rearrangement, T cell clonal expansion, and telomere shortening) with that observed in the context of aging. It is tempting to speculate that chronic infections with other micro-organisms could also lead to this process (De Martinis et al., 2005).

Many studies have tried to collect immune data in older people to establish reliable "biomarkers of aging". However, the literature is full of confusing and conflicting data. There are many difficulties in interpreting immunogerontological observations. The major concern is the way "young" and "old" populations are defined in these studies. On one hand, restricting selection to only "healthy" older people might introduce a bias and not be representative of the general population. On the other hand, comorbidities that are encountered in the geriatric population will certainly affect many parameters of the immune responses. Some studies try to restrict inclusion criteria to better characterize age-associated alterations of immunity such as the SENIEUR protocol (Wikby, 2008; Chen et al., 2009; Ligthart et al., 1984). Unfortunately, it does not represent our geriatric population (only 10% of older people meet the criteria) (Chen et al., 2009). OCTO study was less restrictive for inclusion criteria, admitted 400 octogenarians that were not institutionalized, had no or only mild cognitive dysfunction and were not on drug regimen that might have influenced the immune system. This study predicts the same **immune risk profile (IRP)** of subsequent 2 year-mortality than SENIEUR protocols characterized by high level of CD8 T cells, inversion of the CD4+/CD8+ T cell ratio, poor mitogen stimulated lymphoproliferative responses and loss of CD28 costimulatory molecule (table 1).

Immune Risk Phenotype (IRP)

- Low levels of B cells
- Inversion of the CD4+/CD8+ ratio
- Poor mitogen stimulated lymphoproliferative response
- Increased levels of CD8+ CD28- CD57+ T cells
- Positive serology for Cytomegalovirus

Table 1. The "immune risk phenotype".

Finally, the NONA study did not exclude individuals because of compromised health to place immune risk phenotype in a broader context of health and cognitive dysfunctioning. It confirmed the OCTO study and demonstrated that the immune risk phenotype concept could be generalized to a sample of nonagenarians not specifically selected for good health at baseline (Pawelec et al., 2005; Wikby, 2008). Both studies demonstrated that aging is associated with low-grade inflammation and that inflammatory markers like increase of IL-6, C-reactive protein (CRP) and decrease of albumin are significant predictors of mortality in very old humans independently of disease and comorbidity (Wikby, 2008). The new HEXA study examined the IRP profile in hexagenarians and shows the same characteristics than in the very old. The study has now to examine the impact of the IRP on morbidity and mortality in this age group (Wills et al., 2011).

Herein, we will first review the major changes in adaptive immune responses observed in the geriatric population. We will then focus on what is known about innate immune responses in this age group. Finally, we will discuss the links between the specific clinical context of aging and alterations of immune responses.

2. Adaptative immune responses: thymic involution, T cell exhaustion and persistent infections

2.1 Thymic involution

The thymus is the site of T cells differentiation and maturation and is often referred to as the "immunologic clock" of aging. Age-associated thymic involution is a well-recognized factor associated with immunosenescence, and in particular with reduced vaccine efficacy. The thymus undergoes a progressive involution and the output of new cells falls significantly. Thymic functions already start decreasing after one year of life but the process becomes significant after 40 years of age. The expansion of perivascular space (adipocytes, peripheral lymphocytes, stroma) with age is such that thymic epithelial space represents less than 10% of the total thymic tissue by 70 years of age. When extrapolated, data suggest that the thymus would cease to produce new T cells by 105 years of age (Boren & Gershwin, 2004; Ongradi & Kovesdi, 2010; Gruver et al., 2007). There might be a benefit for the organism to reduce cell proliferation within the thymus, once a T-cell repertoire is established, so that energy can be devoted to other physiological processes (Shanley et al., 2009). Both intrinsic and extrinsic factors are thought to be involved in this process (Boren & Gershwin, 2004). Thymic epithelial cells produce a number of factors that can be thymosuppressive (Interleukin (IL)-6, LIF, OSM) or thymostimulatory (interleukin (IL)-7, Keratinocyte growth factor, Thymic stromal lymphopoïetin, growth hormone, leptin). Thymic atrophy is mediated by upregulation of thymosuppressive and decrease of thymostimulatory cytokines such as IL-7. This cytokine plays an important role for thymus function maintenance; it promotes thymopoiesis by maintaining anti-apoptotic protein Bcl-2 and inducing V-DJ recombination (Ongradi & Kovesdi, 2010; Gruver et al., 2007). Extrathymic factors including zinc, thymulin, cathepsin L, melatonin, thyroid hormone, growth hormone also contribute to thymus function. Stressful events, such as infections, septic shock, malnutrition, pregnancy, chemotherapy or irradiation have been associated with reversible thymic involution. Exogenous administration of leptin prevents this stress-induced thymic involution in mice, suggesting possible therapeutic intervention in aged humans (McElhaney & Effros, 2009; Boren & Gershwin, 2004; Gruver et al., 2007; Gruver et al., 2009; Hick et al., 2006). However, it is unclear whether age-associated and stress-induced thymic involutions result from the same mechanisms (McElhaney & Effros, 2009; Boren & Gershwin, 2004; Gruver et al., 2007). "Thymic rejuvenation" techniques have been sought for many years. Keratinocyte growth factor, IL-7 and ghrelin are interesting candidates (McElhaney & Effros, 2009; Aspinall et al., 2007). Keratinocyte growth factor enhances IL-7 production in the thymus, promoting development and maintenance of T cells following vaccination. IL-7 treatment has been shown to increase thymic output and number of central memory T cells and improve the antibody response to influenza vaccination in aged rhesus macaques (McElhaney & Effros, 2009). Intrathymic infection with IL-10-expressing adenovirus can prevent thymocyte apoptosis induced by sepsis in mice (Ongradi & Kovesdi, 2010; Gruver et al., 2007).

Thymic involution causes a continuous drop in the output of recent thymic emigrants while homeostatic mechanisms attempt to maintain constant peripheral T cell numbers. Consistent with greater proliferative history, naïve T cells from elderly have less T cell receptor excision circle (TREC) numbers and shorter telomere length (see below) (Ferrando-Martinez et al., 2011). However, the total number of T cells shows very little decline with advancing age, except in the very old. Furthermore, the proportion of naïve and memory T cells is well maintained up to the age of 65 years. It has been postulated that the majority of naïve T cells in the adult are generated by cell division of existing T cells, rather than thymic export. The repertoire of naïve CD4 T cells is also very well maintained up to the age of 65 years. It then dramatically dwindles and is found to be severely contracted and undistinguishable from the repertoire of memory T cells at 75-80 years of age. The same phenomenon is shown for naïve CD8 T cells. IL-7 plays an essential role in controlling homeostatic proliferation of naïve CD4+ and CD8+ T cells (Ferrando-Martinez et al., 2011; Arnold et al., 2011; Naylor et al., 2005; Kilpatrick et al., 2008).

Main lymphocyte subsets
T lymphocytes cells (CD3+):
CD4+ helper T cells
CD8+ cytotoxic T cells
CD25+ Regulatory T cells
B lymphocytes cells (CD19+)
Naive B cells
Memory B cells
Plasmatocytes
Natural killer (NK) cells and NKT cells
γδ T cells

Table 2. Main lymphocyte subsets.

2.2 T lymphocytes

Memory and naïve human T cells are distinguished by their expression of members of the CD45 family surface antigens. CD45RA antigen is expressed primarily on naïve T lymphocytes and CD45RO is present on the cell surface of memory T lymphocytes (Figure 1). With normal aging, the slow turnover and long lifespan of naïve T cells are preserved but thymus output diminishes gradually and ultimately becomes insufficient to replace naïve T cells lost from the periphery. Conversely, cumulative chronic exposure to pathogens and environmental antigens promotes the accumulation of memory cells and eventually a state of "exhaustion". This phenomenon is associated with increased complication risk following viral illnesses such as influenza, respiratory syncytial virus and reactivation of herpes viruses (McElhaney & Effros, 2009; Desai et al., 2010).

In aged mice, formation of "immunological synapse" between CD4 T cells antigen presenting cells is hindered. This has been related to altered cholesterol/phospholipid ratio in lymphocyte membranes, leading to impaired T cell receptor (TCR)-dependent recruitment of signal molecules to the immunological synapse. In humans, alteration in the cholesterol/phospholipid ratio of lymphocyte membranes has also been documented and is associated with reduced proliferation rate (Arnold et al., 2011; Huber et al., 1991; Stulnig et al., 1995). With age, human and murine T cells tend to secrete less IL-2, an observation linked to important alterations in the proximal TCR signalling pathway (Boren & Gershwin, 2004; Fulop et al., 2007; Chakravarti & Abraham, 1999). Peripheral blood lymphocytes from aged individuals also display decreased NFAT expression, a key transcription factor implicated in IL-2 gene activation (Rink et al., 1998; Mysliwska et al., 1998; Wikby et al., 1994; Desai et al., 2010; DiPenta et al., 2007). However, when only "healthy older" people are considered (SENIEUR protocol), production of IL-2 was not different from that observed in younger individuals (Chen et al., 2009).

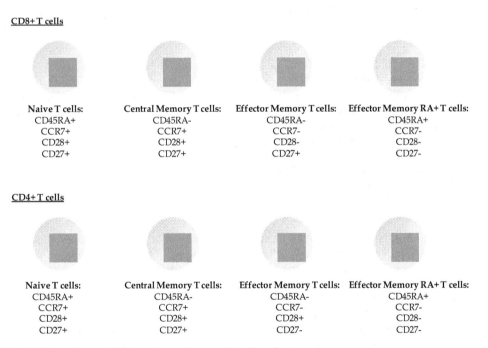

<u>CD8+ T cells</u>

Naive T cells:	Central Memory T cells:	Effector Memory T cells:	Effector Memory RA+ T cells:
CD45RA+	CD45RA-	CD45RA-	CD45RA+
CCR7+	CCR7+	CCR7-	CCR7-
CD28+	CD28+	CD28-	CD28-
CD27+	CD27+	CD27+	CD27-

<u>CD4+ T cells</u>

Naive T cells:	Central Memory T cells:	Effector Memory T cells:	Effector Memory RA+ T cells:
CD45RA+	CD45RA-	CD45RA-	CD45RA+
CCR7+	CCR7+	CCR7-	CCR7-
CD28+	CD28+	CD28+	CD28-
CD27+	CD27+	CD27-	CD27-

Fig. 1. Phenotype of different lymphocytes T cells subsets.

CD4 T lymphocytes from aged mice display decreased CD40L expression. In humans, CD40L expression is also reduced on peripheral blood CD4 T cells upon anti-CD3 stimulation in old people compared to younger individuals (Fernandez-Gutierrez et al., 1999). As this molecule is critical for B-T cell interactions, it could participate to the alteration of humoral responses observed in the old population. The function of "follicular helper T cells" in older people should be revisited in the light of the recent advances in the field (Ongradi & Kovesdi, 2010; Gruver et al., 2007; Crotty, 2011).

2.2.1 Naïve T cells

Naïve T cells from young and old adults differ significantly. Compared to young adults, 40% of human naïve CD8+ CD28+ T cells of older people do not express CD62L and CCR7, two receptors implicated in the migration to peripheral lymphoid tissues (Ongradi & Kovesdi, 2010; Aspinall et al., 2007). In humans, naïve CD8 T cells seem to be more susceptible to death receptor-mediated apoptosis and are more affected by age-related changes than the CD4+ T cell pool (Gupta & Gollapudi, 2006; Gupta & Gollapudi, 2008). CD45RA+CD28+CD8+ T cells from older people produce larger amounts of interferon (IFN)–γ upon polyclonal stimulation than those from young persons (Pfister & Savino, 2008).

As mentioned earlier, IL-7 plays an essential role in controlling homeostatic proliferation of naïve CD4+ and CD8+ T cells and supports the survival of naïve CD8+ T cells. IL-7 acts in conjunction with T cell receptor signals from contact with self-MHC/peptide that sustain the expression of anti-apoptotic molecules. However, this extended lifespan of naïve T cells could be associated with prolonged exposure to unfavourable environmental factors which cause DNA damage and contribute to decreased function in old age (Arnold et al., 2011).

2.2.2 Memory T cells

The three protocols (SENIEUR, OCTO and NONA) compared immune risk phenotype in older people with different state of comorbidities. Aging is associated with an increase of memory cells, a decrease of naïve T cells and a loss of CD28 molecules. Chronic cytomegalovirus (CMV) infection has been proposed as the main stimulus driving the *in vivo* process of "replicative senescence" (see section 4.3). CMV is associated with clonal expansion of CD8 T cells, increased numbers of CD8+ CD28- T cells, largely terminally differentiated effector memory T cells expressing CD45RA CCR7- (effector memory T cells, "EMRA") and inverted CD4:CD8 ratio (McElhaney & Effros, 2009; Pawelec & Derhovanessian, 2011; Pawelec et al., 2005; Derhovanessian et al., 2010). This will be further developed in this chapter.

Much effort has been dedicated to characterize cellular markers of immunosenescence. While T cell receptor repertoire contraction is a characteristic of the aging immune system, there is increasing evidence that clonal T cells of older persons may express a variety of receptors normally found on natural killer (NK) cells such as CD16, CD56, CD57, CD94, CD161, NKG2D and KIR family. NK receptors expression can have profound impact on immunity. Whereas, NK receptors diversity defines functional subsets of NK cells that contribute to normal innate antigen-independent responses, it is proposed that NK receptors expression on T cells from aged individuals is an adaptive mechanism of immunological diversity in the midst of a contracting T cell receptor repertoire. Studies with *in vitro* replicative senescence systems indicate stable NK receptors expression on T cells follows the loss of CD28 (Abedin et al., 2005; Alonso-Arias et al., 2011; Rajasekaran et al., 2010). Expression of CD57 is also found on T lymphocytes, where it is currently considered as a marker for "replicative senescence" (also termed "clonal exhaustion") i.e., a high susceptibility to activation-induced cell death and the inability to undergo new cell-division cycles despite preserved ability to secrete cytokines upon encounter with their cognate antigen. The phenotypes associated with replicative senescent CD8+ T lymphocytes are not well defined but are generally attributed to lack of CD28 or expression of CD57. CD8+CD57+ T lymphocytes have high cytotoxic effector potential including perforin, granzymes and granulysin. At the messenger and protein levels, CD8+CD57+T lymphocytes express more adhesion molecules and fewer chemokine receptors (CCR7 and CXCR4) than CD8+CD57– T lymphocytes but preferentially express CX3CR1. The lower expression level of genes involved in cell-cycle regulation supports the limited proliferation capacities of CD8+CD57+ T lymphocytes, even in response to polyclonal or cytokine stimulation (Focosi et al., 2010).

As detailed below, these CD8+CD57+T lymphocytes are commonly found in individuals with chronic immune activation and increase in frequency with age (from absence in newborns to 15–20% of circulating CD8 T cells), but the percentage of CD8+CD57+ cells increases in a series of clinical conditions whose common denominator is functional immune alteration, including HIV and CMV infections, common variable immunodeficiency, hematological cancers and autoimmune diseases (Pawelec & Derhovanessian, 2011; Focosi et al., 2010). OCTO, NONA and SENIEUR protocols conclude that the number of cells in the CD57+CD28-, CD45RACD27- and CD57+CD56+CD8+ T cells subsets in older people were independent of the individual's health status (disease interfering with immunity were excluded) (Nilsson et al., 2003). In older humans, CD4 T cells also express more NKG2D molecules and are associated with replicative senescence. NKG2D+ CD4+ T cells are mostly CD28- CD4+ T cells and also present cytotoxic properties (Alonso-Arias et al., 2011). These senescent cells resulting from permanent immune activation are potent producers of proinflammatory cytokines and have shorter telomeres than NKG2D- CD4+ T cells (Ongradi & Kovesdi, 2010; Gruver et al., 2007). Immune phenotype of T cells is correlated with individual "fitness" in individuals over 78 years. Unimpaired aged individuals display T cells expressing inhibitory NK receptors (CD158a, CD158e and NKG2a) and functionally impaired aged individuals display T cells expressing stimulatory NK receptors (CD56, CD16, NKG2D) (Vallejo et al., 2011).

It has been shown that high proportions of CD8+ CD25+ memory T cells are associated with healthy aging and are rare or absent in older people with latent CMV infection. The presence of CD8+CD25+ T cells is associated with the maintenance of intact humoral responses. They produce IL-2 and IL-4, assist B memory generation, induce MHC II upregulation on B cells, and promote antibody isotype switching to IgG1 and IgE. These T cells coexpress CD4 molecule and present a highly diverse TCR repertoire and longer telomere compared to the CD8+ CD25- subset (Herndler-Brandstetter et al., 2005).

Aged individuals (more than 65 years) have an increase in peripheral blood regulatory T cells expression. The increase of this population seems to be linked to the healthy state of elderly people. The *in vitro* function of this population is not altered with age (Ongradi & Kovesdi, 2010; Gruver et al., 2007; Gregg et al., 2005).

γδT cells represent a minor population of human peripheral lymphocytes (1-10%). They play a role in antiviral and antitumoral immunosurveillance. They produce high levels of cytokines, mainly TNFα and IFNγ. With increasing age, the absolute number of γδT cells and their proliferation rate is reduced while they express more TNFα. Inversely, they present no change in IFNγ expression and cytolytic activity with age (Argentati et al., 2002).

2.3 B lymphocytes and humoral responses

B cells also present alterations with increasing age. Decreased IL-7 production provokes a reduced ability to support B cell expansion by bone marrow stromal cells (Ongradi & Kovesdi, 2010). Bone marrow contains pluripotent stem cells that mature into bone tissue and cells that form peripheral blood cells, which further develop in specialized secondary compartments into functional immune cells. The stroma matrix of the bone marrow compartment is composed of accessory cells such as megakaryocytes, osteoblasts, osteoclasts, adipocytes, chondrocytes, myoblasts and fibroblasts. The hematopoietic compartment decreases with increasing age and is replaced by adipose tissue. Surprisingly, increased number of bone marrow resident macrophages is observed with age but these cells have decreased ability to secrete TNFα. Both TNFα and IL-1 are essential to promote secretion of other cytokines critical to stromal integrity, such as IL-6, IL-11, M-CSF or GM-CSF. There is no clear evidence that hematopoietic cells number (CD34+) decreases with age. Hematopoietic cells give rise into common lymphoid progenitors like pro-B cells. There are discrepancies about the evolution of pro-B cells with age. Conversely, pre-B cells decrease markedly with age (Gruver et al., 2007).

The proportion and numbers of total B cells (CD19+) decrease with age. Data on specific B cell subsets is less clear. Naïve B cells are defined as IgG- IgA- IgD+ CD27- whereas memory B cell population is very heterogeneous, comprising three subtypes (Figure2): "IgM memory" cells (that are IgD+ IgM+ CD27+, important against bacterial infections), "classical switched memory" (IgG+/IgA+ CD27+) and "double negative" B cells (IgG+/IgA+, IgD-CD27- B cells). This later group could emerge independently from T cell help.

B lymphocytes:

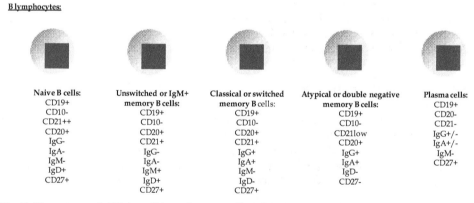

Naïve B cells:	Unswitched or IgM+ memory B cells:	Classical or switched memory B cells:	Atypical or double negative memory B cells:	Plasma cells:
CD19+	CD19+	CD19+	CD19+	CD19+
CD10-	CD10-	CD10-	CD10-	CD20-
CD21++	CD20+	CD20+	CD21low	CD21-
CD20+	CD21+	CD21+	CD20+	IgG+/-
IgG-	IgG-	IgG+	IgG+	IgA+/-
IgA-	IgA-	IgA+	IgA+	IgM-
IgM-	IgM+	IgM-	IgD-	CD27+
IgD+	IgD+	IgD-	CD27-	
CD27+	CD27+	CD27+		

Fig. 2. Phenotype of different B lymphocyte cells subsets.

Proportion of naïve B cells decreases with age. Several reports indicate that the proportion and number of CD27+ (memory) B cells increase but other reports show the opposite (Bulati et al., 2011; Colonna-Romano et al., 2009). The discrepancy probably reflects differences in the subsets definition and study protocols. Naïve B cells exhibit a reduced susceptibility to apoptosis in aged individuals (Chong et al., 2005). B cells produce large amounts of proinflammatory cytokines upon CD40 and IL-4 activation and so could play a role in the generation or in the maintenance of the inflammatory environment of the older people (Buffa et al., 2011). The "IgM memory" subset decreases with age. Other reports indicate a decrease of "switched memory" B cells. Finally the proportion of "double negative" B cells seems to increase with age (Ademokun et al., 2010; Bulati et al., 2011; Colonna-Romano et al., 2003; Colonna-Romano et al., 2009; Chong et al., 2005). This "double negative" population in aged individuals presents reduced expression of CD40, HLA-DR and CD80 and shorter telomeres. These cells are also present in patients with systemic lupus erythematosus (Colonna-Romano et al., 2009). There is a significant increase of anergic, "exhausted" memory cells with CD27 downregulation (CD27-) in older people. In centenarians, naïve B cells (IgD+ CD27-) are more abundant whereas exhausted memory cells (IgD- CD27-) do not show the increase previously demonstrated in healthy older people. Authors conclude that the reservoir of naïve B cells might be one factor of "successfully aging" (Ongradi & Kovesdi, 2010; Fernandez-Gutierrez et al., 1999).

B cells progenitors undergo maturation and differentiation in secondary lymphoid tissue, such as spleen and lymph nodes. Spleen arteries are surrounded by T lymphocytes in the periarteriolar lymphoid sheath. Primary lymphoid follicules containing B cells are adjacent to the periarteriolar lymphoid sheath. Other cell types such as T cells, dendritic cells and macrophages make up the marginal zone. This constitutes the white pulp. Age-associated architectural changes have been documented. Spleen from aged humans demonstrates a decrease in arterial vessels and an increase in stromal cells over lymphocytes. Total splenic weight increases with age due to fibroblastic infiltration (Gruver et al., 2007).

The germinal centre reaction is essential for the generation of high affinity antibody in response to infectious agents. This process is accomplished by two distinct mechanisms: class switch recombination, which enables B cells to change antibody isotype, and somatic hypermutation, the process of introducing mutations into the B cell receptor to increase antigen affinity. Data indicate that there is no change in the fundamental mechanisms of somatic hypermutation with age in man but an impaired ability of class switch recombination has been described in aged mice (Ademokun et al., 2010).

There is also a collapse in B cell receptor repertoire diversity with age and an expansion of monoclonal cells. The incidence of "monoclonal gammopathy of undefined significance" (MGUS) has been shown to increase with age. Sensitive assays reveal that as many as 50% of old mice and 20% of elderly humans have serum monoclonal immunoglobulin. As half of serum monoclonal immunoglobulins reacts with autoantigens, it appears that cells producing monoclonal immunoglobulins are drawn preferentially from the population of "B1 cells" that expand with age in both humans and mice (Weksler & Szabo, 2000). These CD5+CD20+ cells are produced during fetal live and are T-independent (in contrast to CD5- CD20+ "B2 cells" that are produced post-natally and are T-dependent). In humans, approximately 1% of old subjects with serum monoclonal immunoglobulin develop multiple myeloma each year, derived probably from plasma cell clonal expansions. Chronic lymphocytic leukemia, another lymphoid malignancy that occurs late in life, may arise from malignant transformation of the large B-cell clonal expansions. Chronic lymphocytic leukemia is frequently associated with T-cell abnormalities, including an inversion of the normal CD4 to CD8 T cell ratio, expansions of large granular lymphocytes, and clonal expansions of CD4 and CD8 T cells. These T-cell clonal expansions may represent a clonotypic response to transformed B cells or their secreted immunoglobulins. This hypothesis is supported by the finding that T cells from myeloma patients can be activated by monoclonal Ig fragments (Ademokun et al., 2010; Bulati et al., 2011; Colonna-Romano et al., 2003; Weksler & Szabo, 2000). However, in humans, despite the reduced number of B cells and the defects in class-switching, serum IgG, IgA are increased with age; IgD levels decrease with age but IgE and IgM remain unchanged or are decreased. IgG1 and IgG3 (in men) subtypes are also increased with age (Ademokun et al., 2010; Bulati et al., 2011; Colonna-Romano et al., 2003).

The quality of the humoral response also declines with age, characterized by lower antibody responses and decreased production of high affinity antibodies. B cells from aged individuals can be directly activated by cytokine but are weakly activated by anti-CD3 activated PBMCs. This result suggests that poor B cell responses is a consequence of inadequate help from T cells (Ongradi & Kovesdi, 2010; Fernandez-Gutierrez et al., 1999). In mice, aged CD4+ T cells provide poor assistance in germinal centres and promote low-affinity antibody production. Furthermore, overproduction of Th2 cytokines could augment B cell-mediated autoimmune disorders by enhancing the production of autoreactive antibodies. The percentage of naïve follicular B cells declines whereas subsets of antigen-experienced mature B cells with longer life span increase including poly/self reactive subtypes. These cells may be reactivated due to age-associated reduced tolerance or loss of tissue integrity leading to the exposure of neo-self antigens that results in aberrant autoimmune response (Ongradi & Kovesdi, 2010). Taken together, these data indicate that in older people, B cell repertoire diversity is limited while there is an increase of polyspecific and auto-antibodies.

3. Innate immune responses and aging.

3.1 Monocytes and dendritic cells subsets, neutrophils

Monocytes represent about 5-10% of peripheral blood leukocytes in humans. They originate from a myeloid precursor in the bone marrow, circulate in the blood and spleen then enter tissues. Monocytes represent circulating precursors for tissue macrophages and dendritic cells. The differential expression of CD14 (part of the receptor for LPS) and CD16 (also known as FcγRIII) are commonly used to define two major subsets (Figure 3): "classical" CD14++ CD16- cells, representing 95% of monocytes in healthy individuals and the "non-classical" CD14+ CD16+ comprising the remaining fraction. This later population is considered to represent activated cells that have undergone CD16 upregulation and CD14 downregulation and have been implicated in the pathogenesis of atherosclerosis. In healthy older volunteers, there is a shift of "classical" to "non-classical" monocytes. While "classical" monocytes express CCR2, "non-classical" monocytes preferentially express CX3CR1. Expression intensity of CXCR3 tends to decrease with age (Seidler et al., 2010; Sadeghi et al., 1999).

Dendritic cells (DCs) play a key role in the immune system since they orchestrate initiation, amplification and suppression of immune responses. In particular, maturation of DCs is crucial for the initiation of immunity. In fact, immature DCs are extremely efficient in capturing and processing antigens, but their unique ability to potently activate naïve T lymphocytes is acquired after maturation. This process is accompanied by the up-regulation of major histocompatibility complex molecules and the increased expression of membrane molecules that interact with T lymphocytes to enhance cell activation and adhesion. Furthermore, DC maturation leads to the release of high levels of cytokines that are

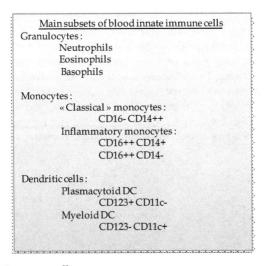

Table 3. Blood innate immune cells.

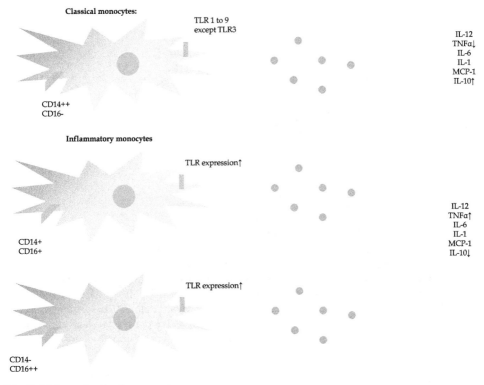

Fig. 3. Major subsets of monocytes.

responsible for the regulation and polarization of both innate and acquired immune responses (Ciaramella et al., 2011; Agrawal et al., 2007a). DCs are heterogeneous and are subdivided into two major categories: those that are present in peripheral blood (myeloid and plasmacytoid DCs) and those that are present in tissue/organs (Langerhans cells, interstitial and interdigitating DCs) (Agrawal et al., 2007b). Myeloid DCs express CD11c+ and low level of CD123 and can be subdivided into CD16+ (40-80%), CD1b/c+ (20-50%) and BDCA3+ (2-3%) subpopulations (Figure 4). Plasmacytoid DCs express low level of CD11c, high level of CD123, BDCA2 and BDCA4 and are specialized for production of type I IFNs in the context of viral infections (MacDonald et al., 2002; Dzionek et al., 2000).

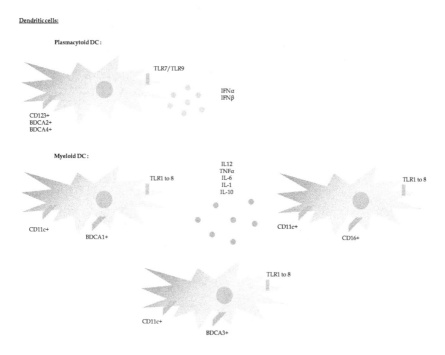

Fig. 4. Major subsets of dendritic cells.

In vitro monocyte-derived DCs, cultured with GM-CSF+IL-4, are closely related to interstitial or myeloid DCs (Agrawal et al., 2007b). Several studies used these *in vitro* cultured cells to assess the phenotype and functions of DCs in aged populations. Monocyte-derived DCs present no clear differences of costimulatory or activatory molecules (HLA-DR, CD80, CD86, CD40, CD83) except for CD25 and ICAM after lipopolysaccharide stimulation in healthy older individuals compared to younger (Agrawal et al., 2007b; Ciaramella et al., 2011; Agrawal et al., 2007a). Monocyte-derived DCs of older people are less efficient for micropinocytosis and phagocytosis of apoptotic cells and are impaired for migration (Agrawal et al., 2007b).

Several reports indicate that there are no significant differences in numbers of circulating myeloid and plasmacytoid DCs between older people and young subjects and that the expression of costimulatory molecules (CD86 and HLA DR) is similar (Agrawal et al., 2007a; Agrawal et al., 2007b; Pietschmann et al., 2000). In contrast, another study showed that numbers of myeloid DCs progressively declined with age while proportion of plasmacytoid DCs was unaffected. Peripheral blood DCs from healthy old subjects expressed CD86 and CD83, two markers of activation, on a higher percentage of cells, in comparison to young subjects. Maturation with lipopolysaccharide was unaffected with age (Della et al., 2007). Other studies showed reduced numbers of plasmacytoid DCs but not of myeloid DCs in healthy aged blood donors. Absolute numbers of circulating myeloid DCs is affected by declining health status (Perez-Cabezas et al., 2007; Panda et al., 2010; Shodell & Siegal, 2002; Jing et al., 2009). The use of Ficoll-enriched cells versus whole blood, differences in sample sizes, age groups, health status, genetic factors and subset definitions may contribute to the inconsistent findings with age in these studies. Taken together these data suggest that many factors, in addition to age itself, probably influence absolute/relative numbers or activation status of circulating DCs in geriatric populations.

Neutrophils are key players for early responses to bacterial infections. They rapidly produce reactive oxygen and nitrogen species when pathogens are encountered and produce many pro-inflammatory mediators. Several studies have shown alterations of neutrophil functions with age. Data remain conflicting in the literature concerning their number and phagocytic functions. One suggested alteration is their propensity to undergo apoptosis because of augmented cell oxidative load and perturbation of anti-apoptotic/proapoptotic mechanisms (Tortorella et al., 2006). Several reports indicate reduced chemotaxis (Fulop et al., 2004), phagocytosis and production of superoxide anion. Negative feedback mechanisms could also be perturbated (Fulop et al., 2004; Wessels et al., 2010). In contrast, centenarians do not present neutrophil defects compare to old people for adherence, chemotaxis, superanion production (Wessels et al., 2010; Alonso-Fernandez et al., 2008); (Crighton & Puppione, 2006).

3.2 Toll-like receptors

Toll-like receptors (TLR) are expressed on a variety of cells including macrophages, monocytes, natural killer cells, DCs, B and T lymphocytes. To date, 10 TLR are functional in humans. Pathogen associated molecular patterns serving as TLR ligands include lipopolysaccharide (LPS) on gram (-) bacteria (TLR4), diacetylated (TLR2/6) and triacetylated (TLR1/2) lipopeptides, peptidoglycan (TLR2), bacterial flagellin (TLR5), nucleic acid and double-stranded RNA (TLR3), single stranded RNA (TLR7 and TLR8) and unmethylated CpG oligodeoxynucleotides (TLR9). Recognition of microbial components by TLR initiates MYD88 and TRIF-dependent signal transduction pathways that culminate in both the elaboration of proinflammatory cytokine responses (via NFκB-dependent pathways) and the upregulation of type I IFNs and IFN-dependent genes. TLR-dependent activation of antigen presenting cells is a crucial step not only for the innate response but also for the ensuing initiation of the adaptive immune response. Inherited defects in TLR signaling are associated with a greater susceptibility to bacterial (especially Streptococcus pneumonia) and mycobacterial infection (Figure 5). Furthermore, TLR ligands as immunogens or adjuvants play an important role in mediating immune response to several human vaccines (Shaw et al., 2011; van Duin & Shaw, 2007).

Several studies in humans and mice have shown that TLR expression and functions tend to decline with age (van Duin & Shaw, 2007). Human monocytes from aged individuals present lower surface TLR1 expression than their younger counterparts (van Duin et al., 2007). These studies revealed an age-associated reduction in TNFα and IL-6 after stimulation of the TLR1/2 heterodimer. Similar observations were also noted for TLR7-induced IL-6 production. There is a significant decrease in TLR-induced upregulation of CD80 in older compared to young for all TLR ligands (van Duin & Shaw, 2007; Shaw et al., 2011). Myeloid DCs show decreased expression of TLR1, TLR3 and plasmacytoid DCs a decrease of TLR7 and TLR9 in older people compared to young individuals (Panda et al., 2010; Jing et al., 2009). DCs from older donors had diminished late phase responses such as the induction of transcription factors STAT1 and IRF7 and lower expression of IRF1,

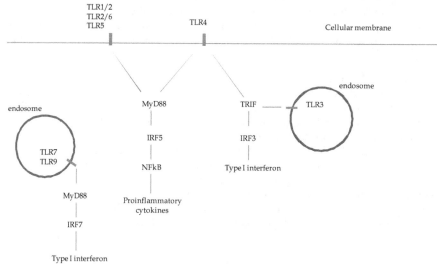

Fig. 5. Toll like receptor signaling.

suggesting a defective positive feedback regulation of type I IFN expression. Responses to TLR ligands may also be influenced by single nucleotide polymorphism within TLR genes. Authors report decreased IFNα, IL-6, IL-8 and TNFα in influenza virus-stimulated or HSV-2-stimulated plasmacytoid DCs from older compared to younger individuals (Shaw et al., 2011; Jing et al., 2009). IFNα production may be restored by zinc supplementation (Rink et al., 1998). Stimulated myeloid DCs and plasmacytoid DCs with different TLR ligands show a reduced expression of TNFα, IL-6, IL-12p40 and IFNα in healthy older people but an increased of the basal levels of this cytokine in older people (Panda et al., 2010). This decrease in TLR-induced cytokine production was strongly associated with the inability to mount protective antibody responses to the trivalent inactivated influenza vaccine currently recommended (Panda et al., 2010). LPS-stimulated monocytes from old people were reported to express less IL-12/23p40 levels in comparison to monocytes from young individuals (Della et al., 2007). However, their capacity to produce either bioactive IL-12 or IL-23 has not been addressed.

In contrast, analysis of monocyte-derived DCs from aged individuals revealed higher production of TNFα, IL-6 and IL-18 in response to LPS- and ssRNA but no difference in IL-

12p40/p70 (Ciaramella et al., 2011). There was no reduction of TLR4 expression with age but it was associated with decreased of phosphor-inositol 3(PI3) kinase, a negative regulator of TLR signalling. It manifested by decreased AKT phosphorylation and increased p38 mitogen activated protein kinase activation. They also present an increased expression of phosphatase and tensin homolog (PTEN), a negative regulator of PI3 kinase signalling pathway (Shaw et al., 2011; Agrawal et al., 2007a; Agrawal et al., 2007b).

Aging is generally associated with increased basal production of inflammatory cytokines but results of studies are often contradictory, depending on study designs and age groups (Beharka et al., 2001). Most studies report augmented plasma/serum levels of IL-6 and TNFα with increasing age, even in "selected" SENIEUR elderly over 85 years of age (Krabbe et al., 2004; Della et al., 2007). An elevated circulating IL-6 level is a strong predictor of thromboembolic complications while elevated TNFα levels are correlated with frailty (Krabbe et al., 2004). Another study shows that high basal IL-6 had a better predictive value for mortality than TNFα and that both cytokines were associated with classical risk factor like smoking, physical inactivity and body mass index (Bruunsgaard et al., 2003). A study confirmed increased serum IL-6, TGFβ and s-ICAM in the older people but IL-6 increased also with poor health status (comparing SENIEUR, OCTO and NONA elderly) (Forsey et al., 2003; Mysliwska et al., 1998). Serum IP-10 and CXCL9 levels have also been reported with increasing age, in contrast to IL-10 and IL-12p40. These chemokines display strong chemoattractant activity for Th1 lymphocytes and have been involved in the pathogenesis of autoimmune disorders, such as Grave's disease or Crohn's disease, and in metabolic disorders, such as diabetes mellitus or atherosclerosis (Shurin et al., 2007). A recent study confirms that "impaired" (poor functional status) older people express higher basal levels of IFNγ, IL-12p70, IL-6 and TNFα while "unimpaired" older people express higher basal levels of IL-5 and IL-13 when compared to each other (Vallejo et al., 2011).

High basal production of pro-inflammatory cytokines is generally associated with poor capacity to respond to TLR stimulation (Bruunsgaard et al., 1999a). Indeed, several studies indicate that reduced responsiveness to LPS stimulation (lower TNFα, IL-1β, IL-6, IL-10 and IL-1Ra production by whole blood cells) from 85-year olds is significantly associated with a worse survival and more risk factors like history of malignancies, chronic illness and elevated CRP levels (van den Biggelaar et al., 2004). Some whole blood studies however suggest that TNFα and IL-6 production upon TLR stimulation is increased in aged individuals, in particular for SENIEUR population under 85 years. This population probably does not display chronic low-grade inflammation (Gabriel et al., 2002). Zinc plasma levels could also represent an important factor to consider (Mariani et al., 2006).

IL-1 and TNFα are the earliest mediators of the acute phase response. Both cytokines induce a strong wave of cytokines including IL-6 and chemokines. In the course of S. *Pneumoniae* infection, inflammatory cytokines levels tend to persist for longer periods in older patients in contrast to younger ones (Bruunsgaard et al., 1999b). This observation could be related to increased pro-inflammatory environment in aged individuals but also to reduced clearing of the bacteria. It should also be interpreted in the light of possible alterations of renal function in the older people.

Taken together, low-grade chronic inflammation ("inflamm-aging") seems to be a cardinal feature of advanced "healthy" aging. The magnitude of this process at a given age is strongly influenced by multiple factors, including metabolic disorders and nutritional status. Indeed, poor health status and frailty will be associated with more intense inflammatory markers but poor responses to stimulation.

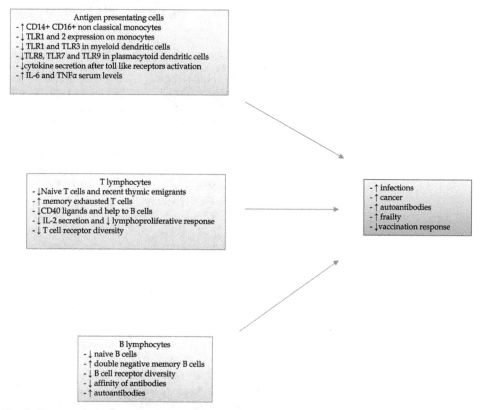

Fig. 6. Changes in immune responses observed in aged individuals.

4. Linking the characteristics of immune responses in the geriatric population to the clinical status.

"Normal" aging is determined genetically. At the cellular level, increased lifetime is associated with replicative-dependent shortening of chromosomal ends, also known as telomeres. In immune cells, this process is linked to immunosenescence. While this phenomenon is the normal destiny of dividing cells, it also reflects the global history of the organism. Here, we will discuss how the different immune parameters of the older people can be linked to the clinical characteristics encountered in the geriatric population.

4.1 Shortening of telomere length, genetic factors and hormonal changes

Telomeres consist of simple tandem DNA repeats (10-20kb) that do not encode for any gene products. The main function of telomeres is to cap the chromosome ends. Telomere capping is necessary to distinguish the chromosome ends from DNA breaks within the genome. DNA breaks within the genome lead to cell cycle arrest and DNA repair or to induction of apoptosis when the damage is too severe. In contrast to DNA breaks, chromosome ends do not provoke DNA damage responses (Ongradi & Kovesdi, 2010; Jiang et al., 2007). Telomeres are regarded as the molecular clock of aging, including that of the immune system, especially for lymphocytes. Telomere shortening is due to the end replication problem of DNA polymerase at each round of cell division and to diminished activity of telomerase that fails to add telomere repeat sequence to the end of chromosomes. Telomerase is active during embryogenesis but is suppressed postnataly in most somatic tissues. In adult humans, telomerase stays only active in germ cells, certain stem cells and progenitor compartment. Telomerase reactivation occurs in activated lymphocytes and human cancer cells (Jiang et al., 2007; Ongradi & Kovesdi, 2010). Regulation of the telomerase activity is complex and is limited by expression of the catalytic subunit hTERT. Many transcription factors act as activators (including c-Myc, SP1, USF1/2, Ets, HIF-1, hALP) or repressors (p53, AP1, Mad1, Wilm's tumor 1, Smad3,...). Oestrogens activate c-myc thereby influencing telomerase activity. Indeed, women present longer telomeres than men. Cortisol inhibits telomerase activity in CD4 and CD8 T cells, suggesting a mechanism by which stress can negatively affect immune response (Andrews et al., 2010; Balasubramanyam et al., 2007). Chronic psychological stress in caregivers of Alzheimer's patients or chronically ill children is associated with telomere loss in peripheral blood lymphocytes, possibly explained by increased cortisol levels. Another study shows reduced telomerase activity related to neuroendocrine and psychosocial data indicative of greater stress (cortisol, epinephrine, norepinephrine) in women but they failed to show an association between telomere shortening and negative mood or education (Andrews et al., 2010; Jiang et al., 2007; Epel et al., 2006). In humans, telomeres shorten by 50-100 base pairs with each cell division. Most human tissues and organs show significant telomere shortening during aging, including peripheral blood mononuclear cells (PBMCs), isolated lymphocytes, kidney epithelium, vascular endothelial cells, hepatocytes, intestinal and lung epithelial cells, muscle but not for brain. Telomere length in PBMCs also correlated inversely with the mortality rate in 60-75 year olds. Individuals with short telomeres have a 3.18-fold higher mortality rates from heart diseases and 8.54-fold higher mortality rates from infectious diseases compared to those with relatively long telomeres but it is not a significant prognostic factor for survival above 85 years. In addition to telomere shortening with aging, accelerated shortening observed in PBMCs occurs in various human diseases such as myelodysplasic syndrome (Jiang et al., 2007; Andrews et al., 2010; Ohyashiki et al., 1999), atherosclerosis and hypertension (Jiang et al., 2007; Andrews et al., 2010; Benetos et al., 2004), coronary artery disease, human immunodeficiency virus, rheumatoid arthritis (Jiang et al., 2007; Andrews et al., 2010; Steer et al., 2007) systemic lupus erythematosus, cognitive decline,... (Jiang et al., 2007; Andrews et al., 2010). Alzheimer patients present reduced telomere length in PBMCs compared to control. There was also a significant correlation between T cell telomere length and MMSE score, CD28 expression and an inverse correlation between serum TNFα production and telomere shortening in T cells (Panossian et al., 2003). Telomere shortening is also correlated with duration of type 1 and type 2 diabetes and systolic blood pressure but not with diabetes complications (Astrup et al., 2010; Sampson et al., 2006). Another study confirms the negative correlation between cardiovascular risk factor or coronary heart disease and telomere length (Spyridopoulos et al., 2009; Brouilette et al., 2007). This study also shows that treatment with statins in patients with high risk on the basis of telomere length results in substantial benefit effect (Brouilette et al., 2007). Oxidative stress is believed to be a major factor of accelerated aging, possible due to an increased pace of telomere shortening resulting from DNA damages observed upon smoking, obesity or cardiovascular diseases (Andrews et al., 2010; Balasubramanyam et al., 2007). The incidence of cancer sharply increases with aging. Telomere shortening appears to have a dual role in cancer formation. It was originally proposed that telomere shortening limits the lifespan of human cells thus acting as a tumor suppressor mechanism. The majority of human cancers exhibit very short telomeres, much shorter than the surrounding non-transformed tissue. However, more than 90% of human cancers show a strong reactivation of telomerase (Jiang et al., 2007).

Early studies showed that human somatic cells have a finite number of replicative cycles. The term "replicative senescence" is used to describe the stage at which telomeres are shortened to a critical length such that a proliferative response can no longer be elicited. One of the approaches to prevent or delay the generation of senescent CD8+ T cells is based on the well-documented link between telomere shortening and overall replicative potential and function of T lymphocytes. Although telomerase is capable of elongating telomeres and is upregulated in concert with T cell activation, the activity of this enzyme is completely turned off in CD8+ T cells that are chronically stimulated in cell culture. One suggested way to improve age-dependent decline of immune function would be to elicit strong cellular immunity by compounds that favour telomerase activity (McElhaney & Effros, 2009).

Other "genetic" factors have also been implicated in the process of immunosenescence. For example, IL-6 gene may be involved in the genetic regulation of longevity. IL-6 VNTR D/D genotypes were associated with increased levels in the blood and brain from Alzheimer's disease patients and IL6 VNTR allele B could be detrimental for reaching extreme longevity (Capurso et al., 2007; Krabbe et al., 2004). It was also reported that -1082 IL-10 promoter polymorphism was increased in male centenarians as compared to younger men and this genotype was associated with increased production of IL-10 (Krabbe et al., 2004).

Age is also characterized by hormone changes. It seems that oestrogens can have powerful immunomodulating effects, albeit mainly during stress. *In vitro* studies have shown that oestrogens deficiency leads to reduced IL-2 expression (Ku et al., 2009). Oestrogens seem to have important effects on B cells. A study shows that the percentage of conventional B cells (B-2, CD5- CD20+ cells) is significantly lower in late post menopause while B-1 cells (CD5+ CD20+) remain unchanged. It suggests that oestrogens may be involved in maintaining peripheral B-2 cell pool in women. Even if oestrogens seem to influence B cells, hormone replacement therapy does not influence the production of antinuclear antibodies or anti-IL-1 antibodies observed with aging (Kamada et al., 2001). Circulating oestradiol in late postmenopausal women without hormonal replacement therapy is positively correlated to CRP and serum level of IL-6 but the association for IL-6 was not significant anymore after adjustement for other clinical factors. Testosterone levels were also positively correlated with C-reactive protein, TNFα and IL-6 even after adjustment for confounders (Maggio et al., 2011).

Dehydroepiandrosterone (DHEA) has been considered for immunorestoration because serum levels dramatically decrease with age in both sexes. No DHEA-specific receptor has been identified in human T lymphocyte and it exerts probably its action indirectly via downstream conversion to other steroids, in particular sex steroid. Furthermore, DHEA exerts also anti-glucocorticoid action. *In vitro*, it increases IL-2 production, NK cell activity. Conversely, *in vivo*, it decreases circulating IL-6 levels. However, no consistent *in vivo* data on immune effect of DHEA supplementation in healthy older humans has been reported. Conversely, it shows a beneficial effect for patients treated in the context of systemic lupus erythematosus (Fulop et al., 2007; Arlt & Hewison, 2004). Other studies show that DHEA negatively correlates with basal IL-6 seric levels in older people but this relation is more complex in younger people. DHEA added in culture of PBMCs inhibits IL-6 secretion (Straub et al., 1998; James et al., 1997).

4.2 Comorbidities and medications

The main confounding factor that might impact on immune functions of the geriatric patient is the occurrence of multiple morbidities. These pathologies have potential direct effect on immune cells but the influence of pharmaceutical treatments should also be kept in mind. Recent research has attempted to identify risk factors for mortality and functional decline in older persons. A 7-year community based cohort study shows that 5% of "high functioning" aged individuals display three or four markers of inflammation (IL-6, cholesterol, albumin, CRP). This was associated with a more than 6-fold increased risk of 3-year mortality and a more than 3-fold risk of 7-year mortality independently of other measures of health status (Reuben et al., 2002). This indicates that innate immune parameters are strongly linked to clinical status.

4.2.1 Cardiovascular diseases and associated metabolic disorder

Atherosclerotic plaques contain smooth muscle cells, activated T lymphocytes and monocyte-derived macrophages. Several epidemiological studies have linked systemic low-grade inflammation in older populations to the prevalence and prognosis of cardiovascular disease. High IL-1β serum levels were associated with congestive heart failure, angina and dyslipidemia. High TNFα serum levels have been correlated with dyslipidemia and a higher prevalence of cardiovascular disease in 80 year olds and with high blood pressure, insulin resistance and common carotid intima media thickness in healthy middle-aged men. IL-6 acts as a marker of subclinical cardiovascular disease in older people and is a predictor of mortality related to cardiovascular disease (Krabbe et al., 2004). TNFα directly causes upregulation of cellular adhesion molecules at the surface of endothelial cells and causes insulin resistance. IL-6 induces procoagulant changes by increasing fibrinogen, tissue factor, factor VIII, von Willebrand factor and platelets. Moreover, both TNFα and IL-6 favour dyslipidemia (Bruunsgaard et al., 2003).

TLRs are expressed throughout the body and are mainly found on professional innate immune cells, including macrophages, dendritic cells and mast cells but also on non-professional immune cells such as endothelial cells and smooth muscle cells. All these cells are present in the atherosclerotic lesion and contribute to the inflammatory response. The expression of several TLRs is increased in atherosclerotic lesions. TLR4 is also increased on circulating monocytes from patients with coronary artery disease compared to controls. Several epidemiologic studies have reported elevated risk of atherosclerosis associated with a large number of infections (Chlamydia pneumonia, Helicobacter pylori, cytomegalovirus (CMV), Epstein-Barr virus (EBV), human immunodeficiency virus (HIV), herpes simplex virus (HSV) 1 and 2, Hepatitis virus A and B, influenza A virus). Studies have shown that vaccination above the age of 65 decreased the risk of acute coronary syndrome (Nichol et al., 2003; Lundberg & Hansson, 2010). The precise mechanism whereby pathogens are able to accelerate atherosclerosis is unclear but TLRs are probably involved in detection and initiation of a subsequent inflammatory response. TLRs also recognise endogenous ligands that are released during necrotic cell death or are derived from the degradation of extracellular matrix (Heat shock protein, oxidative Low density lipoprotein, endogenous mRNA, fibrinogens,...). While TLR signalling pathways activate the genes encoding IL-1β and IL-18, these mediators require a second signal resulting in cleavage of the pro-form to release the active molecules. This is regulated by a cytosolic protein complex (the "inflammasome") that leads to caspase-1 activation (Lundberg & Hansson, 2010). Various molecules can activate the inflammasome: ATP, crystalline structures (explaining the role of inflammasome in gout and pseudogout), aluminium salts (used as adjuvants), amyloid-B (playing important role in Alzheimer disease), fibers (silicosis, asbestosis) or the M2 channel from the influenza virus. Cholesterol crystals also directly activate the inflammasome, a process that is implicated in the pathogenesis of atherosclerosis (Duewell et al., 2010; McIntire et al., 2009). It would therefore be of interest to look at inflammasome activation/regulation in the context of aging. Other signalling pathways, such as those linked to the endoplasmic reticulum (ER) stress also participate to inflammation in the context of metabolic disorders (Hotamisligil, 2010). Whether perturbations in ER stress pathways could also contribute to age-related inflammation should also be further investigated (Naidoo, 2009).

Pravastatin, a 3-hydroxy-3-methylglutaryl coenzyme A reductase inhibitors or statin, has been recognize to have beneficial effects on atherosclerosis. Statins have pleiotropic effects, notably on immune system and dendritic cells. It has been shown that patients treated with pravastatin show decreased expression of CD86 on monocyte-derived dendritic cells, a reduced level of IFNα and IL-1β after four weeks of treatment and an increase of IL-10 and TGFβ in mixed lymphocyte reactions. It also reduces plasma levels of inflammation markers (IL-6, TNFα, CRP) and soluble CD40L without apparent link with the degree of lipid lowering achieved (Li et al., 2009; Schonbeck & Libby, 2004). Fenofibrate and simvastatine in type 2 diabetic patients with mixed dyslipidemia and in patients with hypercholesterolemia or impaired fasting glucose, reduce expression of TNFα, IL-1β, IL-6 and MCP-1 by LPS-stimulated monocytes. Both treatments significantly reduce high-sensitivity CRP levels (Krysiak et al., 2011b; Krysiak et al., 2011a) but there are conflicting results (Coen et al., 2010). Statin and aspirin decrease serum levels of IL-1β and C-reactive protein in hypercholesterolemic patients (Ferroni et al., 2003). Valsartan in hypertension patients also reduces the secretion of IL-1β by LPS-stimulated PBMCs. Angiotensin II is identified as the main mediator of vascular complications of hypertension. It stimulates the expression of vascular cell adhesion molecule-1 and induces IL-1β and MCP-1 production by vascular smooth cells (Li et al., 2005; Ferro et al., 2000).

Type 2 Diabetes mellitus is a serious chronic disease that is very prevalent in the developed world. Several studies have shown that IL-6 and IL-1β levels are independent predictors of type 2 diabetes development. The role of TNFα is more controversial, some studies show a relationship between TNFα and insulin resistance but this might be restricted to obese type 2 diabetic subjects. Higher serum IL-8 levels have also been found in diabetic patients

(DiPenta et al., 2007). Production of IL-6, IL-8, IL-1β upon LPS stimulation could also be influenced by glucose concentrations and insulin levels but *in vitro* results on PBMCs do not take into account the contribution of skeletal muscles, fibroblasts and vascular endothelial cells (Beitland et al., 2009).

Chronic heart failure is a major epidemiological burden in the industrialized world. Approximately 2% of the adult population is diagnosed with moderate or severe left ventricular systolic dysfunction with an incidence rate of 10 per 1000 population over the age of 65. Chronic inflammation interacting with increased oxidative stress, cytokine production, proteolytic matrix degradation and autoimmunity is implicated in heart failure pathophysiology by increasing cardiac injury, fibrosis and dysfunction. There are several sources of systemic inflammation in cardiac heart failure (TNFα, IL-1, IL-6, IL-18, MCP-1) due to release from leukocytes and blood platelets as well as the lungs, liver, endothelium and the failing heart itself. These cytokines are capable of modulating cardiovascular performance in an autocrine, paracrine or endocrine fashion. Inflammatory cytokines may enhance the expression of adhesion molecules and inflammatory chemokines in endothelial cells which in turn may further increase the inflammatory response within the vessel wall, representing a pathogenic loop leading to inappropriate endothelial activation in heart failure. TNF superfamily ligands may directly induce endothelial cell apoptosis (Picano et al., 2010). Aged patients with heart failure present higher IL-6 serum levels in the acute but also the recovery phase of cardiac failure compare to healthy aged controls (Vo et al., 2011).

In summary, these "metabolic disorders" are associated with chronic inflammation that contributes to the pathogenesis. Hence, "inflamm-aging" processes are likely to contribute to the development of these pathologies. Conversely, the increased prevalence of these diseases in the geriatric populations will affect innate immune parameters accordingly and favour the maintenance of low-grade inflammation.

4.2.2 The "Frailty" syndrome

Frailty has been defined as an age-related decline in lean body mass, decreased muscle strength, endurance, balance and walking performance, low activity, weight loss accompanied by a high risk of disability, incident falls, hospitalisation and mortality. Plasma levels of TNFα were strongly associated with impendent death independently of dementia and cardiovascular disease in centenarians. It supports the hypothesis that TNFα has specific biological effects and is a marker of the frailty syndrome in the oldest. Systemic low-grade inflammation has been associated with decreased muscle mass as well as the development of functional disability in older population. TNFα might directly contribute to sarcopenia. Indeed, *in vitro* experiments indicate that TNFα disrupts the differentiation process and promotes catabolism in muscle cells. It is also responsible for increased basal energy expenditure, anorexia, loss of muscle and bone mass *in vivo* and has been associated with cachexia in chronic inflammatory disorders such as rheumatoid arthritis, AIDS and cancer. His role in septic shock is well known. The potential role of IL-6 in sarcopenia is less clear. Age-related sarcopenia is partly reversed by exercise. Muscle contractions induce IL-6 production and release into the blood stream and it has been suggested that muscle-derived IL-6 contributes to the beneficial metabolic effect of exercise (Krabbe et al., 2004). Along the same line, another study shows that fatigue resistance and grip work correlate positively with IL-6 in older male participant. In contrast, the same group shows that older nursing home residents present a worse fatigue resistance and grip work related to high levels of IL-6, Heat shock protein 70 and TNFα (Bautmans et al., 2007; Bautmans et al., 2008). High levels of IL-6, C-reactive protein and TNFα predict an increased incidence of mobility limitation during a 30-month follow-up period in well functioning older people (Penninx et al., 2004).

4.2.3 Neurodegenerative disorders and depression

Cognitive impairment is an important problem with age. Epidemiological studies show an increasing body of evidence on the deleterious association between chronic peripheral cytokine elevation found in aged subjects and cognitive functions. Several studies show an association between serum levels of TNFα, IL-1β and Alzheimer disease. In contrast, IL-6 seems to be associated with vascular dementia (Krabbe et al., 2004; Ravaglia et al., 2007). Studies have suggested that inflamm-aging can be a prodrome for Alzheimer's disease. Alzheimer's disease is connected with a dysregulation in the metabolism of beta amyloid precursor protein with a consequent transient overproduction or a decreased degradation of β-amyloid in the brain. IFNγ and other pro-inflammatory cytokines interact with processing and production of β-amyloid peptides. Neopterin, a blood compound produced by monocyte-derived macrophages upon stimulation with IFNγ is increased in Alzheimer's disease patients compared to age-matched controls. 70% of these patients are seropositive for cytomegalovirus and it correlates with neopterin and C-reactive protein concentrations. It was suggested that elevated neopterin may be a vestigial result of serum immunity to cytomegalovirus (Giunta et al., 2008). IL-1, IL-6 and TNFα have been clearly involved in the local inflammatory process around amyloid plaques, might be cytotoxic when chronically produced and might stimulate the production of β-amyloid peptides (Krabbe et al., 2004; Ravaglia et al., 2007). As for atherosclerosis, inflammasome activation seems to be implicated in Alzheimer's disease. Amyloid β oligomers can disturb the function of K+ channels and decrease intracellular K+ concentration leading to activation of NALP-1 then caspase-1, production of IL-1β and IL-18, and cellular apoptosis through pyroptosis. Fibrillar amyloid β can also lead to the activation of NALP3 and lead to the same phenomenon (Cook et al., 2010). Plasma levels of IL-1β and TNFα are higher in patients with vascular dementia and late onset Alzheimer's disease when compared to control and after adjustment for confounding variables. IL-6 was only increased in patients with vascular dementia (Krabbe et al., 2004; Ravaglia et al., 2007) but not in Alzheimer's patients (Zuliani et al., 2007). Alzheimer's patients present a decrease of CD8+T lymphocytes, a slight increase of CD4+ T lymphocytes and CD19+ B lymphocytes compared to age-matched controls (Giunta et al., 2008). Once again, there is a strong link between this irreversible neurodegenerative process and general chronic inflammation.

Depression is also a cardinal feature of the geriatric population. Comorbidities, such as cardiovascular diseases, atherosclerosis, diabetes, osteoporosis, dementia, cancer or frailty can precipitate depressive states that are further enhanced by poor socioeconomic outcomes. Depression is a risk factor for low resistance to infection and insufficient response to vaccine. The pathogenesis and severity of depression are connected to chronic stress. Chronic diseases, stressfull life events, personal loss, decline in self concepts of efficacy may contribute to this process. Depression in older people is associated with increased exposure to cytomegalovirus in the past and a pro-inflammatory profile demonstrated by elevated

TNFα, IL-6, IFNα, C-reactive protein and deficiency of suppressive IL-10+cells. These changes negatively affect humoral and innate responses in depressed patients (Penninx et al., 2003; Bouhuys et al., 2004; Trzonkowski et al., 2004; Irwin & Miller, 2007). IL-6 and TNFα have the capacity to exert direct effects on the central nervous system by stimulating the hypothalamic-pituitary axis activity and the release of corticotrophin-releasing factor. These direct effects may lead to behavioural and neurochemical changes that may induce depression (Penninx et al., 2003). Depression has been associated with a decreased number of lymphocytes and NK and altered functions, which can be modulated by antidepressant treatment (Bouhuys et al., 2004; Irwin & Miller, 2007). Antidepressant therapy decreases LPS-induced IL-1β and IL-6 in whole blood from depressed patients. IL-1β has been shown to up-regulate hippocampus expression of serotonin transporters and proinflammatory cytokines might play a causative role in the depression-related activation of hypothalamic-pituitary-adrenal system (Himmerich et al., 2010).

4.2.4 Osteoporosis

Postmenopausal osteoporosis is a progressive disorder characterized by a decreased bone mass and increased susceptibility to fractures. It affects one out of three women after menopause (Breuil et al., 2010). Oestrogen deficiency leads to an uncoupling between activity of bone resorbing cells (osteoclasts) and bone forming cells (osteoblasts) responsible for accelerated bone loss. The concept of osteoimmunology recently emerged from increasing evidence of intimate links between bone tissue and the immune system. Indeed, recent studies have suggested that the increase in bone resorption induced by oestrogen deficiency is at least partly mediated by increased paracrine production of bone resorbing cytokines (Breuil et al., 2010). Multiple soluble mediators of immune cell function, including cytokines, chemokines and growth factors also regulate osteoblast and osteoclast activity. This is particularly true in pathological conditions such as rheumatoid arthritis and inflammatory bowel disease (Breuil et al., 2010). IL-1 is one of the most potent stimulators of bone resorption and IL-6 appears to be a potent osteotrophic factor that may play an important role in diseases characterized by increased bone resorption. Oestrogens inhibit IL-6 gene expression (Zheng et al., 1997; De Martinis et al., 2006). TNFα and IL-1 enhance bone resorption by stimulating development of osteoclast progenitors and increasing the activity of mature cells. IFNγ inhibits the process of IL-1 stimulated bone resorption. Some studies do not find any differences in the serum levels of IL-1β, IL-1α and IL-6 between osteoporotic and normal women. In contrast, Il-1β, IL-6, TNFα are significantly higher in whole blood after polyclonal activation in osteoporotic women than controls and negative correlation is found between lumbar bone mineral density and IL-1β, IL-6 or TNFα levels (De Martinis et al., 2005; Zheng et al., 1997). A study performed on osteoporotic women and controls without oestrogen or vitamin D deficiencies shows that osteoporotic women present a decrease in circulating B cells, decreased basal secretion of IFNγ by CD4+ T lymphocytes, a decreased in memory CD4+ T cells expressing RANK+ and CD28+ (Breuil et al., 2010). The TNF-family RANK-L and its receptor RANK are key regulator and essential for the development and activation of osteoclasts. RANK-L is expressed in osteoblasts and can be upregulated by bone resorbing factors such as glucocorticoids, 1,25(OH)2D3, IL-1, IL-6, IL-17, TNFα, PGE2, parathyroid hormone. RANK-L is produced by activated T cells and can directly induce osteoclastogenesis. Several factors can inhibit RANK-l such as osteoprotegerin, IFNγ, IL-12 and IL-18 (De Martinis et al., 2006).

Biphosphonates are currently widely used for the prevention and treatment of osteoporosis as well skeletal metastasis. It has been recently demonstrated that biphosphonates lead to the expansion and activation of γδ T cells, these effects may represent potential novel anti-tumor mechanisms. Another study indicates that low dose zoledronate *in vitro* reduces TNFα production by monocytes, inhibits upregulation of typical maturation markers and NFκB activation in dendritic cells (CD83, CD86, CD40) (Wolf et al., 2006).

4.3 Chronic infections and immune "exhaustion"?

One of the hallmarks of the "immune risk phenotype" (see table 1) in the OCTA/NONA subjects is the accumulation of terminally-differentiated CD8 T cells, (lacking CD27 and CD28) leading to inversion of the CD4:CD8 ratio. An important fraction of these cells are specific for cytomegalovirus (CMV) antigens. These effector memory T cells contain large amount of cytotoxic effector molecules like granzyme and perforin and progressively acquire inhibitory receptors such as KLRG1, CD57 and PD-1 (Pawelec & Derhovanessian, 2011). Similarly, CMV-specific CD4 T cells are highly differentiated, have shorter telomeres and decreased telomerase induction after stimulation. These cells are thought to become dysfunctional and "exhausted" in old individuals (Hadrup et al., 2006). However, these cells are still capable of rapidly producing cytokines upon *in vitro* stimulation and display effector functions (Ouyang et al., 2003). Interestingly, a study performed on individuals genetically enriched for longevity, with a 30% decreased mortality risk, possess immune signatures different from those of the general population. Even if they are CMV-seropositive, they fail to show the CMV-(and age-) associated alterations of immune parameters that CMV-seropositive general population does show (Derhovanessian et al., 2010). As previously mentioned, it has been reported that IL-4 producing T cells with a CD25+ memory phenotype accumulate in a subgroup of healthy elderly people who have an intact humoral immune response after influenza vaccination. These apparently beneficial CD8+ CD25+ T cells are rare or even absent in older persons with latent CMV infection (Herndler-Brandstetter et al., 2005).

Could there be a direct link between this CMV-dependent immune signature and other parameters of immunosenescence? Conceptually, accumulation of these memory oligoclonal cells with age would occupy the "immunological space" and limit homeostatic proliferation of naïve T cells and response to new antigens. It has also been suggested that CMV infection could participate to the inflamm-aging process (Trzonkowski, 2003). Whether accumulation of CMV-specific T cells with age is actually detrimental remains to be established (Wills, 2011). Analysis of several recent cohorts does not support a relationship between CMV status, mortality or inflammatory markers (Wills 2011). Another recent study found a gradual increase in CMV antibody titers with deteriorating functional status in aged individuals (Moro-Garcia et al., 2011). CMV infection is also associated with atherosclerosis and the risk for heart diseases (Stranberg TE 2009). In longitudinal studies of CMV-seropositive patients, antibody levels have been reported to correlate inversely with survival in individuals with stable cardiovascular diseases, cardiovascular risk factors and in older women in their 70's. Furthermore, telomere shortening of CD8 CD28- T cells correlates with cardiac dysfunction in CMV+ patients with coronary heart diseases (Spyridopoulos et al., 2009).

In addition to these unresolved issues related to the association of CMV infection and disease states, the causality links are still unclear. Indeed, if CMV infection were directly implicated in age-dependent deterioration of immune functions and cardiovascular diseases, it would be highly beneficial to consider CMV eradication in the general population through vaccination (Pawelec, 2011).

4.4 How living habits and nutrition status impact on immune functions

Malnutrition is associated with a decrease in immunity and an increase in susceptibility to many infectious diseases, notably due to an inability to meet the energy demands associated with the immune response. Interventions on nutrition could have a large impact on immune functions (Ongradi & Kovesdi, 2010).

It seems that caloric restriction is the only known method to prolong median as well as maximal lifespan in all tested animals, from invertebrates to rodents and non-human primates. It is able to attenuate the natural shift from naive to memory phenotype T cells and maintain a higher number of naive T cells in aged animals. The increase of proinflammatory cytokines such as IL-6, TNFα and IFNγ can be reversed by caloric restriction. Caloric restriction is known to inhibit mTOR and thereby promoting autophagy mechanisms. It allows recycling of the cellular components to gain new building blocks for critical proteins by degrading momentarily unneeded proteins and even organelles (Arnold et al., 2011).

The dietary intake of essential macro and micronutrients is usually inadequate in the elderly and several factors contribute to this deficiency: poor socioeconomic status may lead to a greater consumption of inexpensive foods poor in micronutrients. Nutrient deficiency is exacerbated by loss of appetite, lack of teeth, intestinal malabsorption and decreased energy requirement. Many micronutrients contribute directly or indirectly to the biological activity of some antioxidant enzymes, to the efficiency of immune response and to the maintenance of metabolic functions (Mocchegiani et al., 2011).

Vitamin A contributes to the maintenance of epithelium integrity in the respiratory and gastrointestinal tracts. Pyridoxins, folic acid, vitamin E have been suggested to influence lymphocyte functions. Antioxidant vitamin supplements have been shown to enhance antibody titers upon influenza vaccination and to reduce incidence of infection over a 2-year study period (Lesourd, 2006).

Lipids are also important actors in immune system. High-density lipoprotein (HDL) has anti-inflammatory and anti-oxidative effects and influence proximal T cell signalling. Conjugated linoleic acid has been shown to have anticarcinogenic, antiatherogenic and antidiabetic properties correlating with increased lymphocyte proliferation and decreased proinflammatory cytokine secretion. The most important effect is a decrease of risk and severity of cardiovascular diseases originating from atherosclerosis, a chronic inflammatory condition. Living habits can serve as anti-aging process: aerobic exercise, weight loss and smoking cessation can raise HDL levels and physical activity tends to lower IL-6 and C-reactive protein serum levels (Fulop et al., 2007; Ongradi & Kovesdi, 2010).

The potential role for vitamin D and its active metabolite 1,25(OH)2vitD in modulating the immune response was first appreciated 25 years ago with three important discoveries: The ability of 1,25(OH)2vit D to inhibit T cell proliferation, the ability of disease-activated macrophages to produce 1,25 (OH)2vitD and the presence of vitamin D receptor in activated human inflammatory cells. 1,25(OH)2vitD suppresses proliferation and immunoglobulin production and delays the differentiation of B cell precursors into plasma cells. It shifts the balance to a Th2 cell phenotype and increased CD4/CD25 regulatory T cells. It inhibits Th17 development and appears beneficial for autoimmunity diseases. In innate immunity, vitamin D enhances activation of TLRs. It promotes innate immune responses to TLR activation by Mycobacterium tuberculosis. 1,25(OH)2vit D increases cathelicidin, a antimicrobial peptide after activation of TLR1/2 but inhibits the maturation of monocyte-derived dendritic cells (Bikle, 2009; Hewison, 2010; Schwalfenberg, 2011). By increasing cathelicidin, vitamin D supplementation improves the outcome of many diseases: it reduced dental caries and Helicobacter pylori infections. Vitamin D insufficiency is associated with Crohn's disease, pour outcome in severe pneumonia and urinary tract infections (Schwalfenberg, 2011). Vitamin D improves physical barrier by stimulating gap junctions genes, adherent genes and tight junction genes (Schwalfenberg, 2011). In contrast, a study failed to show influence of a short-term calcium and vitamin D treatment in healthy post menopausal woman on IL-6, TNFα and C-reactive protein serum levels (Gannage-Yared et al., 2003).

Vitamin C is an essential watersoluble nutrient, which primarily exerts its effect on host defence mechanisms and immune homeostasis, by being the most important physiological antioxidant. It has been implicated as having a preventative and therapeutic role in a variety of diseases including scurvy, viral infections and common cold, cancer and atherosclerosis. A study shows that *in vitro*, vitamin C inhibits IL-6 and TNFα production by monocytes after LPS stimulation and an inhibition of IL-2 production by lymphocytes after PMA ionomycin (Hartel et al., 2004).

Zinc is one of the most relevant nutritional factors in aging because it affects immune responses, metabolic harmony and antioxidant activity. The human body contains 2-3 g zinc most of which is bound to proteins. Plasma pool, which is required for the distribution of zinc represents less than one percent of the total body content. A multitude of factors is likely to influence zinc intake: malnutrition, socioeconomic factors, decreased intestinal absorption and medications like diuretics. The recommended daily allowance for zinc in adult in the United States is 11mg/day for men and 8 mg/day for women. In human, the most prominent example of the effect of zinc deficiency on the immune system is acrodermatitis enteropathica, a rare autosomal recessive inheritable disease that causes thymic atrophy and a high susceptibility to bacterial, fungal and viral infections. It is caused by zinc-specific malabsorption. The intracellular concentration of free zinc is regulated by three mechanisms: one is transport through the plasma membrane; another involves storage in zincosomes and finally zinc binding to metallothionein. Metallothioneins are a group of low molecular weight metal binding proteins with high affinity for zinc. It distributes intracellular zinc and has a protective role in transient and acute stress-like conditions. Elevated IL-6 levels observed in aged individual are also associated with increased and persistent metallothioneins expression in peripheral mononuclear cells, leading to an increased sequestration of zinc and immune impairment. Notably, centenarians display low levels of metallothioneins coupled with satisfactory zinc ion availability. *In vitro* studies show that many parameters are affected by zinc: caspases, reactive oxygen species production, NFκB and iNOS activity, superoxide dismutase, catalase, gluthatione peroxidase, telomere length, several cytokines and chemokines expression. The most prominent effect of zinc deficiency is a decline in T cell function, the shift of a Th1 toward Th2 responses. Effect of zinc on cytokine levels is concentration-dependent: it stimulates cytokine production in monocytes in response to lipopolysaccharide with moderated supplementation but higher concentrations can have an antagonistic effect. With regard to older people, inconsistent data exist on the beneficial effect of zinc supplementation upon the immune efficiency due to different doses and duration of treatment. The most important parameter affected by physiological dose (10-25 mg/day from 1 to 3 months) is the innate immunity represented by the natural killer cell cytotoxicity. Zinc treatment at the dose of 15mg a day for 1 month in older people and old infected patients restores thymic endocrine activity, lymphocyte mitogen proliferative response, CD4+ T cell number, peripheral immune efficiency and DNA repair. At clinical level, significant reduction of relapsing infections occurs in these patients (Mocchegiani et al., 2011; Haase & Rink, 2009; Mocchegiani, 2010). In hospitalized geriatric patients, poor zinc status has been associated with higher proportion of congestive cardiopathy, respiratory infections, gastrointestinal diseases and depression (Pepersack et al., 2001).

Protein energy malnutrition is common in elderly population. It is present in 2-4% of home-living self-sufficient older subjects and in more than 50% of institutionalized older subjects. During stress, the body reacts with acute phase responses associated with proinflammatory cytokine release from monocytes-macrophages. The cytokines induce the use of nutritional reserves which is particularly harmful in the older people for several reasons: 1) body reserves are already decreased in older individuals who exhibit osteoporosis and often sarcopenia 2) acute phase responses are long lasting in older people, so that more body reserves are used ; 3) nutritional reserves are never fully replaced in older individuals during recovery, since protein anabolism is decreased; 4) each acute phase response in the older people can therefore leads to lower nutritional reserves, mainly muscle protein reserves which can increase frailty (Lesourd, 2006).

In light of these observations, it is clear that addressing the specific nutritional requirements in advancing age could modulate immune functions. Whey proteins are a mixture of globular proteins isolated from milk. It is left when milk coagulates and contains everything that is soluble in milk. It has been shown that older people receiving whey proteins, in comparison to soy proteins, present greater antibody responses against four serotypes of S. pneumoniae (Freeman et al., 2010). Along the same line, Enprocal, a recently formulated supplementary food has been designed to meet the nutritional needs of frail older people. The ingredients of Enprocal are dairy-based proteins (Whey protein concentrate, skim milk powder, whole milk powder), vitamins and minerals (calcium, zinc, vitamins C, D, B and A), vegetable oils and inulin. An in vitro study suggested that Enprocal displays some immunomodulatory properties on immune cells (Kanwar & Kanwar, 2009). Lactoferrine has also important immune modulator protein. It belongs to the transferrin family and bind two irons ions reversibly. It is synthesized by glandular epithelia and found in milk, tears, bile, respiratory and gastrointestinal secretions. Protein antigens and bacteria within the digestive systems act as stimulating agents in the process. It has pleiotropic effects: bactericidal, anti-fungal and anti-viral effects, anti-oxidant activity, it reduces the production of proinflammatory cytokines, inhibits tumour growth by inhibiting angiogenesis, promoting apoptosis and finally, it promotes bone growth (Pierce et al., 2009).

Exercise has also been shown to have influence on immunological parameter. Studies have found that mitogen- or influenza- induced lymphocyte proliferation was increased, the number of natural killer cells was greater, antibody IgM and IgG response to influenza vaccine two weeks post immunization was greater in active old people. Greater levels of physical activity in terms of walking speed was also associated with lower serum levels of several inflammatory markers such as IL-6, TNFα, and C-reactive protein. In contrast, intervention trials involving frail older people were not promising suggesting that immune alterations in the frail state cannot be reversed (Senchina & Kohut, 2007). A study performed on older men shows that older people with long-term training present reduce levels of IL-6, IL-1ra, IL-10, sTNFRI but an increase of MCP-1 compared to sedentary older people. It was associated with increases of DHEA and IGF-1 levels (Gonzalo-Calvo et al., 2011). Another study shows also that exercise reduces inflammatory monocytes in hypercholesterolemic patients (Coen et al., 2010).

In summary, many different dietary factors are able to influence innate and adaptive immune parameters. It is very difficult from *in vitro* studies to draw hypothesis on how deficiency/supplementation of specific factors impact on the organism. However, clinical studies indicate that these factors should be taken into account and might be beneficial for healthy aging as a whole.

4.5 Erosion of epithelial barriers: susceptibility to infections and potential impact on chronic inflammatory status

Epithelial cells represent the first protective barrier towards invading pathogens. Aging is associated with alteration of these barriers, including the skin, lung, stomach, intestine and urinary tract. Bacteriemic pneumococcal pneumonia in persons older than 70 is associated with a death rate greater than 50 percent. It appears that oropharyngeal colonization with gram-negative bacilli plays an important predisposition role. With age, in the lung, there is a reduced function of the mucociliary tract, a reduced local immunity (T cells and reduced secreted immunoglobulin), and reduced cough reflex. All these factors but also deglutition trouble, reduced production of gastric acid secretion, antibiotics or antiacid treatment, favour the apparition of pneumonia in older people (Cretel et al., 2010; Yoshikawa, 1981).

Older people also present more urinary infections than young people. Urinary tract infection has an incidence of 5-35% in men and 15-50% in women. Poor emptying of the urinary bladder because of reduced muscle tonicity, prostatic hypertrophy, reduced oestrogen and increased pH level that lead to increased bacterial adherence, previous genitorurinary instrumentation and perineal contamination from fecal incontinence are possible reasons for the high incidence (Yoshikawa, 1981; Cretel et al., 2010).

Skin and soft tissue infection is a common complication in aged patients. Even minor trauma to the skin might result in serious skin and soft tissue infections because of skin changes (thinning of epidermis and subcutaneous tissues, decreased glandular secretions and atherosclerosis, pressure injuries). Skin also presents modifications of immune cells such as a decrease of Langerhan's cells (Cretel et al., 2010; Desai et al., 2010; Grewe, 2001; Yoshikawa, 1981).

Older patients are also at higher risk for bacterial meningitis (pneumococci, gram negative bacilli and listeria monocytogenes) and bacterial arthritis (Yoshikawa, 1981).

Gram-negative bacterial infections occur more frequently in patients older than 60 years. Intra-abdominal sepsis is of special importance to the older people. Complications like perforation, wound infection, abscess formation and pneumonia are more common in the older people following appendectomies. The risk of diverticulitis rapidly increases with aging and cholelithiasis is another disease of the aged.

With age, the capacity of the gastrointestinal tract to protect individuals from pathogens is lowered because of reduced gastric pH leading to pneumonia and malabsorption, mechanical trouble like diverticulitis and alteration of the mucosal immune system (Cretel et al., 2010). The mucosal immune system consists of an integrated network of tissues, lymphoid and mucous membrane-associated cells and innate effectors and acquired molecules. The IgA isotype is key players in mucosal immunity and seems to function in synergy with innate immune system. Mucosal inductive sites include the Peyer's patches; gut associated lymphoreticular tissues (GALT), waldeyer's ring of tonsil and adenoid. The mammalian lower intestine contains up to 10^{12} bacteria per gram of intestine. The normal microbiota is essential to maintain appropriate homeostatic conditions providing energy in the form of short chain fatty acids and nutrients and protection against colonization by pathogenic bacteriae. It also plays a role in maturation of the host immune system including intestinal secretory soluble IgA and intraepithelial lymphocyte development. There is some evidence in mice that there are alterations of the mucosal immune system with age. Reduced levels and quality of soluble IgA and alterations of mucosal dendritic cells functions have been reported. Qualitative change in the composition of the microbiota has also been reported (fewer total anaerobes bacteroides and bifidobacterium and higher levels of enterobacteriacea and endotoxin-producing, gram-negative bacteria like fusobacteria, clostridia, eubacteria species). As a direct result of these age-related changes in the microbiota, the quality of the secretary IgA response can be altered, although the absolute amount of these antibodies is generally unchanged (Fujihashi & Kiyono, 2009). Non-pathogenic bacteriae in the intestine play important role for protecting host from pathogens. It has been suggested that limited TLR stimulation will contribute to the physiological, low-level inflammation in healthy intestine. In contrast, true pathogens induce a rapid and more aggressive response that is initiated by microbial danger signals and tissue damage. It is now known that the innate and adaptive immune activation by the microbiota prevents other inflammatory responses and induces cytoprotective responses of the intestine epithelium that are critical for intestinal homeostasis. This is achieved by low expression of pattern recognition receptors on intestinal epithelial cells and limited gene activation via NF-κB. It promotes epithelial integrity through production of cytoprotective molecules such as heat shock proteins. Low-grade bowel inflammation is frequently present in the older population and may account for elevated systemic C-reactive protein and faecal calprotectin. Blood intestinal perfusions and oxygenation are also altered in the aged population. It is possible that the combination of a normally harmless bacterial signal, tissue injury and nutritional deficiency may trigger pathogenic inflammatory response. In the intestinal environment, a loss of barrier integrity may result in heightened exposure to exogenous components derived from the non-pathogenic intestinal microbiota and a breakdown in tolerance mechanisms. Impaired clearance of apoptotic cells by intestinal dendritic cells may lead to the accumulation of necrotic cells that release autoantigens such as nucleic acids, uric acid and the induction of an inflammatory dendritic cells phenotype. This might lead to autoimmune response and abnormal immune response to commensals.

Taken together, it seems that both endogenous signals (cell senescence and cumulative cell damage) and exogenous non-self signals (bacteria translocation through a leaky gut) may both contribute to chronic inflammation (Schiffrin et al., 2010).

5. Immunosenescence and cancer

Epidemiological studies indicate that about 55% of tumours are detected after the age of 65. The most frequent sites in men over 65 are represented by lung, colon, rectum, prostate and bladder; in women by breast, lung, colon-rectum, bladder and pancreas as well as non-Hodgkin lymphoma. The association between age and cancer can be explained by a multitude of factors, including a more prolonged exposure to carcinogens in older individuals and an increasingly favourable milieu for the induction of neoplasm in senescent cells. The immune system counteracts tumour cell growth through different ways:

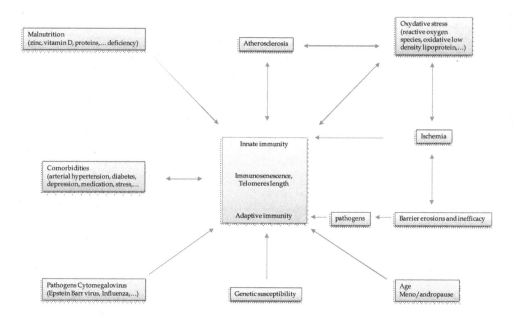

Fig. 7. External factors leading to immunosenescence.

1) protection of the host from virus-induced tumours by eliminating or suppressing viral infections 2) suitable eradication of pathogens and rapid resolution of inflammation thereby preventing the establishment of an inflammatory environment favourable to tumorigenesis 3) specific identification and elimination of tumour cells on the basis of their expression of tumour-specific antigens or molecules induced by cellular stress (a process known as "immunosurveillance"). Hence, reduction of T cell function and cellular immunity as seen in the older people could favour carcinoma development. In older people suffering from different types of cancer, there was a reduced number of CD3 T cells, CD4 T helper cells and

natural killer cells in peripheral blood compared to healthy older people (Malaguarnera et al., 2010; Fulop et al., 2010; Motta et al., 2003). "Inflamm-aging" processes could favour tumour development. For example, IL-1α plays a role in tumorigenesis (and promotes angiogenesis and chemoresistance). TNFα plays an important role in the initiation of tumour by stimulation the production of nitric oxide and reactive oxygen species which can lead to DNA damage. Enhanced TNFα levels are associated with increased risk of multiple myeloma, hepatocellular carcinoma, bladder, gastric and breast cancer. It also correlates with poor prognosis of haematological malignancies. The paracrine secretion of IL-6 acts as a growth factor for multiple myeloma, non-Hodgkin lymphoma, bladder, colorectal and renal cell carcinoma (Malaguarnera et al., 2010; Fulop et al., 2010).

Accumulation of memory CD8 T cells might also participate to cancer development. One of the most intriguing evidences about the role of CD57+ T lymphocytes in cancer comes from the fact that metastasis-free regional lymph nodes draining different human epithelial tumors present a reduction in almost all immune cells, except CD57+ lymphocytes (Kanwar & Kanwar, 2009). CD8+CD28–CD57+ T lymphocyte clones may be the result of persistent stimulation by tumor-associated antigens, combined with a reduced cellular death rate secondary to reduced expression of the apoptosis-related molecule CD95. A long-lived population of CD8+CD57+CD28– perforin+ T lymphocyte clones has been reported in the peripheral blood of patients with multiple myeloma. Despite being more commonly found in patients with progressive and advanced-stage disease, this population was associated with superior survival. In patients with relapsed/refractory multiple myeloma treated with thalidomide, multivariate analysis showed that inferior survival was associated with low pretreatment bone marrow CD57+ cells and overall, CD8+CD57+T lymphocytes account for up to 25% of the marrow T cell population. Such CD8+CD57+ T lymphocytes have been shown to suppress T cell functions in multiple myeloma (Focosi et al., 2010).

CD57+ lymphocytes in the lymph nodes of B-chronic lymphoid leukemia patients have abnormal orthogonal light-scattering signals and an abnormal density of CD57+ receptors in comparison with their peripheral blood CD57+lymphocytes or the CD57+ lymphocytes in the peripheral blood, bone marrow, and tonsils of hematological normal donors. It has been reported that these patients with neutropenia have higher numbers of peripheral blood CD8+CD57+ T lymphocytes than the non-neutropenic ones. An elevated frequency of CD4+CD57+ T cells was correlated with more advanced disease. The role of the CD4+perforin+ T cell population is at present uncertain. However, this potentially cytotoxic T cell population could contribute to enhancing survival of the B-chronic lymphoid leukemia cells through production of IL-4 and to the immunodeficient state seen frequently in patients with this tumor, independent of drug treatment. (Focosi et al., 2010).

Finally, few reports analyzed the impact of immunosenescence on the complications of patients with cancer. Neutropenia is a complication of patients treated by chemotherapy and responsible of infection called febrile neutropenia. In older patients, pyrexia can be absent and little is known about the consequence of neutrophil defect and other immune defects on the increased rate of infections in old cancer patients. It is well known that CSFs enhance bone marrow production and is used to counteract neutropenia. CSFs have proven to be beneficial in old people but they still suffer from increased infection rates compared to younger adults. Finally, the factors influencing immunity (such as malnutrition, alteration of intestinal barriers, depression...) can also negatively influence the outcome of cancer in geriatric patients. So, it will be important to reconsider guidelines and management of old patients suffering from cancer (Crighton & Puppione, 2006).

6. Immunosenescence and autoimmunity

"Inflamm-aging" results in both decreased immunity to exogenous antigens and increased autoreactivity. It is well documented that a significant fraction of older people has low affinity autoantibodies in their serum and the prevalence of autoantibodies associated with autoimmune disease increases with age without clinical significance. Rheumatoid factors are present in up to 5% of young healthy individuals and increase up to five times in older persons such as antinuclear antibodies. A number of hypotheses have been proposed to explain the relationship between aging and the development of autoimmunity: reduced thymic output has been postulated to induce compensatory autoproliferation of T cells which can lead to premature T cell senescence and contribute to autoimmunity; alteration in apoptosis in T cells, expansion of exhausted CD4 and CD8 T cells that have lost the expression of CD28 are associated with autoimmune disease like rheumatoid arthritis, reactivation of self-reactive memory B cells, a shift from Th1 to Th2 cytokine profile that enhances the production of autoreactive antibodies, elevated levels of circulating inflammatory cytokines such as IL-6, TNFα and C-reactive protein is related to age-related diseases such as coronary heart disease and stroke, diabetes mellitus, Alzheimer's disease, lupus, Sjogren's syndrome and rheumatoid arthritis (Grolleau-Julius et al., 2010).

7. Immunosenescence and vaccination

Influenza is the fifth leading cause of death in the developed world after 50 years of age. As such, this group is the major target of vaccination campaigns. While influenza vaccination has 70-90% efficacy in healthy adult in western countries, the success rate falls to 17-53% in older people when determined as specific immune responses. Nevertheless, vaccination campaigns in aged individuals result in 25% reduction of morbidity, 50% of pneumopathies, 20% of hospital care and 70% of mortality (Ongradi & Kovesdi, 2010; Gruver et al., 2007; Bouree, 2003; Nichol et al., 2003). Both humoral and cell-mediated influenza specific responses are lower than in young adults. Upon *in vitro* restimulation, peripheral blood mononuclear cells exhibit a decrease in the proportion of IFNγ+ T cells. Mortality is associated with coexistent bacterial infection in one third of case, which could be a consequence of altered innate immune responses (Ongradi & Kovesdi, 2010; Gruver et al., 2007; Bouree, 2003). In older people, low plasma level of DHEA, decreased TNFα in whole blood after lipopolysaccharide stimulation and increased IL-10 production in whole blood after PHA stimulation is correlated with lower antibody response to influenza vaccination. The increase of IL-10 is likely to inhibit the maturation of antigen presenting cells, together with decreased TNFα production, hampering their migration to draining lymph node, compromising the subsequent induction of the specific immune response. Furthermore, IL-10 can induce antigen-specific CD4 T cells anergy. Thus, it is intriguing that the possession of an anti-inflammatory genotype (high IL-10 and low TNFα production) is increased significantly in centenarians. It is tempting to speculate that the presence of "high IL-10/low TNFα" could be favorable in protecting against age-related diseases, particularly neurodegenerative diseases, but conversely it could hamper the immune response to infections and vaccine (Corsini et al., 2006). As said before, studies show a correlation between the cytomegalovirus seropositive status and non responsiveness to influenza vaccine. They show that majority of volunteers fulfilling the criteria of SENIEUR protocol belonged to responders generating protective titers of antibodies against antigens of the influenza vaccine. Proinflammatory status such as elevated serum IL-6, TNFα was also associated with non-responders. The increase of anti-inflammatory cytokines in non-responders may be seen as a compensation for the inflammatory activity of IL-6 and TNFα. The coexistence of high levels of IL-6 and anti-CMV IgG suggested to the authors that chronic infection may be one of the causes of the proinflammatory status in the non-responding group, shrinking the capacity of immune system (Trzonkowski et al., 2003). Decreased TLR responsiveness of dendritic cell subsets is also associated with the inability to mount protective antibody responses to the trivalent inactivated influenza vaccine currently recommended (Panda et al., 2010).

Infection caused by Streptococcus pneumonia account for 25-35% of bacterial pneumonia resulting in hospitalization, morbidities and mortality in the older people. The current pneumococcal polysaccharide vaccine is recommended for all individuals above 65 years of age and those between 18-65 years of age at risk. The data for efficacy in older people are not as persuasive. Antibodies levels are lower in the older people and in those with chronic disease, except for healthy older adults after the age of 75 (modified SENIEUR protocol) (Chen et al., 2009; Bouree, 2003). Antibody concentrations were found to be similar for six out of seven serotypes for streptococcus pneumonia after vaccination of older and young subjects while opsonization titers were significantly higher in six out of seven serotypes in the younger population. Antibody potency, as measured by the ratio of opsonization titer to antibody concentration was found to be significantly higher for the younger subjects for all serotypes. Effectiveness of antibodies seems to be reduced in the older adult population (Schenkein et al., 2008). Tetanus, diphtheria and pertussis vaccination coverage are low, persons aged of more than 60 years frequently do not have protective antibody. It is the same problem for hepatitis B virus vaccine (Chen et al., 2009; Bouree, 2003).

Widely used adjuvant formulations such as those containing alum are poorly effective in older people compared with young subjects (Fulop et al., 2007). Alteration of TLR function in older adults is particularly relevant in view of the increased development and use of TLR agonist in vaccine. Influenza vaccine formulation in clinical trials employs the TLR5 agonist flagellin that would not require yearly reformulation and administration. CpG-containing oligonucleotides are used as TLR9-dependent vaccine adjuvants in the 7-valent pneumococcal conjugate vaccine and significantly enhanced the proportion of vaccine responders amongst HIV-infected adults. MPL, a derivative of lipid A from lipopolysaccharide is already used as an adjuvant in vaccines against human papillomavirus (Cervarix) (Shaw et al., 2011).

8. Conclusion

The first obvious conclusion is that immunosenescence is a complex phenomenon, which does not only reflect the action of time on immune cells. As discussed herein, many other factors, such as genetics, infection history, nutritional status, co-morbidities, socio-economic factors are likely to contribute to this process and its clinical impact. Geriatric medicine has to take into account all these specific characteristics to provide better care to this age group.

Data from literature and our ongoing study tend to suggest that "inflammaging" appears not only with age but is associated with indicators of frailty and the occurrence of comorbidities. Frail geriatric individuals express higher seric levels of TNFα and IL-6. This persistent chronic inflammation could directly participate to dampened innate immune responses upon stimulation. Indeed, *ex vivo* whole blood response to molecules like LPS tends to be reduced in older people. In intensive care units, old people with high basal levels of TNFα and IL-6 show increased severity of sepsis after community-acquired pneumonia (Mira et al., 2008). Intriguingly, increased IL-6 levels in the course of community acquired-pneumonia, is also associated with more severe sepsis. This might reflect the fact that *ex vivo* blood experiments do not take into account cytokine production by stromal cells such as endothelial cells, adipocytes or muscle cells. Moreover, circulating cytokine levels are also influenced by kidney function that is generally altered in the course of sepsis (Gomez CMH, 2000). Finally, it is possible that in the earlier phase of infections, old people are less efficient to control infection, leading to increased late inflammatory response.

Epidemiological associations do not always reflect causality. It is possible to link altered immunological parameters with frailty and comorbidities (fig 3). Should we conclude that dampened immune responses and exacerbated inflammation contribute to the fragility of the organism or that specific pathologies lead to immunosenescence? It is likely that both hypothesis are valid and reinforce each other. It has important implications in terms of therapeutic interventions. Should we treat or prevent chlamydia, CMV or H. *pylori* that could be responsible for local inflammation within atherosclerotic plaques (Rosenfeld & Campbell, 2011)? Would treatment of metabolic disorders reduce "inflammaging" processes? Should we try to "rejuvenate" the immune system through cytokine or hormonal replacement (Dorshkind et al., 2009)? Is the CMV-associated immune phenotype responsible for increased mortality rate or is it possible that frail individuals undergo more frequent reactivation of CMV, leading to the skewing of the memory response? To answer these crucial questions, clear immunological and biological parameters will have to be used is well-defined populations to overcome the weight of confounding factors.

Finally, to improve geriatric health, it seems clear that one should take into account several features of older people. We cannot imagine improving vaccinal responses without correcting nutritional status, frailty, controlling comorbidities and evaluate the impact of drug treatments. So even in this specific field, geriatric medicine requires multidisciplinary approach.

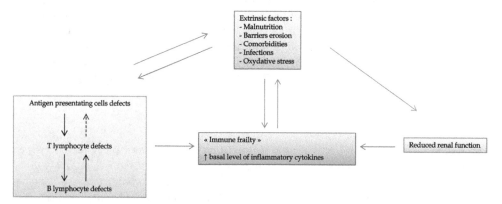

Fig. 8. Potential interplays between immune function and extrinsic factors.

9. References

Abedin,S., Michel, J. J., Lemster, B., & Vallejo, A. N. (2005). Diversity of NKR expression in aging T cells and in T cells of the aged: the new frontier into the exploration of protective immunity in the elderly. *Exp.Gerontol.* Vol.40, No.7, pp.537-548.

Ademokun,A., Wu, Y. C., & Dunn-Walters, D. (2010). The ageing B cell population: composition and function. *Biogerontology.* Vol.11, No.2, pp.125-137.

Agrawal,A., Agrawal, S., Cao, J. N., Su, H., Osann, K., & Gupta, S. (2007a). Altered innate immune functioning of dendritic cells in elderly humans: a role of phosphoinositide 3-kinase-signaling pathway. *J.Immunol.* Vol.178, No.11, pp.6912-6922.

Agrawal,A., Agrawal, S., & Gupta, S. (2007b). Dendritic cells in human aging. *Exp.Gerontol.* Vol.42, No.5, pp.421-426.

Alonso-Arias,R., Moro-Garcia, M. A., Lopez-Vazquez, A., Rodrigo, L., Baltar, J., Garcia, F. M., Jaurrieta, J. J., & Lopez-Larrea, C. (2011). NKG2D expression in CD4+ T lymphocytes as a marker of senescence in the aged immune system. *Age (Dordr.)* .

Alonso-Fernandez,P., Puerto, M., Mate, I., Ribera, J. M., & de la, F. M. (2008). Neutrophils of centenarians show function levels similar to those of young adults. *J.Am.Geriatr.Soc.* Vol.56, No.12, pp.2244-2251.

Andrews,N.P., Fujii, H., Goronzy, J. J., & Weyand, C. M. (2010). Telomeres and immunological diseases of aging. *Gerontology* Vol.56, No.4, pp.390-403.

Argentati,K., Re, F., Donnini, A., Tucci, M. G., Franceschi, C., Bartozzi, B., Bernardini, G., & Provinciali, M. (2002). Numerical and functional alterations of circulating gammadelta T lymphocytes in aged people and centenarians. *J.Leukoc.Biol.* Vol.72, No.1, pp.65-71.

Arlt,W. & Hewison, M. (2004). Hormones and immune function: implications of aging. *Aging Cell* Vol.3, No.4, pp.209-216.

Arnold,C.R., Wolf, J., Brunner, S., Herndler-Brandstetter, D., & Grubeck-Loebenstein, B. (2011). Gain and loss of T cell subsets in old age--age-related reshaping of the T cell repertoire. *J.Clin.Immunol.* Vol.31, No.2, pp.137-146.

Aspinall,R., Del Giudice, G., Effros, R. B., Grubeck-Loebenstein, B., & Sambhara, S. (2007). Challenges for vaccination in the elderly. *Immun.Ageing* Vol.4, pp.9.

Astrup,A.S., Tarnow, L., Jorsal, A., Lajer, M., Nzietchueng, R., Benetos, A., Rossing, P., & Parving, H. H. (2010). Telomere length predicts all-cause mortality in patients with type 1 diabetes. *Diabetologia* Vol.53, No.1, pp.45-48.

Balasubramanyam,M., Adaikalakoteswari, A., Monickaraj, S. F., & Mohan, V. (2007). Telomere shortening & metabolic/vascular diseases. *Indian J.Med.Res.* Vol.125, No.3, pp.441-450.

Bautmans,I., Gorus, E., Njemini, R., & Mets, T. (2007). Handgrip performance in relation to self-perceived fatigue, physical functioning and circulating IL-6 in elderly persons without inflammation. *BMC.Geriatr.* Vol.7, pp.5.

Bautmans,I., Njemini, R., Predom, H., Lemper, J. C., & Mets, T. (2008). Muscle endurance in elderly nursing home residents is related to fatigue perception, mobility, and circulating tumor necrosis factor-alpha, interleukin-6, and heat shock protein 70. *J.Am.Geriatr.Soc.* Vol.56, No.3, pp.389-396.

Beharka,A.A., Meydani, M., Wu, D., Leka, L. S., Meydani, A., & Meydani, S. N. (2001). Interleukin-6 production does not increase with age. *J.Gerontol.A Biol.Sci.Med.Sci.* Vol.56, No.2, pp.B81-B88.

Beitland,S., Opdahl, H., Aspelin, T., Saetre, L., & Lyberg, T. (2009). Blood leucocyte cytokine production after LPS stimulation at different concentrations of glucose and/or insulin. *Acta Anaesthesiol.Scand.* Vol.53, No.2, pp.183-189.

Benetos,A., Gardner, J. P., Zureik, M., Labat, C., Xiaobin, L., Adamopoulos, C., Temmar, M., Bean, K. E., Thomas, F., & Aviv, A. (2004). Short telomeres are associated with increased carotid atherosclerosis in hypertensive subjects. *Hypertension* Vol.43, No.2, pp.182-185.

Bikle,D. (2009). Nonclassic actions of vitamin D. *J.Clin.Endocrinol.Metab* Vol.94, No.1, pp.26-34.

Boren,E. & Gershwin, M. E. (2004). Inflamm-aging: autoimmunity, and the immune-risk phenotype. *Autoimmun.Rev.* Vol.3, No.5, pp.401-406.

Bouhuys,A.L., Flentge, F., Oldehinkel, A. J., & van, d. B. (2004). Potential psychosocial mechanisms linking depression to immune function in elderly subjects. *Psychiatry Res.* Vol.127, No.3, pp.237-245.

Bouree,P. (2003). Immunity and immunization in elderly. *Pathol.Biol.(Paris)* Vol.51, No.10, pp.581-585.

Breuil,V., Ticchioni, M., Testa, J., Roux, C. H., Ferrari, P., Breittmayer, J. P., Albert-Sabonnadiere, C., Durant, J., De Perreti, F., Bernard, A., Euller-Ziegler, L., & Carle, G. F. (2010). Immune changes in post-menopausal osteoporosis: the Immunos study. *Osteoporos.Int.* Vol.21, No.5, pp.805-814.

Brouilette,S.W., Moore, J. S., McMahon, A. D., Thompson, J. R., Ford, I., Shepherd, J., Packard, C. J., & Samani, N. J. (2007). Telomere length, risk of coronary heart disease, and statin treatment in the West of Scotland Primary Prevention Study: a nested case-control study. *Lancet* Vol.369, No.9556, pp.107-114.

Bruunsgaard,H., Ladelund, S., Pedersen, A. N., Schroll, M., Jorgensen, T., & Pedersen, B. K. (2003). Predicting death from tumour necrosis factor-alpha and interleukin-6 in 80-year-old people. *Clin.Exp.Immunol.* Vol.132, No.1, pp.24-31.

Bruunsgaard,H., Pedersen, A. N., Schroll, M., Skinhoj, P., & Pedersen, B. K. (1999a). Impaired production of proinflammatory cytokines in response to lipopolysaccharide (LPS) stimulation in elderly humans. *Clin.Exp.Immunol.* Vol.118, No.2, pp.235-241.

Bruunsgaard,H., Skinhoj, P., Qvist, J., & Pedersen, B. K. (1999b). Elderly humans show prolonged in vivo inflammatory activity during pneumococcal infections. *J.Infect.Dis.* Vol.180, No.2, pp.551-554.

Buffa,S., Bulati, M., Pellicano, M., Dunn-Walters, D. K., Wu, Y. C., Candore, G., Vitello, S., Caruso, C., & Colonna-Romano, G. (2011). B cell immunosenescence: different features of naive and memory B cells in elderly. *Biogerontology.* Vol.12, No.5, pp.473-483.

Bulati,M., Buffa, S., Candore, G., Caruso, C., Dunn-Walters, D. K., Pellicano, M., Wu, Y. C., & Colonna, R. G. (2011). B cells and immunosenescence: a focus on IgG+IgD-. *Ageing Res.Rev.* Vol.10, No.2, pp.274-284.

Capurso,C., Solfrizzi, V., D'Introno, A., Colacicco, A. M., Capurso, S. A., Semeraro, C., Capurso, A., & Panza, F. (2007). Interleukin 6 variable number of tandem repeats

(VNTR) gene polymorphism in centenarians. *Ann.Hum.Genet.* Vol.71, No.Pt 6, pp.843-848.

Chakravarti,B. & Abraham, G. N. (1999). Aging and T-cell-mediated immunity. *Mech.Ageing Dev.* Vol.108, No.3, pp.183-206.

Chen,W.H., Kozlovsky, B. F., Effros, R. B., Grubeck-Loebenstein, B., Edelman, R., & Sztein, M. B. (2009). Vaccination in the elderly: an immunological perspective. *Trends Immunol.* Vol.30, No.7, pp.351-359.

Chong,Y., Ikematsu, H., Yamaji, K., Nishimura, M., Nabeshima, S., Kashiwagi, S., & Hayashi, J. (2005). CD27(+) (memory) B cell decrease and apoptosis-resistant CD27(-) (naive) B cell increase in aged humans: implications for age-related peripheral B cell developmental disturbances. *Int.Immunol.* Vol.17, No.4, pp.383-390.

Ciaramella,A., Spalletta, G., Bizzoni, F., Salani, F., Caltagirone, C., & Bossu, P. (2011). Effect of age on surface molecules and cytokine expression in human dendritic cells. *Cell Immunol.* Vol.269, No.2, pp.82-89.

Coen,P.M., Flynn, M. G., Markofski, M. M., Pence, B. D., & Hannemann, R. E. (2010). Adding exercise to rosuvastatin treatment: influence on C-reactive protein, monocyte toll-like receptor 4 expression, and inflammatory monocyte (CD14+CD16+) population. *Metabolism* Vol.59, No.12, pp.1775-1783.

Colonna-Romano,G., Bulati, M., Aquino, A., Pellicano, M., Vitello, S., Lio, D., Candore, G., & Caruso, C. (2009). A double-negative (IgD-CD27-) B cell population is increased in the peripheral blood of elderly people. *Mech.Ageing Dev.* Vol.130, No.10, pp.681-690.

Colonna-Romano,G., Bulati, M., Aquino, A., Scialabba, G., Candore, G., Lio, D., Motta, M., Malaguarnera, M., & Caruso, C. (2003). B cells in the aged: CD27, CD5, and CD40 expression. *Mech.Ageing Dev.* Vol.124, No.4, pp.389-393.

Cook,G.P., Savic, S., Wittmann, M., & McDermott, M. F. (2010). The NLRP3 inflammasome, a target for therapy in diverse disease states. *Eur.J.Immunol.* Vol.40, No.3, pp.631-634.

Corsini,E., Vismara, L., Lucchi, L., Viviani, B., Govoni, S., Galli, C. L., Marinovich, M., & Racchi, M. (2006). High interleukin-10 production is associated with low antibody response to influenza vaccination in the elderly. *J.Leukoc.Biol.* Vol.80, No.2, pp.376-382.

Cretel,E., Veen, I., Pierres, A., Bongrand, P., & Gavazzi, G. (2010). [Immunosenescence and infections, myth or reality?]. *Med.Mal Infect.* Vol.40, No.6, pp.307-318.

Crighton,M.H. & Puppione, A. A. (2006). Geriatric neutrophils: implications for older adults. *Semin.Oncol.Nurs.* Vol.22, No.1, pp.3-9.

Crotty,S. (2011). Follicular helper CD4 T cells (TFH). *Annu.Rev.Immunol.* Vol.29, pp.621-663.

De Martinis,M., Di Benedetto, M. C., Mengoli, L. P., & Ginaldi, L. (2006). Senile osteoporosis: is it an immune-mediated disease? *Inflamm.Res.* Vol.55, No.10, pp.399-404.

De Martinis,M., Franceschi, C., Monti, D., & Ginaldi, L. (2005). Inflamm-ageing and lifelong antigenic load as major determinants of ageing rate and longevity. *FEBS Lett.* Vol.579, No.10, pp.2035-2039.

Della Bella S., Bierti, L., Presicce, P., Arienti, R., Valenti, M., Saresella, M., Vergani, C., & Villa, M. L. (2007). Peripheral blood dendritic cells and monocytes are differently regulated in the elderly. *Clin.Immunol.* Vol.122, No.2, pp.220-228.

Derhovanessian,E., Maier, A. B., Beck, R., Jahn, G., Hahnel, K., Slagboom, P. E., de Craen, A. J., Westendorp, R. G., & Pawelec, G. (2010). Hallmark features of immunosenescence are absent in familial longevity. *J.Immunol.* Vol.185, No.8, pp.4618-4624.

Desai,A., Grolleau-Julius, A., & Yung, R. (2010). Leukocyte function in the aging immune system. *J.Leukoc.Biol.* Vol.87, No.6, pp.1001-1009.

DiPenta,J.M., Green-Johnson, J. M., & Murphy, R. J. (2007). Type 2 diabetes mellitus, resistance training, and innate immunity: is there a common link? *Appl.Physiol Nutr.Metab* Vol.32, No.6, pp.1025-1035.

Dorshkind,K., Montecino-Rodriguez, E., & Signer, R. A. (2009). The ageing immune system: is it ever too old to become young again? *Nat.Rev.Immunol.* Vol.9, No.1, pp.57-62.

Duewell,P., Kono, H., Rayner, K. J., Sirois, C. M., Vladimer, G., Bauernfeind, F. G., Abela, G. S., Franchi, L., Nunez, G., Schnurr, M., Espevik, T., Lien, E., Fitzgerald, K. A., Rock, K. L., Moore, K. J., Wright, S. D., Hornung, V., Latz, E. (2010). NLRP3 inflammasomes are required for atherogenesis and activated by cholesterol crystals. *Nature* Vol.464, No.7293, pp.1357-1361.

Dzionek,A., Fuchs, A., Schmidt, P., Cremer, S., Zysk, M., Miltenyi, S., Buck, D. W., & Schmitz, J. (2000). BDCA-2, BDCA-3, and BDCA-4: three markers for distinct subsets of dendritic cells in human peripheral blood. *J.Immunol.* Vol.165, No.11, pp.6037-6046.

Epel,E.S., Lin, J., Wilhelm, F. H., Wolkowitz, O. M., Cawthon, R., Adler, N. E., Dolbier, C., Mendes, W. B., & Blackburn, E. H. (2006). Cell aging in relation to stress arousal and cardiovascular disease risk factors. *Psychoneuroendocrinology* Vol.31, No.3, pp.277-287.

Fernandez-Gutierrez,B., Jover, J. A., De Miguel, S., Hernandez-Garcia, C., Vidan, M. T., Ribera, J. M., Banares, A., & Serra, J. A. (1999). Early lymphocyte activation in elderly humans: impaired T and T-dependent B cell responses. *Exp.Gerontol.* Vol.34, No.2, pp.217-229.

Ferrando-Martinez,S., Ruiz-Mateos, E., Hernandez, A., Gutierrez, E., Rodriguez-Mendez, M. M., Ordonez, A., & Leal, M. (2011). Age-related deregulation of naive T cell homeostasis in elderly humans. *Age (Dordr.)* Vol.33, No.2, pp.197-207.

Ferro,D., Parrotto, S., Basili, S., Alessandri, C., & Violi, F. (2000). Simvastatin inhibits the monocyte expression of proinflammatory cytokines in patients with hypercholesterolemia. *J.Am.Coll.Cardiol.* Vol.36, No.2, pp.427-431.

Ferroni,P., Martini, F., Cardarello, C. M., Gazzaniga, P. P., Davi, G., & Basili, S. (2003). Enhanced interleukin-1beta in hypercholesterolemia: effects of simvastatin and low-dose aspirin. *Circulation* Vol.108, No.14, pp.1673-1675.

Focosi,D., Bestagno, M., Burrone, O., & Petrini, M. (2010). CD57+ T lymphocytes and functional immune deficiency. *J.Leukoc.Biol.* Vol.87, No.1, pp.107-116.

Forsey,R.J., Thompson, J. M., Ernerudh, J., Hurst, T. L., Strindhall, J., Johansson, B., Nilsson, B. O., & Wikby, A. (2003). Plasma cytokine profiles in elderly humans. *Mech.Ageing Dev.* Vol.124, No.4, pp.487-493.

Freeman,S.L., Fisher, L., German, J. B., Leung, P. S., Prince, H., Selmi, C., Naguwa, S. M., & Gershwin, M. E. (2010). Dairy proteins and the response to pneumovax in senior citizens: a randomized, double-blind, placebo-controlled pilot study. *Ann.N.Y.Acad.Sci.* Vol.1190, pp.97-103.

Fujihashi,K. & Kiyono, H. (2009). Mucosal immunosenescence: new developments and vaccines to control infectious diseases. *Trends Immunol.* Vol.30, No.7, pp.334-343.

Fulop,T., Kotb, R., Fortin, C. F., Pawelec, G., de Angelis, F., & Larbi, A. (2010). Potential role of immunosenescence in cancer development. *Ann.N.Y.Acad.Sci.* Vol.1197, pp.158-165.

Fulop,T., Larbi, A., Douziech, N., Fortin, C., Guerard, K. P., Lesur, O., Khalil, A., & Dupuis, G. (2004). Signal transduction and functional changes in neutrophils with aging. *Aging Cell* Vol.3, No.4, pp.217-226.

Fulop,T., Larbi, A., Hirokawa, K., Mocchegiani, E., Lesourds, B., Castle, S., Wikby, A., Franceschi, C., & Pawelec, G. (2007). Immunosupportive therapies in aging. *Clin.Interv.Aging* Vol.2, No.1, pp.33-54.

Gabriel,P., Cakman, I., & Rink, L. (2002). Overproduction of monokines by leukocytes after stimulation with lipopolysaccharide in the elderly. *Exp.Gerontol.* Vol.37, No.2-3, pp.235-247.

Gannage-Yared,M.H., Azoury, M., Mansour, I., Baddoura, R., Halaby, G., & Naaman, R. (2003). Effects of a short-term calcium and vitamin D treatment on serum cytokines, bone markers, insulin and lipid concentrations in healthy post-menopausal women. *J.Endocrinol.Invest* Vol.26, No.8, pp.748-753.

Giunta,B., Fernandez, F., Nikolic, W. V., Obregon, D., Rrapo, E., Town, T., & Tan, J. (2008). Inflammaging as a prodrome to Alzheimer's disease. *J.Neuroinflammation.* Vol.5, pp.51.

Gomez CMH. (2000). elimination of cytokines by the kidney: comparison between normal individuals and patients with severe sepsis or the systemic inflammatory response syndrome. *british journal of anesthesia* Vol.84, No.5. sheldon J, Riches P, and Palazo MGA.

Gonzalo-Calvo,D., Fernandez-Garcia, B., Luxan-Delgado, B., Rodriguez-Gonzalez, S., Garcia-Macia, M., Suarez, F. M., Solano, J. J., Rodriguez-Colunga, M. J., & Coto-Montes, A. (2011). Long-term training induces a healthy inflammatory and endocrine emergent biomarker profile in elderly men. *Age (Dordr.)* .

Gregg,R., Smith, C. M., Clark, F. J., Dunnion, D., Khan, N., Chakraverty, R., Nayak, L., & Moss, P. A. (2005). The number of human peripheral blood CD4+ CD25high regulatory T cells increases with age. *Clin.Exp.Immunol.* Vol.140, No.3, pp.540-546.

Grewe,M. (2001). Chronological ageing and photoageing of dendritic cells. *Clin.Exp.Dermatol.* Vol.26, No.7, pp.608-612.

Grolleau-Julius,A., Ray, D., & Yung, R. L. (2010). The role of epigenetics in aging and autoimmunity. *Clin.Rev.Allergy Immunol.* Vol.39, No.1, pp.42-50.

Gruver,A.L., Hudson, L. L., & Sempowski, G. D. (2007). Immunosenescence of ageing. *J.Pathol.* Vol.211, No.2, pp.144-156.

Gruver,A.L., Ventevogel, M. S., & Sempowski, G. D. (2009). Leptin receptor is expressed in thymus medulla and leptin protects against thymic remodeling during endotoxemia-induced thymus involution. *J.Endocrinol.* Vol.203, No.1, pp.75-85.

Gupta,S. & Gollapudi, S. (2006). TNF-alpha-induced apoptosis in human naive and memory CD8+ T cells in aged humans. *Exp.Gerontol.* Vol.41, No.1, pp.69-77.

Gupta,S. & Gollapudi, S. (2008). CD95-mediated apoptosis in naive, central and effector memory subsets of CD4+ and CD8+ T cells in aged humans. *Exp.Gerontol.* Vol.43, No.4, pp.266-274.

Haase,H. & Rink, L. (2009). The immune system and the impact of zinc during aging. *Immun.Ageing* Vol.6, pp.9.

Hadrup,S.R., Strindhall, J., Kollgaard, T., Seremet, T., Johansson, B., Pawelec, G., thor, S. P., & Wikby, A. (2006). Longitudinal studies of clonally expanded CD8 T cells reveal a repertoire shrinkage predicting mortality and an increased number of dysfunctional cytomegalovirus-specific T cells in the very elderly. *J.Immunol.* Vol.176, No.4, pp.2645-2653.

Hartel,C., Strunk, T., Bucsky, P., & Schultz, C. (2004). Effects of vitamin C on intracytoplasmic cytokine production in human whole blood monocytes and lymphocytes. *Cytokine* Vol.27, No.4-5, pp.101-106.

Herndler-Brandstetter,D., Schwaiger, S., Veel, E., Fehrer, C., Cioca, D. P., Almanzar, G., Keller, M., Pfister, G., Parson, W., Wurzner, R., Schonitzer, D., Henson, S. M., Aspinall, R., Lepperdinger, G., & Grubeck-Loebenstein, B. (2005). CD25-expressing CD8+ T cells are potent memory cells in old age. *J.Immunol.* Vol.175, No.3, pp.1566-1574.

Hewison,M. (2010). Vitamin D and the immune system: new perspectives on an old theme. *Endocrinol.Metab Clin.North Am.* Vol.39, No.2, pp.365-79, table.

Hick,R.W., Gruver, A. L., Ventevogel, M. S., Haynes, B. F., & Sempowski, G. D. (2006). Leptin selectively augments thymopoiesis in leptin deficiency and lipopolysaccharide-induced thymic atrophy. *J.Immunol.* Vol.177, No.1, pp.169-176.

Himmerich,H., Milenovic, S., Fulda, S., Plumakers, B., Sheldrick, A. J., Michel, T. M., Kircher, T., & Rink, L. (2010). Regulatory T cells increased while IL-1beta decreased during antidepressant therapy. *J.Psychiatr.Res.* Vol.44, No.15, pp.1052-1057.

Hotamisligil,G.S. (2010). Endoplasmic reticulum stress and atherosclerosis. *Nat.Med.* Vol.16, No.4, pp.396-399.

Huber,L.A., Xu, Q. B., Jurgens, G., Bock, G., Buhler, E., Gey, K. F., Schonitzer, D., Traill, K. N., & Wick, G. (1991). Correlation of lymphocyte lipid composition membrane microviscosity and mitogen response in the aged. *Eur.J.Immunol.* Vol.21, No.11, pp.2761-2765.

Irwin,M.R. & Miller, A. H. (2007). Depressive disorders and immunity: 20 years of progress and discovery. *Brain Behav.Immun.* Vol.21, No.4, pp.374-383.

James,K., Premchand, N., Skibinska, A., Skibinski, G., Nicol, M., & Mason, J. I. (1997). IL-6, DHEA and the ageing process. *Mech.Ageing Dev.* Vol.93, No.1-3, pp.15-24.

Jiang,H., Ju, Z., & Rudolph, K. L. (2007). Telomere shortening and ageing. *Z.Gerontol.Geriatr.* Vol.40, No.5, pp.314-324.

Jing,Y., Shaheen, E., Drake, R. R., Chen, N., Gravenstein, S., & Deng, Y. (2009). Aging is associated with a numerical and functional decline in plasmacytoid dendritic cells, whereas myeloid dendritic cells are relatively unaltered in human peripheral blood. *Hum.Immunol.* Vol.70, No.10, pp.777-784.

Kamada,M., Irahara, M., Maegawa, M., Yasui, T., Yamano, S., Yamada, M., Tezuka, M., Kasai, Y., Deguchi, K., Ohmoto, Y., & Aono, T. (2001). B cell subsets in postmenopausal women and the effect of hormone replacement therapy. *Maturitas* Vol.37, No.3, pp.173-179.

Kanwar,J.R. & Kanwar, R. K. (2009). Gut health immunomodulatory and anti-inflammatory functions of gut enzyme digested high protein micro-nutrient dietary supplement-Enprocal. *BMC.Immunol.* Vol.10, pp.7.

Kilpatrick,R.D., Rickabaugh, T., Hultin, L. E., Hultin, P., Hausner, M. A., Detels, R., Phair, J., & Jamieson, B. D. (2008). Homeostasis of the naive CD4+ T cell compartment during aging. *J.Immunol.* Vol.180, No.3, pp.1499-1507.

Krabbe,K.S., Pedersen, M., & Bruunsgaard, H. (2004). Inflammatory mediators in the elderly. *Exp.Gerontol.* Vol.39, No.5, pp.687-699.

Krysiak,R., Gdula-Dymek, A., & Okopien, B. (2011a). Effect of simvastatin and fenofibrate on cytokine release and systemic inflammation in type 2 diabetes mellitus with mixed dyslipidemia. *Am.J.Cardiol.* Vol.107, No.7, pp.1010-1018.

Krysiak,R., Gdula-Dymek, A., Scieszka, J., & Okopien, B. (2011b). Anti-inflammatory and monocyte-suppressing effects of simvastatin in patients with impaired fasting glucose. *Basic Clin.Pharmacol.Toxicol.* Vol.108, No.2, pp.131-137.

Ku,L.T., Gercel-Taylor, C., Nakajima, S. T., & Taylor, D. D. (2009). Alterations of T cell activation signalling and cytokine production by postmenopausal estrogen levels. *Immun.Ageing* Vol.6, pp.1.

Lesourd,B. (2006). Nutritional factors and immunological ageing. *Proc.Nutr.Soc.* Vol.65, No.3, pp.319-325.

Li,Q.Z., Deng, Q., Li, J. Q., Yi, G. H., & Zhao, S. P. (2005). Valsartan reduces interleukin-1beta secretion by peripheral blood mononuclear cells in patients with essential hypertension. *Clin.Chim.Acta* Vol.355, No.1-2, pp.131-136.

Li,X., Liu, C., Cui, J., Dong, M., Peng, C. H., Li, Q. S., Cheng, J. L., Jiang, S. L., & Tian, Y. (2009). Effects of pravastatin on the function of dendritic cells in patients with coronary heart disease. *Basic Clin.Pharmacol.Toxicol.* Vol.104, No.2, pp.101-106.

Ligthart,G.J., Corberand, J. X., Fournier, C., Galanaud, P., Hijmans, W., Kennes, B., Muller-Hermelink, H. K., & Steinmann, G. G. (1984). Admission criteria for immunogerontological studies in man: the SENIEUR protocol. *Mech.Ageing Dev.* Vol.28, No.1, pp.47-55.

Lundberg,A.M. & Hansson, G. K. (2010). Innate immune signals in atherosclerosis. *Clin.Immunol.* Vol.134, No.1, pp.5-24.

MacDonald,K.P., Munster, D. J., Clark, G. J., Dzionek, A., Schmitz, J., & Hart, D. N. (2002). Characterization of human blood dendritic cell subsets. *Blood* Vol.100, No.13, pp.4512-4520.

Maggio,M., Ceda, G. P., Lauretani, F., Bandinelli, S., Corsi, A. M., Giallauria, F., Guralnik, J. M., Zuliani, G., Cattabiani, C., Parrino, S., Ablondi, F., Dall'aglio, E., Ceresini, G., Basaria, S., & Ferrucci, L. (2011). SHBG, sex hormones, and inflammatory markers in older women. *J.Clin.Endocrinol.Metab* Vol.96, No.4, pp.1053-1059.

Malaguarnera,L., Cristaldi, E., & Malaguarnera, M. (2010). The role of immunity in elderly cancer. *Crit Rev.Oncol.Hematol.* Vol.74, No.1, pp.40-60.

Mariani,E., Cattini, L., Neri, S., Malavolta, M., Mocchegiani, E., Ravaglia, G., & Facchini, A. (2006). Simultaneous evaluation of circulating chemokine and cytokine profiles in elderly subjects by multiplex technology: relationship with zinc status. *Biogerontology.* Vol.7, No.5-6, pp.449-459.

McElhaney,J.E. & Effros, R. B. (2009). Immunosenescence: what does it mean to health outcomes in older adults? *Curr.Opin.Immunol.* Vol.21, No.4, pp.418-424.

McIntire,C.R., Yeretssian, G., & Saleh, M. (2009). Inflammasomes in infection and inflammation. *Apoptosis.* Vol.14, No.4, pp.522-535.

Mira,J.P., Max, A., & Burgel, P. R. (2008). The role of biomarkers in community-acquired pneumonia: predicting mortality and response to adjunctive therapy. *Crit Care* Vol.12 Suppl 6, pp.S5.

Mocchegiani,E. (2010). session 2 : micronutrients and the immune system : zinc, metallothioneins and immunosenescence. *Proc.Nutr.Soc.*

Mocchegiani,E., Costarelli, L., Giacconi, R., Piacenza, F., Basso, A., & Malavolta, M. (2011). Zinc, metallothioneins and immunosenescence: effect of zinc supply as nutrigenomic approach. *Biogerontology.*

Moro-Garcia,M.A., Alonso-Arias, R., Lopez-Vazquez, A., Suarez-Garcia, F. M., Solano-Jaurrieta, J. J., Baltar, J., & Lopez-Larrea, C. (2011). Relationship between functional ability in older people, immune system status, and intensity of response to CMV. *Age (Dordr.)* .

Motta,M., Ferlito, L., Malaguarnera, L., Vinci, E., Bosco, S., Maugeri, D., & Malaguarnera, M. (2003). Alterations of the lymphocytic set-up in elderly patients with cancer. *Arch.Gerontol.Geriatr.* Vol.36, No.1, pp.7-14.

Mysliwska,J., Bryl, E., Foerster, J., & Mysliwski, A. (1998). Increase of interleukin 6 and decrease of interleukin 2 production during the ageing process are influenced by the health status. *Mech.Ageing Dev.* Vol.100, No.3, pp.313-328.

Naidoo,N. (2009). ER and aging-Protein folding and the ER stress response. *Ageing Res.Rev.* Vol.8, No.3, pp.150-159.

Naylor,K., Li, G., Vallejo, A. N., Lee, W. W., Koetz, K., Bryl, E., Witkowski, J., Fulbright, J., Weyand, C. M., & Goronzy, J. J. (2005). The influence of age on T cell generation and TCR diversity. *J.Immunol.* Vol.174, No.11, pp.7446-7452.

Nichol,K.L., Nordin, J., Mullooly, J., Lask, R., Fillbrandt, K., & Iwane, M. (2003). Influenza vaccination and reduction in hospitalizations for cardiac disease and stroke among the elderly. *N.Engl.J.Med.* Vol.348, No.14, pp.1322-1332.

Nilsson,B.O., Ernerudh, J., Johansson, B., Evrin, P. E., Lofgren, S., Ferguson, F. G., & Wikby, A. (2003). Morbidity does not influence the T-cell immune risk phenotype in the elderly: findings in the Swedish NONA Immune Study using sample selection protocols. *Mech.Ageing Dev.* Vol.124, No.4, pp.469-476.

Ohyashiki,J.H., Iwama, H., Yahata, N., Ando, K., Hayashi, S., Shay, J. W., & Ohyashiki, K. (1999). Telomere stability is frequently impaired in high-risk groups of patients with myelodysplastic syndromes. *Clin.Cancer Res.* Vol.5, No.5, pp.1155-1160.

Ongradi,J. & Kovesdi, V. (2010). Factors that may impact on immunosenescence: an appraisal. *Immun.Ageing* Vol.7, pp.7.

Ouyang,Q., Wagner, W. M., Voehringer, D., Wikby, A., Klatt, T., Walter, S., Muller, C. A., Pircher, H., & Pawelec, G. (2003). Age-associated accumulation of CMV-specific CD8+ T cells expressing the inhibitory killer cell lectin-like receptor G1 (KLRG1). *Exp.Gerontol.* Vol.38, No.8, pp.911-920.

Panda,A., Qian, F., Mohanty, S., van Duin, D., Newman, F. K., Zhang, L., Chen, S., Towle, V., Belshe, R. B., Fikrig, E., Allore, H. G., Montgomery, R. R., & Shaw, A. C. (2010). Age-associated decrease in TLR function in primary human dendritic cells predicts influenza vaccine response. *J.Immunol.* Vol.184, No.5, pp.2518-2527.

Panossian,L.A., Porter, V. R., Valenzuela, H. F., Zhu, X., Reback, E., Masterman, D., Cummings, J. L., & Effros, R. B. (2003). Telomere shortening in T cells correlates with Alzheimer's disease status. *Neurobiol.Aging* Vol.24, No.1, pp.77-84.

Pawelec,G., Akbar, A., Caruso, C., Solana, R., Grubeck-Loebenstein, B., & Wikby, A. (2005). Human immunosenescence: is it infectious? *Immunol.Rev.* Vol.205, pp.257-268.

Pawelec,G. & Derhovanessian, E. (2011). Role of CMV in immune senescence. *Virus Res.* Vol.157, No.2, pp.175-179.

Penninx,B.W., Kritchevsky, S. B., Newman, A. B., Nicklas, B. J., Simonsick, E. M., Rubin, S., Nevitt, M., Visser, M., Harris, T., & Pahor, M. (2004). Inflammatory markers and incident mobility limitation in the elderly. *J.Am.Geriatr.Soc.* Vol.52, No.7, pp.1105-1113.

Penninx,B.W., Kritchevsky, S. B., Yaffe, K., Newman, A. B., Simonsick, E. M., Rubin, S., Ferrucci, L., Harris, T., & Pahor, M. (2003). Inflammatory markers and depressed mood in older persons: results from the Health, Aging and Body Composition study. *Biol.Psychiatry* Vol.54, No.5, pp.566-572.

Pepersack,T., Rotsaert, P., Benoit, F., Willems, D., Fuss, M., Bourdoux, P., & Duchateau, J. (2001). Prevalence of zinc deficiency and its clinical relevance among hospitalised elderly. *Arch.Gerontol.Geriatr.* Vol.33, No.3, pp.243-253.

Perez-Cabezas,B., Naranjo-Gomez, M., Fernandez, M. A., Grifols, J. R., Pujol-Borrell, R., & Borras, F. E. (2007). Reduced numbers of plasmacytoid dendritic cells in aged blood donors. *Exp.Gerontol.* Vol.42, No.10, pp.1033-1038.

Pfister,G. & Savino, W. (2008). Can the immune system still be efficient in the elderly? An immunological and immunoendocrine therapeutic perspective. *Neuroimmunomodulation.* Vol.15, No.4-6, pp.351-364.

Picano,E., Morales, M. A., del Ry, S., & Sicari, R. (2010). Innate inflammation in myocardial perfusion and its implication for heart failure. *Ann.N.Y.Acad.Sci.* Vol.1207, pp.107-115.

Pierce,A., Legrand, D., & Mazurier, J. (2009). [Lactoferrin: a multifunctional protein]. *Med.Sci.(Paris)* Vol.25, No.4, pp.361-369.

Pietschmann,P., Hahn, P., Kudlacek, S., Thomas, R., & Peterlik, M. (2000). Surface markers and transendothelial migration of dendritic cells from elderly subjects. *Exp.Gerontol.* Vol.35, No.2, pp.213-224.

Rajasekaran,K., Xiong, V., Fong, L., Gorski, J., & Malarkannan, S. (2010). Functional dichotomy between NKG2D and CD28-mediated co-stimulation in human CD8+ T cells. *PLoS.One.* Vol.5, No.9.

Ravaglia,G., Forti, P., Maioli, F., Chiappelli, M., Montesi, F., Tumini, E., Mariani, E., Licastro, F., & Patterson, C. (2007). Blood inflammatory markers and risk of dementia: The Conselice Study of Brain Aging. *Neurobiol.Aging* Vol.28, No.12, pp.1810-1820.

Reuben,D.B., Cheh, A. I., Harris, T. B., Ferrucci, L., Rowe, J. W., Tracy, R. P., & Seeman, T. E. (2002). Peripheral blood markers of inflammation predict mortality and functional decline in high-functioning community-dwelling older persons. *J.Am.Geriatr.Soc.* Vol.50, No.4, pp.638-644.

Rink,L., Cakman, I., & Kirchner, H. (1998). Altered cytokine production in the elderly. *Mech.Ageing Dev.* Vol.102, No.2-3, pp.199-209.

Rosenfeld,M.E. & Campbell, L. A. (2011). Pathogens and atherosclerosis: Update on the potential contribution of multiple infectious organisms to the pathogenesis of atherosclerosis. *Thromb.Haemost.* Vol.106, No.5, pp.858-867.

Sadeghi,H.M., Schnelle, J. F., Thoma, J. K., Nishanian, P., & Fahey, J. L. (1999). Phenotypic and functional characteristics of circulating monocytes of elderly persons. *Exp.Gerontol.* Vol.34, No.8, pp.959-970.

Sampson,M.J., Winterbone, M. S., Hughes, J. C., Dozio, N., & Hughes, D. A. (2006). Monocyte telomere shortening and oxidative DNA damage in type 2 diabetes. *Diabetes Care* Vol.29, No.2, pp.283-289.

Schenkein,J.G., Park, S., & Nahm, M. H. (2008). Pneumococcal vaccination in older adults induces antibodies with low opsonic capacity and reduced antibody potency. *Vaccine* Vol.26, No.43, pp.5521-5526.

Schiffrin,E.J., Morley, J. E., Donnet-Hughes, A., & Guigoz, Y. (2010). The inflammatory status of the elderly: the intestinal contribution. *Mutat.Res.* Vol.690, No.1-2, pp.50-56.

Schonbeck,U. & Libby, P. (2004). Inflammation, immunity, and HMG-CoA reductase inhibitors: statins as antiinflammatory agents? *Circulation* Vol.109, No.21 Suppl 1, pp.II18-II26.

Schwalfenberg,G.K. (2011). A review of the critical role of vitamin D in the functioning of the immune system and the clinical implications of vitamin D deficiency. *Mol.Nutr.Food Res.* Vol.55, No.1, pp.96-108.

Seidler,S., Zimmermann, H. W., Bartneck, M., Trautwein, C., & Tacke, F. (2010). Age-dependent alterations of monocyte subsets and monocyte-related chemokine pathways in healthy adults. *BMC.Immunol.* Vol.11, pp.30.

Senchina,D.S. & Kohut, M. L. (2007). Immunological outcomes of exercise in older adults. *Clin.Interv.Aging* Vol.2, No.1, pp.3-16.

Shanley,D.P., Aw, D., Manley, N. R., & Palmer, D. B. (2009). An evolutionary perspective on the mechanisms of immunosenescence. *Trends Immunol.* Vol.30, No.7, pp.374-381.

Shaw,A.C., Panda, A., Joshi, S. R., Qian, F., Allore, H. G., & Montgomery, R. R. (2011). Dysregulation of human Toll-like receptor function in aging. *Ageing Res.Rev.* Vol.10, No.3, pp.346-353.

Shodell,M. & Siegal, F. P. (2002). Circulating, interferon-producing plasmacytoid dendritic cells decline during human ageing. *Scand.J.Immunol.* Vol.56, No.5, pp.518-521.

Shurin,G.V., Yurkovetsky, Z. R., Chatta, G. S., Tourkova, I. L., Shurin, M. R., & Lokshin, A. E. (2007). Dynamic alteration of soluble serum biomarkers in healthy aging. *Cytokine* Vol.39, No.2, pp.123-129.

Spyridopoulos,I., Hoffmann, J., Aicher, A., Brummendorf, T. H., Doerr, H. W., Zeiher, A. M., & Dimmeler, S. (2009). Accelerated telomere shortening in leukocyte subpopulations of patients with coronary heart disease: role of cytomegalovirus seropositivity. *Circulation* Vol.120, No.14, pp.1364-1372.

Steer,S.E., Williams, F. M., Kato, B., Gardner, J. P., Norman, P. J., Hall, M. A., Kimura, M., Vaughan, R., Aviv, A., & Spector, T. D. (2007). Reduced telomere length in rheumatoid arthritis is independent of disease activity and duration. *Ann.Rheum.Dis.* Vol.66, No.4, pp.476-480.

Straub,R.H., Konecna, L., Hrach, S., Rothe, G., Kreutz, M., Scholmerich, J., Falk, W., & Lang, B. (1998). Serum dehydroepiandrosterone (DHEA) and DHEA sulfate are negatively correlated with serum interleukin-6 (IL-6), and DHEA inhibits IL-6 secretion from mononuclear cells in man in vitro: possible link between endocrinosenescence and immunosenescence. *J.Clin.Endocrinol.Metab* Vol.83, No.6, pp.2012-2017.

Stulnig,T.M., Buhler, E., Bock, G., Kirchebner, C., Schonitzer, D., & Wick, G. (1995). Altered switch in lipid composition during T-cell blast transformation in the healthy elderly. *J.Gerontol.A Biol.Sci.Med.Sci.* Vol.50, No.6, pp.B383-B390.

Tortorella,C., Simone, O., Piazzolla, G., Stella, I., Cappiello, V., & Antonaci, S. (2006). Role of phosphoinositide 3-kinase and extracellular signal-regulated kinase pathways in granulocyte macrophage-colony-stimulating factor failure to delay fas-induced neutrophil apoptosis in elderly humans. *J.Gerontol.A Biol.Sci.Med.Sci.* Vol.61, No.11, pp.1111-1118.

Trzonkowski,P., Mysliwska, J., Godlewska, B., Szmit, E., Lukaszuk, K., Wieckiewicz, J., Brydak, L., Machala, M., Landowski, J., & Mysliwski, A. (2004). Immune consequences of the spontaneous pro-inflammatory status in depressed elderly patients. *Brain Behav.Immun.* Vol.18, No.2, pp.135-148.

Trzonkowski,P., Mysliwska, J., Szmit, E., Wieckiewicz, J., Lukaszuk, K., Brydak, L. B., Machala, M., & Mysliwski, A. (2003). Association between cytomegalovirus infection, enhanced proinflammatory response and low level of anti-hemagglutinins during the anti-influenza vaccination--an impact of immunosenescence. *Vaccine* Vol.21, No.25-26, pp.3826-3836.

Vallejo,A.N., Hamel, D. L., Jr., Mueller, R. G., Ives, D. G., Michel, J. J., Boudreau, R. M., & Newman, A. B. (2011). NK-Like T Cells and Plasma Cytokines, but Not Anti-Viral Serology, Define Immune Fingerprints of Resilience and Mild Disability in Exceptional Aging. *PLoS.One.* Vol.6, No.10, pp.e26558.

van den Biggelaar,A.H., Huizinga, T. W., de Craen, A. J., Gussekloo, J., Heijmans, B. T., Frolich, M., & Westendorp, R. G. (2004). Impaired innate immunity predicts frailty in old age. The Leiden 85-plus study. *Exp.Gerontol.* Vol.39, No.9, pp.1407-1414.

van Duin,D., Mohanty, S., Thomas, V., Ginter, S., Montgomery, R. R., Fikrig, E., Allore, H. G., Medzhitov, R., & Shaw, A. C. (2007). Age-associated defect in human TLR-1/2 function. *J.Immunol.* Vol.178, No.2, pp.970-975.

van Duin,D. & Shaw, A. C. (2007). Toll-like receptors in older adults. *J.Am.Geriatr.Soc.* Vol.55, No.9, pp.1438-1444.

Vo,T.K., Saint-Hubert, M., Morrhaye, G., Godard, P., Geenen, V., Martens, H. J., Debacq-Chainiaux, F., Swine, C., & Toussaint, O. (2011). Transcriptomic biomarkers of the response of hospitalized geriatric patients admitted with heart failure. Comparison to hospitalized geriatric patients with infectious diseases or hip fracture. *Mech.Ageing Dev.* Vol.132, No.3, pp.131-139.

Weksler,M.E. & Szabo, P. (2000). The effect of age on the B-cell repertoire. *J.Clin.Immunol.* Vol.20, No.4, pp.240-249.

Wessels,I., Jansen, J., Rink, L., & Uciechowski, P. (2010). Immunosenescence of polymorphonuclear neutrophils. *ScientificWorldJournal.* Vol.10, pp.145-160.

Wikby,A. (2008). Immune risk phenotypes and associated parameters in very old humans. Ferguson, F., Strindhall, J., Forsey, R. J., Fulop, T., Hadrup S.R., Straten PT, Pawelec, G., and Johansson, B. *Immunosenescences, 2007 .* landes biosciences and springer sciences.

Wikby,A., Johansson, B., Ferguson, F., & Olsson, J. (1994). Age-related changes in immune parameters in a very old population of Swedish people: a longitudinal study. *Exp.Gerontol.* Vol.29, No.5, pp.531-541.

Wills,M., Akbar, A., Beswick, M., Bosch, J. A., Caruso, C., Colonna-Romano, G., Dutta, A., Franceschi, C., Fulop, T., Gkrania-Klotsas, E., Goronzy, J., Griffiths, S. J., Henson, S., Herndler-Brandstetter, D., Hill, A., Kern, F., Klenerman, P., Macallan, D., Macualay, R., Maier, A. B., Mason, G., Melzer, D., Morgan, M., Moss, P., Nikolich-Zugich, J., Pachnio, A., Riddell, N., Roberts, R., Sansoni, P., Sauce, D., Sinclair, J., Solana, R., Strindhall, J., Trzonkowski, P., van Lier, R., Vescovini, R., Wang, G., Westendorp, R., & Pawelec, G. (2011). Report from the Second Cytomegalovirus and Immunosenescence Workshop. *Immun.Ageing* Vol.8, No.1, pp.10.

Wolf,A.M., Rumpold, H., Tilg, H., Gastl, G., Gunsilius, E., & Wolf, D. (2006). The effect of zoledronic acid on the function and differentiation of myeloid cells. *Haematologica* Vol.91, No.9, pp.1165-1171.

Yoshikawa,T.T. (1981). Important infections in elderly persons. *West J.Med.* Vol.135, No.6, pp.441-445. Zheng,S.X., Vrindts, Y., Lopez, M., De Groote, D., Zangerle, P. F., Collette, J., Franchimont, N., Geenen, V., Albert, A., & Reginster, J. Y. (1997). Increase in cytokine production (IL-1 beta, IL-6, TNF-alpha but not IFN-gamma, GM-CSF or LIF) by stimulated whole blood cells in postmenopausal osteoporosis. *Maturitas* Vol.26, No.1, pp.63-71.

Zuliani,G., Ranzini, M., Guerra, G., Rossi, L., Munari, M. R., Zurlo, A., Volpato, S., Atti, A. R., Ble, A., & Fellin, R. (2007). Plasma cytokines profile in older subjects with late onset Alzheimer's disease or vascular dementia. *J.Psychiatr.Res.* Vol.41, No.8, pp.686-693.

2

Immune System and Environmental Xenobiotics - The Effect of Selected Mineral Fibers and Particles on the Immune Response

Miroslava Kuricova et al.[*]
Slovak Medical University, Bratislava
Slovak Republic

1. Introduction

Mineral fibers and particles are finding growing applications in industry and thus entering into the human environment. The utility of using such products for various purposes is promising but detailed information related to immune safety is needed. Immunotoxic effects may be displayed as immunosuppression, immunostimulation, hypersensitivity and autoimmunity. Humans may be exposed to fibers and particles from a variety of sources, including occupational settings, ambient air, consumer products, drinking water and food. This chapter is dedicated to the effect of inhalation exposure to asbestos, rock wool, glass wool, ceramic fibers and nickel oxide particles on the immune system.

Findings of *in vitro* studies, *in vivo* animal experiments and molecular epidemiological studies conducted during the period of several years are summarized. *In vitro* studies comprised studies on alveolar macrophages and alveolar epithelial type II cells. Refractory ceramic fibers, asbestos and stone wool fibers were tested *in vitro*. *In vivo* testing involved both inhalation and intratracheal instillation studies using amosite, wollastonite, rock wool and glass fibers. Moreover, three population based studies in workers occupationally exposed to asbestos, rock wool and glass fibers were performed.

Finally, options and pitfalls to the use of immune assays as sensitive biomarkers of possible immunotoxic effects are discussed. Since, in human studies, specimens from living people used to examine the effects of particles and fibers on the immune response are typically limited to minimally invasive (whole blood, plasma or serum by venipuncture, sputum) or moderately invasive techniques (bronchoalveolar lavage or nasal lavage), human blood

[*] Jana Tulinska[1], Aurelia Liskova[1], Mira Horvathova[1], Silvia Ilavska[1], Zuzana Kovacikova[1],
Elizabeth Tatrai[2], Marta Hurbankova[1], Silvia Cerna[1], Eva Jahnova[1], Eva Neubauerova[1],
Ladislava Wsolova[1], Sona Wimmerova[1], Laurence Fuortes[3], Soterios A. Kyrtopoulos[4]
and Maria Dusinska[1,5]
[1] *Slovak Medical University, Bratislava, Slovak Republic*
[2] *Department of Pathology, National Institute of Occupational Health, Budapest, Hungary*
[3] *University of Iowa, College of Public Health, Iowa City, Iowa, USA*
[4] *National Hellenic Research Foundation, Institute of Biological Research and Biotechnology, Athens, Greece*
[5] *NILU Norwegian Institute for Air Research, Kjeller, Norway*

leukocytes are the most appropriate specimens for *in vitro* cellular assays. Macrophages and lymphocytes are appropriate models for examining the effects of xenobiotics on cell functions. Serum cytokines, chemokines or soluble adhesion molecules have potential to contribute to the panel of biomarkers used to assess immunotoxicity.

1.1 Immunotoxicology

Immune dysregulation resulting from inhalation, skin exposure or ingestion of chemicals in the workplace and general environment is an important health problem in industrialized an industrializing societies (National Research Council, 1992). Immunotoxicity is an important aspect of the safety evaluation of drugs and chemicals (Descotes, 2005). It has been generally accepted that all new chemicals require safety evaluation before marketing and sale. This is a difficult task due to the large number of chemicals directly consumed by man, such as drugs and food additives, and those that are widely used such as pesticides, household chemicals, and industrial products (De Rosa et al., 2002; IPCS/WHO, 1999).

Immunotoxicity refers to any adverse effect on the structure or function of innate and adaptive immunity. It can be divided into immunosuppression, immunostimulation, hypersensitivity and autoimmunity (Duramad & Holland, 2011; Descotes, 2005; Fig. 1). The outcome of immunotoxicity is influenced by the dose of the immunotoxicant as well as mechanism of action of exposure to other agents, such as bacteria, viruses, parasites, or chemicals normally harmless. Direct immunotoxic effects of xenobiotics including particles and fibers can lead to the suppression or stimulation of immune response. Immunosuppression can result in increased occurrence of infectious diseases or and neoplasias, in particular lymphomas, as shown in both transplant and cancer patients treated with potent immunosuppressive drugs (Descotes, 2000; Vial & Descotes, 1996). Immunosuppression caused by chemicals, may make the course of infections more severe, atypical and or likely to relapse. The target organ systems affected could be the respiratory, gastrointestinal tracts, CNS or the skin (Descotes, 2005). Flu-like reactions, autoimmune diseases and hypersensitivity reactions to unrelated allergens are among the adverse effects related to immunostimulation (Descotes, 2005). Hypersensitivity reactions are the most frequently detected immunotoxic effects of chemicals. They include immune-mediated ('allergic') and non immune-mediated ('pseudoallergic') reactions. Particles and mineral fibers are recognized causes of hypersensitivy reactions provoked mostly within respiratory tract and skin (D'Amato et al., 2005; Di Giampaolo et al., 2011). A large number of drugs and an increasing number of environmental agents can result in the appearance of a number of autoantibodies or even autoimmune diseases. Systemic lupus erythematosus, scleroderma or dermal vasculitis have been associated with exposure to a variety of chemical agents (Hess, 2002; Van Loveren et al., 2001).

1.2 Models and methods in immunotoxicology

The immune system is a complex network comprised of several cell types (i.e., lymphocytes, macrophages, granulocytes, and natural killer cells) whose diversity of functions includes maintaining homeostasis and health (Luster et al., 1989). Scientists use immunocompetent cells as models for studying the toxic mechanisms of xenobiotics at the cellular and

Immune System and Environmental Xenobiotics - The Effect of Selected Mineral Fibers and
Particles on the Immune Response

51

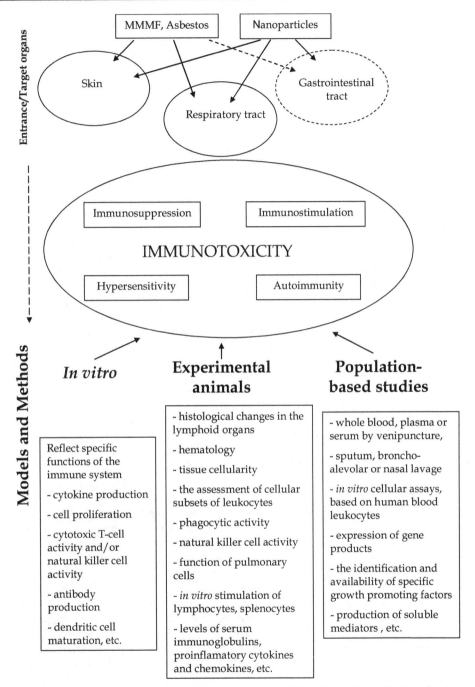

Fig. 1. Strategy for immunotoxicity testing in particle and fiber toxicology. Options for *in vitro, in vivo* and population studies.

molecular levels. In general, biological effects of xenobiotics (including particles and fibers) depend on several factors, e.g., chemical composition and physico-chemical properties such as solubility, chemical reactivity, size, length:width ratio, persistence in the organism, surface properties, dose, duration of exposure, the ability of a material to interact with body proteins etc. Host factors such as underlying health status, individual susceptibility to xenobiotics, metabolism, age, nutrition status, life style (smoking, etc.), presence of immune disease (asthma, allergic rhinitis, immunosuppression etc.) and other factors are also important determinants of immunotoxicity.

Increasing evidence that the immune system is a frequent target of xenobiotics following chronic, subchronic, or acute exposure underlines the need for development of models and immune assays suitable for use in screening potential immunotoxic compounds. For hazard assessment of xenobiotics, *in vitro* studies, experimental studies in laboratory animals, as well as epidemiological studies may provide necessary information (Fig. 1). Recently, several review papers have been published on design and methods used in immunotoxicological studies (Dietert & Holsapple, 2007; Lankveld et al., 2010; Oostingh et al., 2011). Haley published best practice guidelines for routine pathology evaluation of the immune system (Haley et al., 2005). Study methods of immunotoxicology have been reviewed and guidance documents developed by United States and European regulatory agencies (Committee for Proprietary Medicinal Products, 2000; Food and Drug Administration, 2004; Gopinath, 1996; ICICIS 1998; Kuper et al., 2002; Schuurman et al., 1994). In addition, harmonization of immunotoxicity guidelines in the ICH (International Conference on Harmonisation) process has been discussed by Ruehl-Fehlert (2005). One of the first steps in planning and conducting immunotoxicity studies is the identification and characterization of fibers/particles of interest. Secondly, attention must be paid to choosing proper *in vitro* immune cell models, sensitive animal models or occupationally or environmentally exposed human populations to assess the effect of xenobiotics on the immune system. Furthermore the selection of suitable immune assays as sensitive biomarkers of immunotoxic effect is also important.

In vitro assessment of immunotoxicity

In vitro testing has several advantages over *in vivo* animal testing. Among others, 3R requirements - reduction, refinement, and replacement of animal experiments are fulfilled, detailed mechanistic understanding of target immune cell/molecule is a clear benefit to consider and costs are lower. Most assays that are currently used to analyze immunotoxicity were originally designed for diagnostic purposes to examine hereditary or acquired immune disease in humans. Subsequently, these methods have been adapted for analysis of immunotoxicity of xenobiotics. *In vitro* assays may reflect specific functions of the immune system (cytokine production, cell proliferation, cytotoxic T-cell activity, natural killer cell activity, antibody production, and dendritic cell maturation). To avoid inter-species extrapolation, assays should preferably use human primary cells. They reproduce the response of normal cells of normal individuals. However, the use of primary cells is not always feasible (e.g., in the case of primary lung epithelial cells). As an alternative, the use of animal primary cells or human cell lines (transformed or tumor cells with unrestrained proliferative capacity) is applicable to first line screening of immunomodulatory effects. Furthermore, whole blood has the advantage of comprising multiple cell types in their natural proportion and environment (Lankveld et al., 2010).

Immune System and Environmental Xenobiotics - The Effect of Selected Mineral Fibers and
Particles on the Immune Response

53

In vivo models in experimental animals

In investigating potential effects of compounds on the immune system in experimental animals, a tiered approach is recommended. Studies aimed on the identification of histologic changes in the lymphoid organs and functional immune alterations in laboratory animals are useful for detecting probable immunotoxicants and may play an important role as a first indicator of direct immunotoxicity, i.e. immunosuppression (De Jong & Van Loveren, 2007). First tier, general toxicity studies may include parameters for detection of relatively gross toxic effects on the immune system. Hematology, tissue cellularity and the assessment of cellular subsets of T- and B-leukocytes by flow cytometry as non-functional assay are common initial tests. Some authors consider such bioeffects as insensitive indicators of immunotoxicity.

Second tier consists of studies of immune function. Phagocytic activity and determination of Natural Killer (NK) cell activity may be used in evaluation of direct immunotoxicity. In animal models, there is no limitation to obtain cell suspensions from lung tissue or bronchoalveolar lavage to look at function of pulmonary cells affected by particles and fibers. Several other possibilities are presented by thymus, bone marrow or spleen tissues for *in vitro* stimulation of lymphocytes by potential mitogens. These methods may indicate effects of xenobiotics on the functionality of splenic cell populations. Concanavalin A (Con A) and phytohemagglutinin (PHA) activate T-cells, while lipopolysaccharide (LPS) activates primarily B-cell populations. In addition, serum can be obtained for determination of serum immunoglobulins or proinflamatory cytokines and chemokines. Comparison of treated and control groups may give a first indication of possible direct immunotoxic effects (De Jong & Van Loveren, 2007).

Population-based studies

Biological endpoints used in molecular epidemiology are called biomarkers. Several definitions of biomarkers as tools used in human or animal studies to assess exposure and disease risks have been published (Benford et al., 2000). Bottrill defined biomarkers as "parameters which can be evaluated quantitatively, semi-quantitatively or qualitatively and which provide information on exposure to a xenobiotic or on the actual or potential effects of that exposure in an individual or in a group" (Bottrill, 1998). There is a high degree of complexity of the immune system and an enormous variety of responses and mechanisms involved in immunotoxic injury. Therefore it is a challenge to identify a key parameter to develop as a biomarker. The inclusion of several immune endpoints applicable to man is thus essential. Specimens from living people to examine the effects of particles and fibers on the immune response are typically limited to minimally invasive (whole blood, plasma or serum by venipuncture, sputum) or moderately invasive techniques (bronchoalveolar or nasal lavage). *In vitro* cellular assays are typically based on human blood leukocytes. In particular, macrophages and lymphocytes are appropriate models for examining the effects of various agents on cell maturation and function. The expression of gene products can be used as markers of differentiation, the identification and availability of specific growth promoting factors (e.g., interleukins), and their potential to undergo terminal differentiation resulting in production of soluble mediators (e.g., monokines, lymphokines, or antibodies) or indicating effector function (e.g., tumor target cell killing) (Luster et al., 1989).

1.3 Immunotoxicity studies of mineral fibers

The adverse effects that arise from exposure to asbestos have stimulated the development of substitute materials, man-made mineral fibers. However, little is known about the health effects of these fibers. The potentially harmful effects of all types of respirable fibers are at present one of the most important fields of interest in industrial toxicology. The production, sale and use of asbestos are no longer permitted in Europe. Some of the properties of asbestos (e.g. as an insulation material) can be substituted by alternative man-made fibers. In view of the importance of the possible biological effects of fibers we have conducted *in vitro*, animal and a molecular epidemiology studies to examine the relationship between relevant biomarkers and exposure to asbestos, mineral wool and glass fibers. We have measured a range of biomarkers of exposure, effects and individual susceptibility. In this chapter, biomarkers of immunotoxicity will be presented.

1.3.1 Asbestos

Asbestos has long been recognized as a cause of both benign and malignant lung disease (interstitial and pleural fibrosis, lung cancer and mesothelioma). Asbestos refers to a group of naturally occurring mineral fibers with a $\geq$ 3:1 length to diameter ratio. These fibers once inhaled and displaced by various means to lung tissues, can cause a spectrum of diseases including cancer and disorders related to inflammation and fibrosis (American Thoracic Society, 2004; Mossman et al., 1996). Mechanisms of asbestos-induced carcinogenesis are thought to be multiple, including generation of reactive oxygen (ROS) and nitrogen species (RNS), alteration of mitochondrial function, physical disturbance of cell cycle progression, and activation of several signal transduction pathways (Jaurand, 1997; Nymark et al., 2008). Asbestos fibers having iron (or even chrysotile) and producing ROS/RNS can cause DNA damage to nearby cells, and fibers are sometimes directly inserted into the cells and injure chromosomes, while retained fibers may adsorb other carcinogens on their surface (known asbestos bodies) (Toyokuni, 2009a, 2009b).

The extrapulmonary consequences of asbestos exposure were discussed in Bunderson-Schelvan et al., (2011). Authors used several hundred epidemiological, *in vivo* and *in vitro* studies and finally they supported a strong association between asbestos exposure and peritoneal neoplasm. On the other hand, the correlations between asbestos exposure and immune-related disease were less conclusive and effects of asbestos exposure to the GIT (gastrointestinal tract) appeared to be minimal. Immunomodulatory effects of asbestos have been well established in patients with asbestosis and mesothelioma (American Thoracic Society, 2004; Corsini et al., 1994; Mascagni et al., 2003; Rosenthal et al., 1999) however there is limited information on effects in individuals with minimal evidence for asbestos related lung disease or exposure only. Our study offered an opportunity to assess biomarkers which may represent individual susceptibility to and/or early evidence for asbestos related health effects.

1.3.2 Man made fibers

Rock wool, glass fibers and ceramic fibers

The evidence for adverse health effects following exposure to asbestos has prompted a drastic reduction in the use of asbestos, resulting in the increased use of substitutes composed of both naturally occurring and synthetic materials which are thought to have lower toxicity. Man-made mineral fibers include glass fibers (used in glass wool and continuous glass filament), rock (stone)/slag wool and refractory ceramic fibers. Rock (stone) wool, slag wool and glass wool are used extensively in thermal and acoustic insulation, typically in buildings, vehicles and appliances. Refractory ceramic fibers are designed for high-temperature applications, mainly in industrial settings. Continuous glass filament is used primarily in reinforced composite materials for the insulation, electronics and construction industries (IARC, 2002; National Toxicology Program, 2009). Man-made vitreous fibers have some physical similarities to asbestos, in particular, their fibrous character which gives them the same aerodynamic properties and leads to their deposition throughout the respiratory tract. Unlike amphibole asbestos, however, they are synthetic and amorphous, and generally have a lower biopersistence in lung tissues. Also, unlike serpentine asbestos, they tend to break transversely rather than cleaving along the fiber axis (IARC, 2002).

Data on respiratory cancer of man-made mineral (MMMFs) and vitreous fibers (MMVFs) are not consistent. Statistically significant increases in respiratory cancer mortality were observed among glass wool-exposed workers in unadjusted analyses in the United States (Marsh et al., 2001), European (Boffetta et al., 1997), and Canadian cohorts (Shannon et al., 2005). Excesses of lung cancer incidence were observed among the European workers (Boffetta et al., 1997) and Canadian workers (Shannon et al., 2005), but not among French workers (Moulin et al., 1986). Marsh et al., (2001) concluded that the US cohort study of man-made vitreous fiber workers has not provided consistent evidence of a relationship between man-made vitreous fiber exposure and mortality from malignant or non-malignant respiratory disease. Gillissen et al. (2006) stated that MMMFs or MMVFs including glass wool, rock wool, slag wool, glass filaments, microfibers, refractory ceramic fibers are bioactive under certain experimental conditions. Although it has been shown that MMMFs may cause malignancies when injected intraperitoneally in high quantities in rodents, inhalation trials and human studies have not shown such effects. The amorphous structure of synthetic vitreous fibers facilitates designing fibers with low biopersistence. In 2001, IARC reclassified these fibers from Category 2b to Category 3 (with RCF and special purpose fibers remaining in 2b) based on epidemiological data and the animal studies database indicating that there is little if any health risk associated with the use of SVFs of low biopersistence (Bernstein, 2007).

Occupational or environmental exposures to many inhaled particles and fibers have been linked with immunotoxicity. First of all, silica and silicates have been associated with the development of lung inflammation, interstitial fibrosis, bronchitis, small airway disease, emphysema, and vascular diseases as well as immunologic reactions (Song & Tang, 2011). Recent studies showed that Th1 and Th2 cytokines may be involved in silicosis and regulatory T-cells (Treg cells) have crucial role in modulation of immune homeostasis by regulating Th1/Th2 polarization. Studies in animals provided knowledge that depletion of Tregs may attenuate the progress of silica-induced lung fibrosis and enhance Th1 response and decelerate Th1/Th2 balance toward a Th2 phenotype in silica-induced lung fibrosis (Liu et al., 2010). Exposure to diesel exhaust particles (Inoue & Takano, 2011), coal dust (Ates et al., 2011), soil dust (Schenker et al., 2009), beryllium (Martin et al., 2011; Mikulski et al., 2011; Sood, 2009), heavy metal fumes (Montero et al., 2010) can evoke new or facilitate existing immune-mediated pulmonary inflammation.

1.3.3 NiO nanoparticles

Nickel and nickel compounds are widely used in industry. In occupational settings, exposure to nickel and nickel compounds occurs primarily during nickel refining, electroplating, and welding. In addition to nickel, workers in metal mining and processing are exposed to diesel emissions, oil mists, blasting agents and also to various other substances prevalent in the mine or industry (Lightfoot et al., 2010). Some of them, such as silica (Costantini et al., 2011; Huaux, 2007), radon (Chauhan et al., 2011) or arsenic (Burchiel at al. 2009) are known to be potent immunotoxic agents thus implicating possible synergistic effects on the immune response. The most common airborne exposures to nickel in the workplace are to insoluble nickel species, such as metallic nickel, nickel sulfide, and nickel oxides from dusts and fumes. The chemical and physical properties of nickel and nickel compounds strongly influence their bioavailability and toxicity. The lung and the skin are the principal routes of entry and target organs of occupational exposure. The most serious adverse health effects due to occupational exposure to nickel and its compounds are lung fibrosis and lung cancer, nickel is also hematotoxic, hepatotoxic and nephrotoxic. Allergic skin reactions are relatively common in individuals who are exposed to nickel (Brüske-Hohlfeld, 2009; Das & Buchner, 2007; Panizza, 2011; Zhao, 2009).

Recently, nickel nanoparticles are increasingly used in modern industries such as catalysts, sensors and electronic applications (Ahamed, 2011). Due to known toxic effects of "bulk" nickel products, caution in industrial applications of new nickel nanoproducts is important. Several *in vivo* studies in rats demonstrated that nickel oxide nanoparticles (NiO NP) have inflammatory effects in lungs by transient increase in cytokine expression (IL-1alpha, IL-1beta in lung and monocyte chemotactic protein-1 in bronchoalveolar lavage fluid) and persistent increase in CC chemokine (macrophage inflammatory protein-1alpha in lung and bronchoalveolar lavage fluid - BALF) (Morimoto et al., 2010). Cytokine-induced neutrophil chemoattractant-1 (CINC-1), CINC-2 alpha, beta, and CINC-3 were involved in the persistent pulmonary inflammation by NiO NP (Nishi et al., 2009) but NiO NP did not induce the gene expression of MMP-2 and TIMP-2 mRNA in rat lungs (Morimoto et al., 2011). *In vitro* assessment of the toxic effect of nickel nanoparticles in human lung epithelial A549 cells showed reduced mitochondrial function, induction of the leakage of lactate dehydrogenase (LDH) and induction of oxidative stress in dose and time-dependent manner (Ahamed, 2011).

Other airborne and engineered nanoparticles in addition to nickel, such as carbon nanotubes (He et al., 2011), titanium dioxide (Morimoto et al., 2011), cobalt - Co_3O_4 (Cho et al., 2011a) or quantum dots (Jacobsen et al., 2009) has been reported to induce lung inflammation. Anoher example is ZnO nanoparticles (ZnO NP) discovered to induce eosinophilia, proliferation of airway epithelial cells, goblet cell hyperplasia, and pulmonary fibrosis. Fibrosis was associated with increased myofibroblast accumulation and transforming growth factor-beta positivity. Serum IgE levels were up-regulated by ZnO NP along with the eosinophilia whilst serum IgA levels were down-regulated by ZnO NP (Cho et al., 2011b).

1.4 Hazard assessment of mineral fibers and particles

Humans may be exposed to fibrous particles from a variety of sources, including occupational settings, ambient air, consumer products, drinking water and food (De Vuyst et al., 1995). Potential effects of airborne fibers in humans can only occur after a complex process of inhalation, deposition, elimination, retention and translocation. The biological effects of inhaled fibers are highly dependent on dose (fiber exposure concentration - numbers of long fibers), fiber size (diameter/length), (Donaldson & Tran, 2004; Kohyama et al., 1997; Yamato et al., 1998), durability of material in the organism (biopersistence) (Mossman et al., (2011), duration of exposure, chemical composition and properties, solubility, chemical reactivity, surface properties of the material, ability of a material to interact with body proteins etc. Host factors such as efficiency of defense mechanisms of the respiratory tract between the initial deposition and the ultimate contact of the fibers with the target cell, individual susceptibility to xenobiotics, metabolism, age, nutrition status, life style (smoking), presence of immune disease (asthma, allergic rhinitis, immunosuppression etc.) and other factors influence the development of immunotoxicity.

2. *In vitro* studies on lung cells

The lung consists of more than 40 different cell types; each type has its special function, localization and morphology. From the toxicological point of view, the most important cell types being alveolar macrophages (AM - free living cells, whose function is to phagocyte the inhaled particles and maintain the alveoli clean and sterile) and alveolar epithelial type II cells (TII - localized on the inner surface of lung alveoli and which play an important role in tissue renewal). For this reason we focused on these cell types, isolated them from rats and maintained them in cell culture (Hoet et al., 1994; Richards et al., 1987). After 20 h cultivation the cells were exposed to different dose (1, 5, 10 µg.ml^{-1}) of mineral fibers and the cultivation was prolonged for another 20 h period when the experiment was terminated and the analyses were done.

2.1 Lectin histochemistry

Bandeiraea simplicifolia agglutinin (BSA) and *Maclura pomifera* agglutinin (MPA) are able to bind to the terminal N-acetyl-α-galactosaminyl or α-D-galactose/galactosamine residues in the membranes of AM and TII cells which makes them suitable for detection of cell membrane injuries (Tatrai et al., 1994). Control cells showed regular, linear staining with BSA or MPA. Stone wool at the concentration 5 µg.ml^{-1} caused moderate injury to membranes of AM and incomplete phagocytosis in a small fraction of AM. Alveolar epithelial type II cells did not develop detectable membrane damage at any tested fiber dose. Refractory ceramic fibers (RCF) evoked changes in both cell types only at the highest dose: the membranes were not continuous and reduplicated. Wollastonite caused a decreased reaction in the membranes only at the highest dose. After exposure to the lowest dose of crocidolite the membranes of both cell types were fragmented irregularly and frustrated phagocytosis could be found in AM (Tátrai et al., 2004; 2006a; 2006b).

2.2 Effect of mineral fibers on cells using TEM

The control cells and those exposed to fibers at a dose of 1 µg.ml^{-1} were examined. TII cells did not show any alterations after RCF or stone wool exposure. AM cells phagocyted RCF fibers without injuries of cell organelles, intact organelles remained also after exposure to stone wool. In both cell types crocidolite evoked severe damage in the organelles and necrobiosis of whole cells (Tátrai et al., 2004; 2006a; 2006b).

2.3 Immunological studies

Production of proinflammatory peptides MCP-1 and MIP-1α was assayed in growth media after termination of cell cultivation. Exposure to wollastonite did not change production of MCP-1 and MIP-1α in TII cells, but in AM the production was significantly enhanced: MCP-1 at the concentration 10 µg.ml^{-1}, MIP-1α at the concentration 5 µg.ml^{-1}. The results after exposure to stone wool were different: in TII cells the production of MCP-1 was enhanced at all concentrations, MIP-1α at doses of 5 and 10 µg.ml^{-1}; in AM the production of both cytokines was statistically significantly enhanced after doses of 5 and 10 µg.ml^{-1}. Crocidolite evoked statistically significant dose dependent enhancement of the production of MCP-1 in AM, for MIP-1α and both cytokines in TII at doses of 5 and 10 µg.ml^{-1} in all cases (Tátrai et al., 2004; 2006a; 2006b). Comparing the results from different fibers on 2 various primary cell types the following differences are clearly seen: crocidolite (asbestos) evoked the greatest changes, both morphologically and functionally. Effects of wollastonite were seen more significant comparing to stone wool. AM cells are more sensitive to the fibers exposure than TII cells.

3. Animal model

3.1 Intratracheal instillation studies in rat model

Four types of fibers: asbestos and three types of ASMF fibers (asbestos substitute mineral fibers): wollastonite, rock wool and glass fibers were intratracheally instilled at 2 doses (2 mg or 8 mg of fibers) to Fisher 344 rats. Dose of 2 mg was suspended in 0.2 ml of saline solution per animal or control group with 0.2 ml saline only. A dose of 8 mg was divided and instilled 4 times (weekly 2 mg/0.2 ml saline solution). The assays were performed 4 or 16 weeks after last instillation of the fibers. After sacrifice, markers of immune response and hematology were analyzed. Immunotoxic effects were examined using a panel of immune and hematological assays. Phenotypic analysis of leukocytes (T-lymphocytes, activated T-cells, B-lymphocytes, NK-cells, T-helpers, T-cytotoxic cells) and expression of adhesion molecules (CD11b, CD54) were performed by flow cytometry. Immune functions were evaluated by proliferative activity of T and B-lymphocytes *in vitro* stimulated with mitogens and antigen and phagocytic activity of leukocytes.

Our findings demonstrate the immunomodulatory effect of mineral fibers in the rat animal model 4 and 16 weeks after intratracheal exposure to amosite, wollastonite, rock wool and glass fibers. Significant changes were observed in total white blood cell count and percentages neutrophils in all fiber-treated, especially high-dosed, animals after 4 weeks of exposure. The percentage of lymphocytes was altered in rock wool fiber-treated especially in high-dosed animals after 4 weeks of exposure (Table 3.1-1).

Analysis of lymphocyte subsets showed significantly increased percentage of T-lymphocytes, mainly cytotoxic cells and decreased percentage of B-lymphocytes in peripheral blood of animals exposed to amosite. Rats exposed to wollastonite had increased percentage of T-helper cells. Exposure to mineral fibers decreased expression of adhesion molecule CD54 (ICAM-1) on granulocytes (amosite, glass fibers) and monocytes (rockwool). Suppressed expression of adhesion molecules CD11b was found on granulocytes (wollastonite, glass fibers) and monocytes (glass fibers) (data not shown).

Immune System and Environmental Xenobiotics - The Effect of Selected Mineral Fibers and
Particles on the Immune Response

59

		Amosite	Wolastonite	Rock wool	Glass Fibers
White blood cells (10^9/l)	4 weeks, 2mg				
	4 weeks, 8mg	↓ *	↓ *		↑ *
	16 weeks, 2mg			↓ *	
	16 weeks, 8mg	↓ *			
Neutrophils (%)	4 weeks, 2mg				
	4 weeks, 8mg	↑ *	↑ *	↑ *	↑ *
	16 weeks, 2mg		↑ *		
	16 weeks, 8mg				
Lymphocytes (%)	4 weeks, 2mg				
	4 weeks, 8mg			↓ *	
	16 weeks, 2mg				
	16 weeks, 8mg				

* p<0.05; **p<0.01; ***p<0.001; ↓ - decrease ↑ - increase in comparison with relevant control;

Table 3.1-1. White blood cell (WBC) count and differential WBC in Fisher 344 rats
administered with 2 mg or 8 mg of amosite, wollastonite, rock wool or glass fibers.

Although amosite seems to be most potent suppressor of T- and B-lymphocyte proliferation,
especially in high-dosed animals, wollastonite and rock wool also interfered with
lymphocyte proliferation and suppressed the response of T-lymphocytes. The opposite
stimulative effect on proliferative capacity of B-cells was found in animals exposed to glass
fibers (Table 3.1-2). Phagocytic activity was dramatically affected by exposure to rock wool
and glass fibers. A highly significant dose-dependent suppression was found in neutrophils
and monocytes. Rats exposed to wollastonite fibers also had decreased phagocytic activity
of peripheral blood phagocytes 4 weeks after instillation of either dose. Surprisingly, the
phagocytic activity of animals exposed to amosite was affected only in high dosed rats
(Table 3.1-2).

In conclusion, animal exposure to mineral fibers leads to alterations in systemic immune
response. Immune dysregulation consisted of changes of the main lymphocyte subsets.
Moreover, the function of immunocompetent cells that are responsible for the specific
immune response (T- and B-lymphocytes) and phagocytic cells was impaired. Our results
correspond with the hypothesis of Hurbánková (1994), who observed that the phagocytic
activity of granulocytes and monocytes is altered in asbestos-treated rats up to one year
following treatment, displaying a two-phase progress: an initial increase (phase I) followed
by a decrease below the average values of the control animals (phase II).

3.2 Inhalation studies in rat model

The effects of industrial fibrous dusts on the respiratory system represent a potential
environmental and occupational health hazard for humans. Chronic asbestos exposure can
cause pleural plaques, asbestosis and cancer diseases. These effects stimulated research
activities aiming at the study of the health effects of fibrous substitutes as well as combined
effects with other noxious materials respectively (Boor et al., 2009; Donald & Gardner, 2006;
IARC, 2002; 2004). This study gives information about the dose-response relationships after

Function of lymphocytes		Amosite	Wolastonite	Rock wool	Glass Fibers
Proliferative activity of T-lymphocytes	4 weeks, 2mg	↑ Con A *		↓ PHA **	
	4 weeks, 8mg	↓ Con A *** ↓ PHA **	↓ Con A *** ↓ PHA ***		
	16 weeks, 2mg			↓ CD3 *	
	16 weeks, 8mg	↓ Con A **			
Proliferative activity of B-lymphocytes	4 weeks, 2mg				↑ PWM ***
	4 weeks, 8mg	↓ PWM *			↑ STM *
	16 weeks, 2mg				
	16 weeks, 8mg	↓ PWM ***			
Function of phagocytes					
Phagocytic activity of neutrophils	4 weeks, 2mg		↓ *	↓ ***	↓ ***
	4 weeks, 8mg	↓ ***	↓ **	↓ **	↓ ***
	16 weeks, 2mg			↓ *	↓ *
	16 weeks, 8mg			↓ **	↓ *
Phagocytic activity of monocytes	4 weeks, 2mg		↓ *	↓ ***	↓ ***
	4 weeks, 8mg	↓ ***	↓ *	↓ ***	↓ ***
	16 weeks, 2mg			↓ *	
	16 weeks, 8mg			↓ **	↓ *

* $p < 0.05$; **$p < 0.01$; ***$p < 0.001$; ↓ - decrease in comparison with relevant control; ↑ - increase in comparison with relevant control

Table 3.1-2. Activity of immune cells measured via lymphocyte proliferation test and phagocytic test in Fisher 344 rats administered with 2 mg or 8 mg of amosite, wollastonite, rock wool or glass fibers.

inhalation of two concentration levels of amosite asbestos and wollastonite alone or combined with daily exposure to cigarette smoke together with the basic lung inflammation and cytotoxic parameters. Male Fisher 344 rats were exposed for 6 months. Animals inhaled amosite asbestos or wollastonite fibers in a nose-only inhalation device (In-Tox, USA). Amphibole asbestos - amosite and wollastonite fibers belong to naturally occurring silicate inorganic fibers. Wollastonite is used as a substitute of asbestos. Dust aerosol was produced at two dosages: 30 mg/m³ air and 60 mg/m³ air for one hour per exposure. Exposure of animal groups to dusts proceeded every second day, 5 days per week. Six groups, each of 11 animals were exposed to:

- 60 mg/m³ amosite fibers for one hour every two days; combined with exposure to mainstream smoke from three cigarettes daily;

- 60 mg/m³ amosite fibers for one hour every two days;
- 30 mg/m³ amosite fibers for one hour every two days, combined with exposure to mainstream smoke from three cigarettes daily;
- 30 mg/m³ amosite fibers for one hour every two days;
- exposure to mainstream smoke from three cigarettes daily plus immobilization stress as for animals exposed to dust;
- immobilization stress as for animals exposed to dust.

Cigarette smoke exposure: Standard research cigarettes of the 1R1 type (Tobacco and Health Research Institute - THRI, Lexington, KY, USA) were used in all experiments. A whole-body actively ventilated exposure chamber was used, with a cigarette smoke generator and pumps (THRI, Lexington, KY, USA) allowing all smoker animal groups to breathe at the same time diluted main-stream tobacco smoke at the target concentration 30 mg of total particulate matter (TPM)/m³ air for one hour daily (an exposure requiring to burn three cigarettes).

Length [μm]	%	Diameter [μm]
< 20	5	
20 – 30	75	0.71
>30	20	

Diameter [μm]	%
= 1	47
<1	22
<3	21
=3	6
>3	4
Length [μm]	%
1 – 10	48
11 – 30	40
>30	12

Tables 3.2-1. and 3.2-2. Length, diameter and percentage of wollastonite fibers (top) and amosite fibers (bottom).

The aim of our study was to find and compare the combined effect of amosite or wollastonite (asbestos substitute) with cigarette smoke on the selected immune, inflammatory and cytotoxic parameters. The rats inhaled two doses: 30 and 60 mg/m³ of amosite (asbestos) and wollastonite fibers (mineral asbestos substitute) for 1 hour every 2 days and cigarette smoke from 3 cigarettes/day. They were sacrificed after 6 months exposure.

3.2.1 Combined effect of mineral fibers and tobacco smoke on respiratory tract

Six months after the beginning of the inhalation exposures, the animals were anesthetized and BAL was performed.

The following BAL parameters were examined:

Inflammatory response biomarkers
- Total cell count/ml BAL (bronchoalveolar lavage) fluid
- AM count/ml BAL fluid
- Differential cell count (alveolar macrophages - AM, lymphocytes - Ly, granulocytes - Gr)

Cytotoxic parameters
- Phagocytic activity of AM
- Viability of AM
- Lactate dehydrogenase activity (in the cell - free lavage fluid)
- Acid phosphatase activity (in the cell- free lavage fluid and in the BAL cell suspension)
- The cathepsin D activity (in the cell - free lavage fluid and in the BAL suspension)

Methods are described in papers of Hurbánková & Kaiglová (1999) and Černá et al. (2004). The results were statistically evaluated using Mann-Whitney test.

	Fibers alone			Fibers/Tobacco smoke		
	Control	30 mg/m³	60 mg/m³	Tobacco smoke alone	Tobacco smoke + fibers 30 mg/m³	Tobacco smoke + fibers 60 mg/m³
N	7	7	7	7	7	6
Total cell count/ml BALF ($10^3 \cdot ml^{-1}$)						Am ↑ **
AM count/ml BALF ($10^3 \cdot ml^{-1}$)						Am ↓ **
Ly %		Am ↑ *	Am ↑**			Am ↑ ***
AM %		Am ↓ *	Am ↓ *	Am ↓ *	Am ↓ **	Am ↓ ***
PMN %			Am ↑ *		Am ↑ *	Am ↑ **
Immature forms of AM (%)		Am ↑ *		Am ↑ **	Am ↑ *	Am ↑ **
Multinucleated cells (%)			Am ↑**			

Comparison of exposed group with the control group; *p<0.05, **p<0.01, ***p<0.001; ↑ - increase against compared group; ↓ - decrease against compared group; abbreviations: Le - leukocytes; AM - alveolar macrophages; PMN – polymophonuclear leukocytes, BAL - bronchoalveolar lavage

Table 3.2-3. Amosite – inhalation exposure - with/without tobacco smoke; inflammatory response parameters in BAL.

Increased numbers of bronchoalveolar lavage fluid (BALF) cells after asbestos or other fiber-exposure as a result of inflammatory response have been described by numerous authors (Hurbankova & Kaiglova, 1999; Greim et al., 2001; Morimoto & Tanaka, 2001; Osinubi et al., 2000). In our study, a significantly increased number of BALF cells after exposure to amosite in comparison with the control group was observed in the smoker plus 60 mg/m³ fiber group (by 11.4 %) as well as in the corresponding-dose, non-smoker group (by about 16%). This increase could be ascribed to the increase of lymphocyte population proportions. These changes were accompanied by an inverse change in the AM count in BALF, which significantly decreased in the same group exposed to combined higher dust plus cigarette smoke. A very similar but shorter exposure only to cigarette smoke has been reported to lead to a higher (35%) difference of BALF cell counts in comparison with the control values (Hurbánková et al., 2010; Ishihara et al., 1997; Nelson & Kelsey, 2002). The higher

Immune System and Environmental Xenobiotics - The Effect of Selected Mineral Fibers and
Particles on the Immune Response

63

	Fibers alone			Fibers/tobacco smoke		
	Control	30 mg/m³	60 mg/m³	Tobacco smoke alone	Tobacco smoke + fibers 30 mg/m³	Tobacco smoke + fibers 60 mg/m³
N	7	7	7	7	7	6
Phagocytic activity of AM (%)				Am ↓** Woll ↓**	Am ↓**	Am ↓*
Viability of living AM (%)		Am ↓*				Am ↓*
LDH µkat.g prot.⁻¹						
ACP nkat.g prot.⁻¹					Woll ↑*	
ACP nkat.10⁻⁶ cells						
Cathepsin D U$_{tyr}$.mg prot.⁻¹					Am ↑* Woll ↑*	Woll ↑*
Cathepsin D U$_{tyr}$.10⁻⁶ cells		Woll ↑*	Am ↑* Woll ↑*	Am ↑ **	Am ↑ **	Am ↑ **

Comparison of exposed groups with the control group: *p<0.05, **p<0.01, ***p<0.001; ↑ - increase
against compared group, ↓ - decrease against compared group; (1) enzyme activity expressed as µmol
of p-nitrophenol.hour⁻¹ mg protein⁻¹; abbreviations: LDH: lactate dehydrogenase; ACP: acid
phosphatase; U$_{tyr}$: µg of thyrosine released in an hour time

Table 3.2-4. Amosite and wollastonite - inhalation exposure - with/without tobacco smoke;
cytotoxic parameters in BAL.

proportions of PMN and lymphocytes in the BALF than control values indicate the presence
of inflammation in the lungs at sacrifice. The magnitude of the increase of these parameters
was dose-dependent. AM are the predominant cells present in BALF and changes in their
number or function are important factors determining the lung inflammatory response and
characterizing the pathogenesis of such response. A decrease in macrophage number or
phagocytic capacity may result in the reduction of the clearance of inhaled materials and
thus can lead to an increase of the effective dose of the potentially injurious agent (Aoshiba
et al., 2001; Dziedzic et al., 1993). A significant reduction in the number of AM after
intratracheal instillation of amosite has been observed also in our previous experiments
(Hurbankova & Kaiglova, 1999). Associated with inflammatory changes, a dose-dependent
increase in multinuclear cells (MNC) proportions was found in the BALF as well as in the
lung tissue suspensions. MNC were increased after exposure (separate or in combination) to
tobacco smoke as well as both fiber concentrations but significantly only after higher dose
without smoking. Similarly, immature forms of AM in all exposed groups were increased in
comparison with control (Beňo et al., 2005). Strongly dose dependent decrease of AM
viability (higher dose with and without smoking) as well as phagocytic activity of AM (all
group with smoking) was found in this experiment. That is in accordance with previously
described effect of asbestos (Hurbánková & Kaiglová, 1999).

Increased LDH and ACP activity in extracellular fluids are generally accepted as good
markers of cell or tissue injury and used for evaluation of the cytotoxic effect. We did not

find significant changes in activities of measured enzymes in our experiment. Cathepsin D activity was significantly changed after amosite inhalation. These results are in good accordance with study of Sjörstrand et al. (1989). Wollastonite inhalation confirmed the lower cytotoxicity in comparison with asbestos. Significant changes were found only by measurement of cathepsin D activity in BAL cells (increased levels), decreased percentage of phagocytic activity of AM in "tobacco smoke alone" group and increased levels of ACP in "tobacco smoke + wollastonite fibers 30mg/m³"group.

Amosite

- Inflammatory parameters were mostly changed after 60mg/m³ in combined group (amosite exposure and tobacco smoke).
- Tobacco smoke alone induced changes in inflammatory parameters. It confirms that smoking alone might play an important role in inflammatory processes.
- Smoking alone caused some changes of cytotoxic parameters and intensified the harmful effect of amosite exposure.
- Mild dose dependence between 30mg/m³ and 60mg/m³ in groups without tobacco smoke was seen.

Wollastonite

- No dose dependence of inflammatory parameter changes in this study was recorded in groups without smoking and very weak in combined exposure groups.
- Mild dose dependence of cytotoxic parameters changes in groups without or with tobacco smoke was observed.
- Influence of tobacco smoke on cytotoxic parameters was not explicit.

3.2.2 Combined effect of mineral fibers and tobacco smoke on immune parameters

Cellular immunity was examined by phenotypic analysis of leukocytes (CD3⁺, MHC II, CD4⁺, CD8⁺, CD161⁺, B-lymphocytes) and by expression of adhesion molecules (CD11b, CD54) on leukocytes (Table 3.2-5). Inhalation of high dose of amosite fibrous dust resulted in a significantly increased percentage of B-lymphocytes and elevated expression of adhesion molecule CD11b on lymphocytes of peripheral blood in non-smoking rats. Similarly, inhalation of high dose of wollastonite increased the percentage of B-lymphocytes, and this elevation was reinforced with combined exposure to lower dose of wollastonite and tobacco smoke. Moreover, the combined exposure to wollastonite and smoking caused a significant, dose-dependent increase of the percentage of cytotoxic cells and enhanced expression of adhesion molecule CD11b on granulocytes in peripheral blood. On the other hand, cigarette smoke and higher dose of wollastonite resulted in decrease of T-cells (CD3⁺). The stimulative effect of exclusive exposure to smoking on the immune system was shown as significantly elevated percentage of some lymphocyte subsets (T-cytotoxic, T-helper lymphocytes, B-lymphocytes) and elevated expression of adhesion molecule CD11b in comparison with non-smoking animals.

Immune function assays included proliferative response of T- and B-lymphocytes and phagocytic activity of blood leukocytes (Table 3.2-6). The proliferative activity of T-lymphocytes stimulated with CD3 antigen and T-dependent B-cell response in rats exposed to amosite was significantly decreased. The immunosuppressive effect was more pronounced

Immune System and Environmental Xenobiotics - The Effect of Selected Mineral Fibers and
Particles on the Immune Response

65

Proportion of lymphocyte subsets in peripheral blood	30 mg/m³	60 mg/m³	Tobacco smoke alone	Tobacco smoke + fibers 30 mg/m³	Tobacco smoke + fibers 60 mg/m³
CD3+ - T-lymphocytes (%)					Woll ↓ a
CD3+/MHC II - activated T-lymphocytes (%)					
CD4+ - T-helper lymphocytes (%)		↑ **			
CD8+ - T-cytotoxic lymphocytes (%)		↑ *		Woll ↑ *	Woll ↑ *
CD161+- Natural killer cells (%)					
B-Lymphocytes (%)	Am ↑ * Woll ↑ *	↑ *		Woll ↑ *	
Adhesion molecules on leukocytes					
Expression of CD11b on lymphocytes (%)	Am ↑ * Woll ↑ **	↑ *			
Expression of CD11b on monocytes (%)					
Expression of CD11b on granulocytes (%)	Am ↑ *				Woll ↑ *
Expression of CD54 on lymphocytes (%)					
Expression of CD54 on monocytes (%)					
Expression of CD54 on granulocytes (%)					

Ly – lymphocytes; Mono – monocytes; Gr – granulocytes; */a p<0.05; **/aap<0.01; ***/aaap<0.001; *– significant level calculated in exposed rats in comparison with control rats without tobacco smoke exposure; a – significant level calculated in exposed rats in comparison with control rats with tobacco smoke exposure; ↓ - decrease in comparison with relevant control; ↑ - increase in comparison with relevant control; Am – amosite; Woll – wollastonite

Table 3.2-5. Cellular immunity of rats treated via inhalation exposure with two doses of amosite/wollastonite fibers and with/without tobacco smoke.

in low-dosed rats. No effect of exposure to amosite fibers alone on proliferative activity of B-cells stimulated with STM (lipopolysacharide from *Salmonella typhimurium*) was seen in non-smoking rats, while a moderate enhancement was recorded in animals exposed to amosite and tobacco smoke. A marked suppressive effect of amosite on phagocytic activity of leukocytes was also found. Stimulation of the immune system was observed as increased phagocytic activity of leukocytes in animals exposed to cigarette smoke. Animals exposed to wollastonite or cigarette smoke alone caused enhancement of proliferative activity of T-lymphocytes stimulated with concanavalin A. All animals exposed to wollastonite fibers had suppressed phagocytic activity of monocytes and granulocytes. Moreover, decrease of phagocytosis was recorded also in combined exposure to wollastonite and cigarette smoke. In conclusion, inhalation of amosite and wollastonite mineral fibers resulted in marked changes in specific and non-specific immunity. Moreover, findings indicate mutual

Function of lymphocytes	30 mg/m³	60 mg/m³	Tobacco smoke alone	Tobacco Smoke + fibers 30 mg/m³	Tobacco smoke + fibers 60 mg/m³
Proliferative activity of T-lymphocytes stimulated with Con A (cpm)		Woll ↑ *	↑ *		
Proliferative activity of T-lymphocytes stimulated with PHA (cpm)					Am ↓ ᵃ
Proliferative activity of T-dependent B-lymphocytes stimulated with PWM (cpm)	Am ↓ *				
Proliferative activity of B-lymphocytes stimulated with STM (cpm)					Am ↑ *
Proliferative activity of T-lymphocytes stimulated with CD3 (cpm)	Am ↓ *	Am ↓ *			
Function of phagocytes					
Phagocytic activity of neutrophils (%)	Woll ↓ *	Am ↓ ** Woll ↓ *	↑ *	Am ↓ ᵃ	Am ↓ ᵃᵃᵃ
Phagocytic activity of monocytes (%)	Am ↓ ** Woll ↓ *	Am ↓ *** Woll ↓ **		Am ↓ ᵃᵃᵃ Woll ↓ *	Am ↓ ᵃᵃᵃ Woll ↓ *

*/ᵃ $p<0.05$; **/ᵃᵃ$p<0.01$; ***/ᵃᵃᵃ$p<0.001$; *– significant level calculated in exposed rats in comparison with control rats without tobacco smoke exposure; ᵃ– significant level calculated in exposed rats in comparison with control rats with tobacco smoke exposure; ↓ - decrease in comparison with relevant control; ↑ - increase in comparison with relevant control; Woll – wollastonite; Am – amosite; Con A-concanavalin A; PHA-phytohemmagglutinin; PWM-pokeweed mitogen; STM-lipopolysaccharide from *Salmonella typhimurium*; CD3-alloantigen

Table 3.2-6. Proliferative activity of lymphocytes and phagocytic activity in rats treated via inhalation exposure with two doses of amosite/wollastonite fibers and with/without tobacco smoke.

interference of mineral fibers and smoking in the modulation of the systemic immune response during combined exposure.

3.3 Assessment of Immunotoxicity of ceramic fibers and NiO nanoparticles

The aim of the study was the assessment of immune effects of exposure to ceramic fibers and/or NiO nanoparticles in experimental animals – male Sprague-Dawley rats. Rats were treated by intratracheal instillation with 1 mg of refractory ceramic fibers and/or 1mg NiO nanoparticles. Controls were treated with 1 ml physiological saline (1ml per animal). One and six months after instillation, the animals were killed. The blood samples were taken and the spleen was aseptically removed and placed into RPMI medium. Panel of immune assays was performed. The phagocytic activity of blood monocytes and granulocytes was assessed by ability to ingest bacteria *Staphylococcus aureus* (Tulinska et. al., 2005). One month after exposure of animals to ceramic fibers and/or NiO nanoparticles no alterations in phagocytic activity and respiratory burst was shown. However 6 months after exposure, situation was

Immune System and Environmental Xenobiotics - The Effect of Selected Mineral Fibers and
Particles on the Immune Response

67

different. Exposure to NiO nanoparticles and combined exposure to ceramic fibers and NiO nanoparticles caused significantly increased phagocytic activity of granulocytes, as well as percentage of cells with respiratory burst (Table 3.3-1). NiO nanoparticles and combined exposure of ceramic fibers and NiO nanoparticles stimulated this important function of nonspecific immune response.

Function of phagocytes	Ceramic fibers 1 month	NiO nanoparticles 1 month	Ceramic fibers and NiO nanoparticles 1 month
Phagocytic activity of monocyes (%)			
Phagocytic activity of granulocytes (%)			
% of phagocytic cells with respiratory burst			
	Ceramic fibers 6 months	NiO nanoparticles 6 months	Ceramic fibers and NiO nanoparticles 6 months
Phagocytic activity of monocyes (%)			
Phagocytic activity of granulocytes (%)		↑ *	↑ ***
% of phagocytic cells with respiratory burst		↑ *	↑ **

* $p<0.05$, ***$p<0.001$; ↑ - increase in comparison with relevant control

Table 3.3-1. Phagocytic activity and respiratory burst of peripheral blood cells in male Sprague-Dawley rats administered with 1 mg refractory ceramic fibers, NiO nanoparticles and combined exposure to both elements.

Function of T- and B-lymphocytes was studied using lymphoproliferation assay in spleen cells derived from rats exposed to ceramic fibers and/or NiO nanoparticles. Cells were *in vitro* stimulated with mitogens - concanavalin A (Con A), phytohemagglutin (PHA) and pokeweed (PWM) mitogen. One month after exposure, significant decrease of proliferative activity of lymphocytes stimulated with all three mitogens was found in animals exposed to ceramic fibers. To the contrary, 6 months after exposure, significant increase of lymphocyte proliferation stimulated with phytohemagglutin and pokeweed mitogen was recorded. The effect of combined exposure to ceramic fibers and NiO nanoparticles on spleen cells was manifested as significant increase of proliferative activity of T-lymphocytes after stimulation with Con A. Moreover, significant increase of basal proliferative response of spleen cells derived from rats 1 month after exposure to NiO nanoparticles alone and combined exposure to fibers and nanoparticles was seen. (Table 3.3-2).

Immunophenotypic analysis of leukocytes was examined using panel of surface markers: CD3, CD4, CD8, CD161 and MHC II. Six months after exposure, immunophenotypic analysis of leukocytes performed by flow cytometry revealed statistically significant decrease of expression of marker for T-lymphocyte subpopulations (CD4, CD8) in rats administered with ceramic fibers. On the other hand, increase of expression of CD4 marker after combined exposure was observed. 6 months after exposure to NiO nanoparticles, significant increase of expression of molecule MHC II on lymphocytes, monocytes and granulocytes was shown. Similar effect of combined exposure on expression MHC II on monocytes and granulocytes was found (Table 3.3-3).

Function of lymphocytes	Ceramic fibers 1 month	NiO nanoparticles 1 month	Ceramic fibers and NiO nanoparticles 1 month
Proliferative activity of T-lymphocytes stimulated with Conncanavalin A – Con A (cpm)	↓ *		↑ *
Proliferative activity of T- lymphocytes stimulated with Phytohemmagglutinin - PHA (cpm)	↓ ***		
Proliferative activity of T-dependent B-lymphocytes stimulated with Pokeweed mitogen - PWM (cpm)	↓ *		
Basal proliferative activity (cpm)		↑ ***	↑ ***
	Ceramic fibers 6 months	NiO nanoparticles 6 months	Ceramic fibers and NiO nanoparticles 6 months
Proliferative activity of T- lymphocytes stimulated with Con A (cpm)			
Proliferative activity of T- lymphocytes stimulated with PHA (cpm)	↑ *		
Proliferative activity of T- dependent B-lymphocytes stimulated with PWM (cpm)	↑ *		
Basal proliferative activity of lymphocytes (cpm)			

* $p<0.05$, ***$p<0.001$; cpm-counts per minutes after ^3H incorporation into lymphocytes, ↓ - decrease in comparison with relevant control; ↑ - increase in comparison with relevant control

Table 3.3-2. Proliferative response of lymphocytes in male Sprague-Dawley rats administered with 1 mg refractory ceramic fibers, NiO nanoparticles and combined exposure to both elements.

Proportion of leukocyte subsets in peripheral blood	Ceramic fibers 6 months	NiO nanoparticles 6 months	Ceramic fibers and NiO nanoparticles 6 months
CD3+ – T-lymphocytes (%)			
CD4+ – T-helper lymphocytes (%)	↓ *		↑ **
CD8+ – T-cytotoxic lymphocytes (%)	↓ *		
CD4+/CD8+ lymphocytes (%)	↓ *		
Expression of MHCII marker on lymphocytes (%)		↑ *	
Expression of MHCII marker on monocytes (%)		↑ **	↑ *
Expression of MHCII marker on granulocytes (%)		↑ **	↑ ***

* $p<0.05$; **$p<0.01$; ***$p<0.001$; ↓ - decrease in comparison with relevant control; ↑ - increase in comparison with relevant control

Table 3.3-3. Proportion of leukocyte subsets in peripheral blood in male Sprague-Dawley rats administered with 1 mg refractory ceramic fibers, NiO nanoparticles and combined exposure to both elements.

Phagocytosis is a major host defense mechanism of the innate immune system. The specific molecular pathways that direct the process of ingestion depend on the size of the particle (Hazenbos & Brown, 2006). Several other mechanisms, such as release of inflammatory mediators, antigen presentation (Garcia-Garcia & Rosales, 2005; Rabinovitch, 1995) and expression of different membrane receptors (Garcia-Garcia, 2005; Johansson et. al., 1997) are also involved. It is known that different pulmonary macrophages (airway, alveolar, interstitial, pleural, intravascular) are an important part of the lung's defenses against particles deposited by inhalation (Oberdorster, 1994). After phagocytic stimulation, macrophages release various chemotactic factors for neutrophils and other inflammatory cells including TNF, neutrophil chemotactic factor and many proinflammatory mediators such as prostaglandins, leukotrienes, thromboxane. Apart from that, macrophages produce free radical oxygen and release lysosome enzymes which may cause lung tissue injury. Published literature, studying influence ceramic and metal nanoparticles *in vitro,* showed that ceramic nanoparticles had effect on production of cytokines in monocytes. This effect resulted to the shift of cytokine balance towards inflammation. Moreover, obtained results showed that nanoparticles have significant effects on the expression of some TLR molecules, suggesting that they could affect cell reactivity to infections by altering the expression of innate receptors. Particularly interesting is the finding that ceramic nanoparticles can enhance expression of TLR chains important for viral-dependent stimulation (Lucarelli et al., 2004). Another study (Yagil-Kelmer et al., 2004) compared influence of ceramic particles on monocytes of peripheral human blood and human monocytes cell line U937. They found out the higher variability of expression of cytokines of primary human blood monocytes from donors in compared with cell line. Importantly, studies consistently demonstrated that smaller, sub-micrometer ceramic particles provoke relatively larger amounts of the cytokines IL-l alpha, IL-I beta, IL-8, TNF-alpha and IL-10 when compared to 1.5 um particles. The variation in the reactivity of different human individuals to particle stimulation may have highlighted another major contributory factor - genetic capacity of an individual to express related cytokines with their susceptibility to, and subsequently, the severity of, a particular disease (Matthews et al., 2000). Nkamgueu et al., (2000) recorded suppression of phagocytic activity and respiratory burst after *in vitro* exposure of cells to ceramic particles. The results of another study indicated that refractory ceramic fibers 6 months after intratracheal instillation significantly changed the majority of examined BAL parameters. The presence of inflammatory and cytotoxic response in lung may signalize beginning or developing disease process (Hurbankova et al., 2005).

Observations that nickel oxide-induced changes may contribute to significant immunodysfunction are known from immunotoxicity studies examining "bulk" nickel oxide aerosols. 65-day inhalation study in mice showed, that exposure to nickel oxide resulted in increased numbers of lung-associated lymph nodes (LALN), enhanced numbers of nucleated cells in lavage samples, increased antibody-forming cells (AFC) in LALN, but decreased $AFC/10^6$ spleen cells and suppressed alveolar macrophage phagocytic activity (Haley et al., 1990). Significant alterations of humoral immune system and alveolar macrophages were found also in rats after 4 weeks or 4 months of exposure to nickel oxide aerosols, respectively (Spiegelberg et al., 1984). Nanoform might have substantial impact on toxic effects including immunotoxicity. *In vitro* studies demonstrated that ultrafine NiO particles showed higher cytotoxicities toward human keratinocyte HaCaT cells and human lung carcinoma A549 cells *in vitro* than fine NiO particles (Horie et al., 2009). Transmission electron microscope observations revealed uptake of both ultrafine and fine NiO particles into HaCaT cells. Cellular uptake of NiO nanoparticles (NiO NP) was found to be associated with the release of Ni^{2+} ions after 24-48 h (Pietruska et al., 2011). The intracellular Ni^{2+} release could be an important factor that determines the cytotoxicity of NiO. Pathological features of different sizes of nickel oxide following intratracheal instillation in rats were studied by Ogami et al. (2009). Submicrometer nano-nickel oxide was associated with greater toxicity, as for crystalline silica, than micrometer-sized nickel oxide. Biological effects of factors of particle size reduction, when dealing with finer particles such as nanoparticles, were reconfirmed to be important in the evaluation of respirable particle toxicity.

In vivo studies in experimental animals showed persistent high level of inflammation in lungs even at low doses of NiO NP. Cho et al. (2010) described chronic neutrophilic/lymphocytic cytotoxic inflammation in rats 4 weeks after instillation NiO NP accompanied by increased MIP-2, IFN-γ, and LDH in BALF. The alveolar lipoproteinosis evident in NiO NP-exposed lungs was reflected in very high protein and LDH levels in the BALF. Increased levels of neutrophils and macrophages have been observed from 3 days to 3 months after instillation of agglomerated NiO NP suspended in distilled water in Wistar rats (Nishi et al., 2009; Ogami et al., 2009). Gene expression profiling of the rat lung after whole-body inhalation exposure to ultrafine NiO particles induced high expression of genes associated with chemokines, oxidative stress, and matrix metalloproteinase 12 (Mmp12), suggesting that Uf-NiO particles lead to acute inflammation (Fujita et al., 2009). *In vitro* studies conducted to test the possible toxic effects (Ada et al., 2010) bring evidence that one of the contributing underlying mechanisms is oxidative stress. The levels of intracellular reactive oxygen species and lipid peroxidation in A549 cells enhanced with increasing exposure to NiO nanoparticles and growth in gene expressions of HO-1 and SP-D were observed in A549 cells (Horie et al., 2011).

Our data of suppressed proliferative activity of T-lymphocytes and decreased T-dependent B-cell response indicate fiber-induced changes in systemic immune response. The hypothesis that inhaled particles or fibers can exert adverse effects outside of the lung is supported by several studies. Although, most of findings refer to systemic effect of particles, similar influence of fibers can be assumed. For example, ultrafine particles were found to decrease the number of blood PMNs and increase the intracellular oxidation of a fluorescent dye (DCFD) in blood PMNs (Elder et al., 2004). Diesel exhaust particles and carbon black particles had significant adjuvant effect on the local immune-mediated inflammatory response in the draining popliteal lymph node and on the systemic specific IgE response to model allergen ovalbumin in BALB/c mice (Lovik et al., 2003). The data of van Eeden (van Eeden et al., 2002) showed the effects of particulate air pollution on bone-marrow stimulation in animals. Acute exposure to ambient particles accelerates the transit of polymorphonuclear leukocytes (PMN) through the marrow whereas chronic exposure expands the size of the bone marrow pool of PMN. A communication between the fiber-induced processes in the pulmonary compartment and peripheral tissues can be mediated by: 1) leakage of reactive oxygen species and stress-induced cytokines directly into the peripheral blood, 2) (pre)activation of peripheral blood leukocytes that can result in aberrant homing and activation of inflammatory cells in distant tissues, and 3) the liberation of proinflammatory mediators by leukocytes and/or stromal cells present in the pulmonary tissues (Oudijk et al., 2003).

Immune System and Environmental Xenobiotics - The Effect of Selected Mineral Fibers and
Particles on the Immune Response

71

4. Molecular epidemiological studies in human population

The possible immunomodulatory effects of mineral fibers, in workers occupationally exposed to asbestos, rock wool and glass fibers, were examined in the context of a large-scale molecular epidemiology study (Ilavska et al., 2005; Tulinska et al., 2004). In addition to biomarkers of immunotoxicity, biomarkers of genotoxicity (Beňo et al., 2005; Dusinska et al., 2004; Horská et al., 2006; Topinka et al., 2004; 2006), oxidative damage and antioxidant defense (Staruchova et al., 2008) were also examined in the same cohorts. The studies involved workers with at least 5 years' exposure to asbestos, rock wool and glass fibers, respectively, at 3 industrial plants in Slovakia. A control group of clerical workers, matched for sex, age, smoking habits and alcohol use were also studied. All workers underwent clinical examination, including functional spirometry testing, and radiological examination.

Exposure: Fiber samples were used for asbestos fiber and ASMF identification, fiber morphology and quantification, using a microscope with phase contrast (Nikon, Japan) according to the Reference Method for the Determination of Airborne Asbestos Fiber Concentration at Workplaces by Light Microscopy (Membrane Filter Method), AIA 1979, London, UK. Exposure assessment had been based on personal and environmental monitoring.

Subjects and health status: In each plant, 61, 98 and 80 exposed workers and 21, 43 or 36 control clerical subjects, respectively, were recruited. In the case of the asbestos-exposed subjects, an additional town-control group of 49 people was included. Evidence of pulmonary fibrosis was found in 42% of the asbestos-exposed workers, while evidence of pleural fibrosis was found in 24%. The asbestos-exposed cohort had significantly decreased forced vital capacity of lungs as well as forced expiratory volume per first second.

Immune parameters: Markers of lymphocyte function were found to differ significantly between fiber-exposed cohorts and corresponding controls. Workers from the former asbestos cement plant had significantly decreased proliferative capacity of lymphocytes stimulated by T-cell mitogen PHA. In contrast, the proliferative activity of T-lymphocytes in subjects from the rock wool and glass fiber factories was stimulated (Table 4). A significant *in vitro* stimulatory effect was observed in cultured B-lymphocytes stimulated with PWM from peripheral blood obtained from the glass fiber workers, while no such effect was found in workers from the asbestos and rock wool plants in comparison with the corresponding controls (Table 4). Although no other published data on functional changes of lymphocytes has been published in rock wool and glass fiber workers, depression of cell mediated immune response with a clear relationship between defective T-cell function and pulmonary fibrosis was seen in asbestos-exposed individuals. *In vitro* studies have clarified that asbestos fibers inhibit proliferation at an early stage (G_0 phase) of the cell cycle of PHA-stimulated cells. Besides the evidence for an important role of specific immunity in chemically induced pulmonary disease, including asbestosis, and published results on the protective role of T-lymphocytes especially in asbestos-induced pulmonary inflammation, our data also suggest immunomodulatory effects for two man-made fibers. We propose that the different patterns of T-cell proliferative activity found in workers exposed to asbestos versus rock wool and glass fibers may be due to differences in the duration of exposure to the different fibers as well as differences in the underlying health status of the populations studied. In contrast to the relatively good clinical status, shorter duration and low level of fiber exposure in rock wool and glass fiber workers, the former asbestos cement workers had historically high levels of exposure to fibrogenic dust and showed clinical evidence of asbestosis and a high prevalence of low forced vital capacity. It is notable that a biphasic immune response has been reported with silica exposure. In a rat model two distinct phases were noted in development of silicosis: in early stages, silica activates both humoral and cellular immunity; however, in late phases no activated adaptive immune system effects were observed.

The phagocytic activity of polymorphonuclear leukocytes and monocytes as well as respiratory bursts of cells did not differ significantly between the exposed and control groups. Similarly, the results of the natural killer cell assays indicated no significant differences in cytotoxic activity of NK-cells between exposed and controls in the cohort exposed to asbestos and rock wool (cytotoxicity assays were not done in the glass fiber workers). Phenotypic analysis of peripheral blood leukocytes was performed to assess the proportions of the main lymphocyte subsets. Flow cytometry analysis revealed significantly decreased expression of markers CD16$^+$56$^+$ (natural killer cells) in exposed workers from the glass fiber plant in comparison with the corresponding controls (Table 4). No significant alterations between workers exposed to asbestos, rock wool and glass fibers exposed and controls have been found in proportion of CD3$^+$, CD4$^+$, CD8$^+$, CD19$^+$ cells in peripheral blood.

Table 4	Parameters	Asbestos	Rock wool	Glass Fibers
Hematology	White blood cell count (x10^9/l)			↓ *
	Lymphocytes (%)			
	Basophils and eosinophils (%)			
	Neutrophils (%)			
	Lymphocyte count (x10^9/l)			↑ **
	Basophil and eosinophil count (x10^9/l)			↑ *
	Neutrophil count (x10^9/l)			
	Erythrocyte count (x10^{12}/l)			
	Hemoglobin (g/l), hematocrit (%)			
	Mean cell volume (fl)			↓ *
	Platelets (x10^9/l)			
Function of lymphocytes	Proliferative activity of T-lymphocytes stimulated with Concanavalin A – ConA (cpm)		↑ *	↑ **
	Index Con A		↑ **	↑ **
	Proliferative activity of T-lymphocytes stimulated with Phytohemagglutinin - PHA (cpm)			↑ *
	Index PHA	↓ *	↑ **	↑ **
	Proliferative activity of T-dependent B-lymphocytes stimulated with Pokewed mitogen - PWM (cpm)			↑ *
	Index PWM			

Immune System and Environmental Xenobiotics - The Effect of Selected Mineral Fibers and
Particles on the Immune Response

73

Table 4	Parameters	Asbestos	Rock wool	Glass Fibers
	Proliferative activity of T-lymphocytes stimulated with CD3 antigen (cpm), Index CD3			
	Proliferative activity of lymphocytes stimulated with Tetanus antigen - TET (cpm), Index TET			
	Basal proliferative activity of lymphocytes (cpm)			↑ **
Function of phagocytes	Phagocytic activity of monocytes and granulocytes (%)			
	Respiratory burst of granulocytes (%)			
Function of NK cells	Natural killer cell activity (%)			not done
Proportion of lymphocyte subsets in peripheral blood	CD3⁺ – T-lymphocytes (%) CD3⁺/HLA DR – activated T-cells (%)			
	CD4⁺ - T-helper lymphocytes (%)			
	CD8⁺ - T-cytotoxic lymphocytes (%)			
	CD16⁺56⁺ - Natural killer cells (%)			↓ *
	CD 19⁺ - B-lymphocytes (%)			
	CD25, CD81 – activated T-lymphocytes (%)			
Adhesion molecules on leukocytes	Expression of CD62L on lymphocytes (%)	↑ **		
	Expression of CD62L on granulocytes (%)	↑ ***		
	Expression of CD62L on monocytes (%)	↑ ***		
	Expression of adhesion molecules CD11b, CD11c, CD18, CD49d and CD54 – ICAM on lymphocytes, granulocytes and monocytes (%)			
Activation markers on eosinophils	Expression of CD66b on eosinophils (%)	↑ ***		↑ *
	Expression of CD69 on eosinophils (%)	↑ ***		
Soluble adhesion molecules	E-Selectin (ng/ml)			↑ ***
	Intercellular Adhesion Molecule - ICAM (ng/ml)	↑ *	↑ ***	
Immunoglobulins	Immunoglobulin A – IgA (mg/dl)	↑ **		
	Immunoglobulin E – IgE (U/ml)	↑ **	↑ *	
	Immunoglobulin G – IgG (mg/dl)			
	Immunoglobulin M - IgM (mg/dl)		↓ **	
Complement	C3 and C4 Components of Complement (mg/dl)			
Proinflammatory cytokines	Interleukin 1 beta – IL1β (pg/ml)			
	Interleukin 6 – IL6 (pg/ml)	↑ **		
	Interleukin 8 - IL-8 (pg/ml)	↑ ***	↑ ***	↑ ***

* $p < 0.05$; ** $p < 0.01$; *** $p < 0.001$; ↓ - decrease ↑ - increase in comparison with relevant control;

Table 4. Immune parameters measured in population study- humans occupationally exposed to asbestos and two man-made mineral fibers (rock wool and glass fibers).

The expression of adhesion molecules on blood leukocytes was analyzed using flow cytometry. In workers from the former asbestos cement plant, expression of adhesion molecule CD62L (L-selectin) on monocytes and granulocytes was significantly increased (Table 4). Increased levels of soluble adhesion molecules ICAM-1 were found in sera from the cohorts who worked with asbestos and rock wool (Table 4). The chi square test confirmed a significantly increased proportion of people with high levels of soluble ICAM-1 (>306 ng/ml) not only among the asbestos cohort but also in glass fiber workers (asbestos p<0.02, glass fibers p<0.03) compared with the controls. Exposure to glass fibers enhanced the level of soluble E-selectin in workers' sera (Table 4). Pathologically relevant increases in the expression and function of adhesion molecules have been observed in humans with such pulmonary disease/conditions as bronchial hyperreactivity, allergic rhinitis, idiopathic pulmonary fibrosis or neoplasia.

Analysis of serum levels of proinflammatory cytokines revealed increased serum concentrations of interleukin 6 (IL-6) in former asbestos workers. Significantly elevated serum concentrations of IL-8 were found in workers exposed to all three types of fibers, while no changes in IL-1β were recorded in exposed populations. Inflammatory cytokines are rapidly induced and expressed early in a disease or injury process. They mediate and modulate the healing processes but, if overexpressed, may exacerbate the severity of a disease condition as well as give rise to oxidative stress. Up-regulation of IL-8 secretion has been found in patients with fibrosing lung disease and, because IL-8 is the main chemotactic and activation factor for neutrophils, secretion of IL-8 was associated with neutrophil accumulation in the lower respiratory tract. Since the presence of neutrophils in BAL fluid is frequently reported in humans with asbestosis changes in levels of inflammatory cytokines were examined in the context of the present study.

Exposure to asbestos and rock wool was associated with significantly increased levels of immunoglobulin E. The results of the analysis of expression of markers CD66b and CD69 on eosinophils are summarized in Table 4, where it can be seen that workers from the former asbestos cement plant and glass fiber factory had significantly elevated expression of marker CD66b, while significantly increased expression of CD69 on eosinophils was found only in asbestos workers. Immunoglobulin E is well known as being involved in the mechanisms of development of allergic diseases. The observation of significantly increased levels of total immunoglobulin E in asbestos workers is in agreement with published results of Rosenthal et al., (1999) who concluded that asbestos appears to produce a hyperresponsive state, with chronically exposed individuals manifesting an elevation in circulating immunoglobulins (IgG, IgM, IgE). No data are available on populations occupationally exposed to rock wool for comparison.

5. Biomarkers

5.1 Proliferative activity of lymphocytes (lymphocyte transformation test)

Lymphocytes are important cells of the adaptive immune response. T-cells are involved in cell-mediated immunity whereas B-cells are primarily responsible for humoral immunity (relating to antibodies). The function of T-cells and B-cells is to recognize specific "non-self" antigens, during a process known as antigen presentation. Our study revealed high sensitivity of T-lymphocyte response to exposure to mineral fibers. Meanwhile in workers exposed to asbestos, significant suppression of proliferative response of T-cells *in vitro* stimulated with phytohemagglutinin was found, stimulative effect of rock wool and glass fibers on activity of T-lymphocytes in peripheral blood of exposed population were recorded. Our findings indicate that one of the immune targets of mineral fiber exposure seems to be specific cellular immunity. Proliferative activity of lymphocytes might be a sensitive indicator of immunomodulatory effects of mineral fibers; however the limitations of use it as a biomarker of individual susceptibility are interindividual differences.

5.2 Phagocytic activity of leukocytes

Pulmonary macrophages are crucial cells in contact with mineral fibers and nanoparticles representing the first line of defense in the lung alveoli. Expansion of macrophages in the lung is a typical characteristic of that type of exposure in both humans and experimental animals. Total macrophage numbers in the lung may increase by migration of blood monocytes, local proliferation of the alveolar macrophages or induced generation of chemotaxins (Rosenthal et al., 1998). Phagocytosis of asbestos fibers has been shown to be accompanied by the activation of macrophages, which results in the generation of ROS as well as a variety of chemical mediators and cytokines. These mediators amplify the local inflammatory reaction. Persistence of asbestos fibers in the lung interstitium or in the sub-pleural connective tissue may lead to a sustained chronic inflammatory reaction accompanied by fibrosis and proliferation of epithelial and mesenchymal cells (Branche, 2009). Surprisingly, in contrast to a marked suppressive effect of mineral fibers on the activity of phagocytes observed in our animal studies, no dramatic influence was found in worker populations. A statistically significant deterioration of phagocytic activity of monocytes was observed only among smoking workers exposed to asbestos, in comparison with exposed non-smokers (Tulinska et al., 2004).

5.3 Percentage of CD16$^+$56$^+$ cells (natural killer cells – NK cells) and cytotoxic activity of NK cells

Natural killer cells (NK cells) are crucial members of innate immunity responsible for killing of virus infected cells, overseeing of mutated or other way transformed cells and as a first defense line toward cancer cells. They kill cells by releasing small cytoplasmic granules of proteins called perforin and granzyme that cause the target cell to die by apoptosis (programmed cell death). Several authors have reported increased numbers of circulating NK cells and their reduced activity in asbestos exposed humans (Froom et al., 2000; Rosenthal et al., 1999). The results from our study do not confirm these findings. Neither asbestos cement nor rock wool workers were noted to have significant changes in NK-cell activity or the percentage of cells with NK phenotype. However, significantly decreased expression of marker CD16$^+$56 was found in glass fiber-exposed workers in comparison with controls. Although the effect was not dramatic, this observation suggests that exposed workers need to be screened preventively for this marker. This finding is surprising because glass fiber exposure has not as yet been connected with malignant tumors as has asbestos. Synthetic vitreous fibers (that include insulation glass wool and continuous glass filament) were reclassified by International Agency for Research on Cancer (IARC) commission from category 2b (*possibly carcinogenic to humans*) to category 3 (*not classifiable as to their carcinogenicity to humans*) in 2001 (Bernstein, 2007; IARC, 2002). Regardless, that in our study population no significant differences in cytotoxic activity of natural killer cells were found between workers exposed to asbestos and rock wool and corresponding controls (assay in glass fiber workers not done), the assay is considered an important member of a panel to assess antitumor immunity in workers exposed to probable, possible or susceptible carcinogens. We assume that both numbers and activity of NK cells are important in individual health surveys of workers exposed to mineral fibers.

5.4 The phenotypical analysis of peripheral blood leukocytes

T-lymphocytes, CD3, CD4, CD8, HLA DR markers

Published data suggest that asbestos may affect immunocompetent cells such as CD4+ responder T-cells, CD4+ regulatory T-cells, Th17 T-cells, CD8+ cytotoxic T-cells (CTL) or dendritic cells (DC). Continuous exposure to chrysotile produces a stronger Treg function, at least with the capacity to produce soluble functional factors (i.e., IL-10 and TGF-β) (Kumagai-Takei et al., 2011). Recent research indicates that asbestos is able to act as a superantigen (Otsuki et al., 2007). The increased expression of T-cell receptor Vβ without a clonal expansion of T-lymphocytes has been demonstrated after asbestos exposure. This is in line with our results. We did not detect changes either in absolute or relative number of T-lymphocytes and activated T-lymphocytes in the asbestos exposed workers in comparison to controls. Previous papers referred changes in Th/Ts ratio as well as decreased relative and absolute number of circulating T-lymphocytes (Kagan et al., 1977; Tsang et al., 1988). These parameters were without change also in case of rock wool or glass fiber exposure.

Expression of CD81 and CD25 on activated T-lymphocytes

In spite of inhibition of T-cell proliferation observed in the case of asbestos or stimulation in case of glass fibers and rock wool we did not find changes in expression of early activation markers CD81 and CD25 on CD4+ and CD8+ T-cells after PHA stimulation (data not published). Their spontaneous stimulation was not damaged either. Chronic exposure to all of three fibers had no effect on these tested parameters. Similar results were recorded by Wu et al. (2000). The marker CD81 was not expressed on peripheral T-lymphocytes after *in vitro* cultivation with chrysotile asbestos. Dysregulation and long-term T-cell activation can lead to survival of self-recognizing cells, and consecutively to initiation of autoimmune responses. We assume that synthetic mineral fibers do not impact the human organism in the same manner as in the case of asbestos. The expression of T-cells activation markers was not changed after glass fibers and rock wool exposure.

B- lymphocytes, CD19 marker, and immunoglobulins IgG, IgA, IgM, IgE

An increased number of B-cells have been reported in patients with asbestosis, fibrosis or malignant diseases after asbestos exposure (Gaumer et al., 1981; Ozesmi et al., 1988). We did not detect this change after asbestos, glass fiber or rock wool exposure. However, among those with asbestos exposure we confirmed a hyperresponsive B-lymphocytes as seen by Rosenthal et al., (1999) with increased levels of immunogloulins IgE and IgA. Exposure to rock wool was also associated with increased IgE levels and in contrast with decreased levels of IgM. Exposure to glass fibers did not affect these parameters. An elevation in serum immunoglobulins (IgA, IgG, IgM, IgE) and mucosal (salivary) IgA and the presence of autoantibodies, antinuclear antibody and rheumatoid factor is one of the most consistent findings in individuals chronically exposed to asbestos (Doll, 1983). IgE is well known for being a central regulator in the allergic reactions. The increased level of IgE and a higher production of proinflammatory interleukins, IL-6 and IL-8, suggest inflammation with a shift from Th1 to Th2 immune response. Our findings correspond to other studies which confirm a shift towards a Th2 mediated immune response in BAL fluid after asbestos exposure (elevated levels of cytokines IL-1b, Il-4, Il-5, IL-6, Il-13) (Sabo-Attwood et al., 2005; Shukla et al., 2007).

Activation markers on eosinophils

Eosinophils are known for their participation on allergic reactions. Pulmonary diseases as asthma or allergic rhinitis are associated with elevated number of circulating eosinophils (Venarske & deShazo, 2003). The expression of activation markers on eosinophils can indicate a growing allergic status. Workers from the World Trade Center crash (with high exposure to asbestos and synthetic mineral fibers) had enormously increased numbers of eosinophils in BAL fluid but circulating eosinophils were not changed (Rom et al., 2002). Also in our study, we did not detect increased number of peripheral blood eosinophils after mineral fibers exposure, but we observed evidence of their activation. The expression of CD69 and CD66b markers was associated primarily with asbestos exposure, and glass fibers enhanced only CD66b. Rock wool did not have impact on these parameters.

Expression of adhesion molecules CD11b, CD11c, CD18, CD54, CD62L, and CD49d on lymphocytes, monocytes and granulocytes

Transendothelial migration of leukocytes into tissues is a multistep process. Leukocytes express adhesion molecules as mediators. We evaluated the expression of adhesion molecules CD11b, CD11c, CD18, CD54, CD62L and CD49d on leucocytes and detected the increased expression of L-selectin (CD62-L) on monocytes and granulocytes in workers exposed to asbestos. Selectins mediate the rolling of leukocytes on the stimulated endothelium. Increased numbers of alveolar macrophages in the lower human airways is a typical finding after asbestos exposure (Rosenthal et al., 1999). Circulating monocytes transmigrate to tissue in response to chemotactic factors and become tissue macrophages. The over-expression of CD62L as well as IL-8, a chemotactic factor for neutrophils, may be an important part of this process.

5.5 The assessment of soluble markers

Complement components C3 and C4

Sabo-Attwood et al., (2005) showed changes in the gene expression of C1 complement component in a mouse model. The incubation of human plasma with asbestos fibers induced production of C5a fragment of C5 component of complement (Governa et al., 2000). We did not detect any changes of C3 and C4 complement components in human serum of workers exposed to mineral fibers (data not published).

Interleukins IL-1β, IL-6, and IL-8

Asbestosis is accompanied by persistent inflammation and by production of mediators of inflammation. Certain asbestos substitute fibers, e.g. wollastonite fibers are potential angiogenic agents that can induce regenerative cytokine (IL-6, IL-8) and angiogenic factor production (VEGF-A) resulting in the formation of new blood vessels (Carbonari et al., 2011). Many *in vitro* studies showed that measurement of interleukin levels is equally sensitive for testing of cell activation after air-transmitted particles exposure *in vitro*

(Mitschik et al., 2008). In connection with asbestosis, there are cytokines, mainly IL-1β, IL-6, IL-8, which appear to have a role in pathology of this disease (Mossman & Churg, 1998; Tsuda et al., 1997). In spite of the fact that IL-1β is a proinflammatory cytokine required for the synthesis of others cytokines (e.g. IL-8), we did not detect differences in exposed groups in comparison to controls. Our findings were in accordance to observations of Simeonova and Luster (Simeonova & Luster et al., 1996) who noted an enhancement of IL-8 without IL-1β stimuli. IL-6 was previously known as a factor for B-cell differentiation and immunoglobulin production. The increased level of IL-6 may be associated with the increased IgE and IgA levels seen in asbestos exposed individuals. Monitoring of IL-8 in peripheral blood could serve as an early and sensitive marker of developing pulmonary inflammation in consequence of asbestos, glass fibers and rock wool exposure. Across all three exposed groups we observed an increase of cytokine IL-8. Despite the highly significant ($p < 0.001$) differences in IL-8 between exposed workers and human control subjects, these interleukin levels were still in normal reference range.

Soluble adhesion molecules sICAM-1, sVCAM-1 and sE-selectin

The soluble adhesion molecules are products of activated endothelial cells. They are known for their involvement in processes of inflammation. Ciebiada et al., (2011) declared that concentrations of sICAM-1 are significantly higher in patients with asthma, and are dependent on a seriousness of disease. Our observations of increased adhesion molecules are in agreement with findings of Kristovich who stated that in the context of the pulmonary microenvironment, TNF-α elaborated by particulate-laden alveolar monocytes could act upon proximal septal capillary endothelial cells, inducing their expression of endothelial leukocyte adhesion molecules ICAM-1, vascular cell adhesion molecule (VCAM -1 and E-selectin (Kristovich et al., 2004). Based on this fact we can speculate that levels of sICAM-1 corresponded with inflammation of the airways. Levels of sICAM-1 were increased in the asbestos exposed group. This was not surprising because asbestos fibers are persistent and insoluble in the lungs and are known as causative factor of inflammation. Although in the case of rock wool was a rather disturbing finding for a reason of better elimination of these inhaled synthetic mineral fibers from organism. Usually they have a high solubility and short-term durability in the airways. Among others, there was a shorter duration and lower concentration of fiber in the case of rock wool than asbestos exposure. We noted a statistically significantly higher elevation of sICAM-1 levels in individuals exposed to rock wool compared to the group exposed to asbestos. Glass fibers were not associated with differences in sICAM-1 levels. Adhesion molecules seem to be a sensitive indicator of activation of the immune system and inflammatory response in humans exposed to mineral fibers. Oxidative stress and production of ROS is an important component of the multiple effects of asbestos on human airways (Manning et al., 2002; van Helden et al., 2009). ROS modulate receptor signals and immune responses under physiological conditions, but their overproduction mediates endothelial damage through growth and migration of inflammatory cells, over-expression of inflammatory cytokines and adhesion molecules such as ICAM-1, VCAM-1, and E-selectin (Urso et al., 2011). The elevated production of IL-8, sICAM-1 (rock wool exposure) and sE-selectin (glass fibers exposure) signify immunotoxic effects of synthetic fibers from the airways and increased production of ROS.

6. Summary

This chapter addresses the effects of asbestos, man made mineral fibers (rock wool, glass wool, ceramic fibers) and nickel oxide nanoparticles on the immune system using *in vitro* model, animal model and molecular-epidemiological studies. Data from *in vitro* studies contained results of experiments on alveolar macrophages (AM) and alveolar epithelial type II cells (TII). Stone wool, refractory ceramic fibers (RCF), asbestos (crocidolite) and wollastonite have been tested by lectin histochemistry. Stone wool caused moderate membrane injury of AM and incomplete phagocytosis in a small fraction of AM. RCF caused gaps and reduplicated changes in membranes of both cell types (high dose). Wollastonite caused a decreased reaction in the membranes (high dose). After exposure to the lowest dose of asbestos (crocidolite), the membranes of both cell types were fragmented irregularly and frustrated phagocytosis could be found in AM. Analysis using transmission electron microscopy found severe damage in the organelles and cell death of both cell types exposed to crocidolite. No alterations were found after RCF or stone wool exposure. Analysis of proinflammatory peptides showed that exposure to wollastonite did not change production MCP-1 and MIP-1α in TII cells but in AM the production was significantly enhanced. Different doses of stone wool enhanced production of both peptides in TII cells and AM cells. Crocidolite evoked statistically significant dose dependent enhancement of the production of MCP-1 in AM, for MIP-1α; and both cytokines in TII cells. Comparing the results from different fibers on 2 various primary cell types the following differences are clearly seen: crocidolite (asbestos) evoked the greatest changes, both morphologically and functionally. Increased effects in wollastonite were seen when compared to stone wool. AM cells are more sensitive to the fiber exposure than TII cells.

Intratracheal instillation studies in rat model

Four types of mineral fibers were administered intratracheally to rats. Four (4w) and 16 weeks (16w) later, immune parameters were examined. Amosite, wollastonite (4w) and rock wool (16w) significantly decreased number of white blood cells; while opposite effect of glass fibers was seen (4w). A consistent increase in percentage of neutrophils was found in animals exposed to all fibers (4w) while decreased percentage of lymphocytes was observed only in rock wool fiber-treated rats (4w). Analysis of lymphocyte subsets in amosite exposed rats showed significantly increased percentage of T-lymphocytes (4w, 16w), mainly cytotoxic cells (4w) and decreased percentage of B-lymphocytes (4w). An increased percentage of T-helper cells was seen in wollastonite group (4w). Exposure to mineral fibers decreased expression of adhesion molecule CD54 (ICAM-1) on peripheral blood leukocytes (amosite, glass fibers and rockwool; all 4w) and CD11b (glass fibers, wollastonite; 4w). Although amosite (4w, 16w) seems to be most potent suppressor of T- and B-lymphocyte proliferation, especially in high-dosed animals, wollastonite (4w) and rock wool (4w, 16w) also interfered with lymphocyte proliferation and suppressed the response of T-lymphocytes. The opposite, stimulative, effect on proliferative capacity of B-cells was found in animals exposed to glass fibers (4w). A highly significant dose-dependent suppression of phagocytic activity of neutrophils and monocytes was found mainly in rock wool and glass fiber exposed animals (4w, 16w), but present also in wollastonite and amosite group (4w).

Inhalation studies in rat model - combined effect of mineral fibers and tobacco smoke on inflammatory response and cytotoxicity

In rats administered with amosite, weak dose-dependence was seen in simple exposure to fibers without smoking but inflammatory parameters were mostly changed in animals with combined exposure to high dose of fibers and tobacco smoke. In case of wollastonite exposure, no clear dose-dependence in changes of inflammatory parameters was recorded in those administered with fibers alone and very weak in combined exposure groups (fibers and tobacco smoke). Additionally, mild dose dependence of cytotoxic parameters changes in groups without or with tobacco smoke was observed. Tobacco smoke alone induced changes predominantly in inflammatory parameters; alterations in cytotoxic parameters were not explicit.

Combined effect of mineral fibers and tobacco smoke on immune parameters

Inhalation of high dose of both fibers (amosite and wollastonite) resulted in a significantly increased percentage of B-lymphocytes in peripheral blood of exposed rats. Except the percentage the B-cells, the combined exposure to wollastonite and smoking caused a significant, dose-dependent increase of cytotoxic cells, but total T-lympocytes were decreased. Exposure to amosite and wollastonite increased expression of adhesion molecule CD11b on peripheral blood leukocytes. The proliferative activity of T-lymphocytes and T-dependent B-cell response in animals exposed to amosite in simple or combined exposure with smoking was mostly suppressed. The only exception was combined exposure to amosite fibers and smoking resulting in significant increase of proliferative activity of B-cells. Enhanced proliferative reponse of T-cells was found in animals given high dose of wollastonite. A marked suppressive effect of amosite and wollastonite on phagocytic activity of leukocytes was observed. Moreover, decrease of phagocytosis was recorded in combined exposure to wollastonite and cigarette smoke.

Assessment of immunotoxicity of ceramic fibers and NiO nanoparticles

Immunophenotypic analysis of leukocytes was examined only 6 months after exposure to fibers and nanoparticles. Analysis revealed statistically significant decreased expression of marker for T-lymphocyte subpopulations (CD4+, CD8+) in rats administered with ceramic fibers. On the other hand, increased expression of CD4+ marker after combined exposure was observed. Exposure to NiO nanoparticles significantly increased expression of MHC II on leukocytes. A similar effect was found on expression of MHC II with combined exposure. A significant decrease of proliferative activity of lymphocytes stimulated with all three mitogens was found in animals exposed to ceramic fibers one month after exposure. To the contrary, 6 months after exposure, opposite effect was seen. Moreover, significant increase of basal proliferative response of spleen cells derived from rats was seen 1 month after exposure to NiO nanoparticles alone and combined exposure to fibers and nanoparticles. Combined exposure to nickel oxide nanoparticles manifested a significant increase of proliferative activity of T-lymphocytes after stimulation with Con A. No alterations in phagocytic activity and respiratory burst were shown one month after exposure of animals to ceramic fibers and/or NiO nanoparticles. However 6 months after exposure, situation was different. Exposure to NiO nanoparticles and combined exposure to ceramic fibers and NiO nanoparticles caused significantly increased phagocytic activity of granulocytes, as well as percentage of cells with respiratory burst.

Molecular epidemiological studies in human population

In the context of a large-scale molecular epidemiology study, the possible immunomodulatory effects of mineral fibers, in workers occupationally exposed to asbestos, rockwool and glass fibers, were examined. Results of hematological evaluation shown decreased white blood cell count and increased number of lymphocytes and (common) eosinophil and basophil count in glass fiber exposed population. Our findings indicate that exposure to all three types of fibers examined the modulation of immune response to a different degrees. Suppression of T-cell immunity was found in the workers from a former asbestos cement plant, while stimulation of T-cell response was observed in rockwool workers. In addition to an elevated T- lymphocyte response, stimulated T-dependent B-cell response and basal proliferative activity of lymphocytes was seen in workers from glass fiber factory. Changes in lymphocyte subpopulation of CD 16+56 (natural killer cells) in peripheral blood may indicate negative effects of glass fibers on natural cellular immunity. No significant alterations between workers exposed to asbestos, rock wool and glass fibers and controls were found in proportion of CD3+, CD4+, CD8+, CD19+ cells in peripheral blood. Significantly increased serum levels of immunoglobulins IgA (asbestos), IgE (asbestos, rockwool) and decreased levels of IgM (rockwool) were recorded in people exposed to fibers. Increased levels of proinflammatory cytokines (IL-6 asbestos; IL-8 all three fibers), expression of adhesion molecule L-selectin on granulocytes and monocytes (asbestos), levels of soluble adhesion molecules in sera (ICAM-1 asbestos, rockwool; E-selectin glass fibers), increased levels of immunoglobulin E (asbestos and rockwool) and elevated expression of activation markers on eosinophils (CD66b asbestos, glass fibers; CD69 asbestos) may indicate hypersensitivity and an elevated inflammatory status in workers exposed to mineral fibers.

7. Conclusions

With the increasing commercial needs for substitutes of asbestos fibers, a number of man-made and other naturally occurring mineral fibers will appear as a part of living and occupational environments. Fibers discussed in this chapter can enter the human body mainly via the lungs, significance of exposure through digestive tract is less clear. Asbestos has long been recognized as a cause of both benign and malignant lung disease. Man made mineral fibers, once inhaled and displaced to lung tissues, can cause respiratory diseases related to inflammation and fibrosis. Skin diseases have been also reported. In reference to nanoparticles besides the lung and digestive tract, penetration via the skin also occurs (Fig. 1). Knowledge from air pollution showing increased risk of cardiopulmonary, respiratory, hypersensitivity disease and cancer requires specific assessments to be performed for newly produced nanoparticles. The assays currently used to test the safety of materials might be applicable to identify hazards of nanoparticles. Special attention is needed for nanoparticles designed for drug delivery or food components.

To optimize risk assessment for immune system toxicity, it is still necessary to increase our understanding of the underlying immunomodulatory mechanisms which cause negative effects and the quantitative relationships between the immunological tests conducted in the laboratory and manifestation of disease in human populations. There is no universal "consequence of exposure", each type of immunotoxicant should be treated individually when health risks are expected. As mentioned throughout this chapter, the immune system has been identified as a potential target organ for chemicals including particles and fibers. The immune system plays a critical role in host defense from disease as well as in normal homeostasis; thus identification of immunotoxic risk is important in the protection of human, animal and wildlife health. Clear understanding of normal development of cellular components of the immune system, the means by which they interact, and the known parameters by which their structure and function can be modified is necessary for designing investigations into how environmental agents may affect health through the immune system.

A growth of knowledge in immunology and cell biology connected with an explosion in methodologic and technologic capabilities is very promising for the science of immunotoxicology. There are several challenges yet to be solved within the discipline of immunotoxicology: (1) to improve traditional tests and establish a new tests, which reflect the variety of potential impacts of immunotoxicity; (2) to identify valid, sensitive human biomarkers of immunotoxicity; (3) to interpret minor, moderate, or significant immunotoxic effects in animal models in relation to human risk assessment; (4) better integration of methods of exposure assessment and immunotoxicological risk assessment, especially for simultaneous exposure to multiple agents ; (5) to design better human studies to assess the impact on the immune system in the species of the greatest interest in the context of risk assessment and (6) the better understanding of the role of genetic predisposition and susceptibility in identifying sensitive subpopulations to immune-altering agents (Kaminiski et al., 2008). These challenges are not unique to immunotoxicology, but they are critical, and need to be addressed through intensive and systematic efforts to improve human immune testing strategies.

8. Acknowledgment

The work was supported by EU grant, contract No. QLK4-CT-1999-01629-FIBRETOX; NIEHS grants of University of Iowa, Iowa, USA: IMUGENFIB, US NIH # 2 D43 TW00621-006 and NIEHS # 510 20 5240 00000 1 15010 9220; Hungarian-Slovak grants: NKFP-1/B-047/2004, OTKA 046733, ETT 154/2003-6 (Hungarian Medical Research Council), NILU internal grant 106170, EC FP7 [Health-2007-1.3-4, Contract no: 201335].

We would like to express our gratitude to Viera Vachalkova, Helena Turazova, Maria Valentova, Edita Mrvikova, Olga Liskova, Mikulas Krnac, Adriana Paulikova, Darina Cepcova, Jarmila Jantoskova and Lubica Mikloskova and for their excellent technical help.

This article was created by the realization of the project ITMS No.24240120033, based on the supporting Operational research and development program financed from the European Regional Development Fund.

9. References

Ada, K.; Turk, M.; Oguztuzun, S.; Kilic, M.; Demirel, M.; Tandogan, N.; Ersayar, E. & Latif, O. (2010). Cytotoxicity and apoptotic effects of nickel oxide nanoparticles in cultured HeLa cells. *Folia Histochem Cytobiol*. 2010 Dec;48(4):524-9, ISSN (printed): 0239-8508. ISSN (electronic): 1897-5631

Ahamed, M. (2011). Toxic response of nickel nanoparticles in human lung epithelial A549 cells. *Toxicol In Vitro*. 2011 Jun;25(4):930-6. Epub 2011 Mar 3, ISSN: 0887-2333

American Thoracic Society. (2004). Diagnosis and initial management of nonmalignant diseases related to asbestos. *Am J Respir Crit Care Med.* 2004, Vol.170, pp. 691-715, ISSN: 1073-449X

Aoshiba, K.; Tamaoki, J. & Nagai, A. (2001). Acute cigarette smoke exposure induces apoptosis of alveolar macrophages, *Am J Physiol Lung Cell Mol Physiol*, Vol.281, pp. 1392-1401, ISSN: 1040-0605

Ates, I.; Yucesoy, B.; Yucel, A.; Suzen, SH.; Karakas, Y. & Karakaya, A. (2011). Possible effect of gene polymorphisms on the release of TNFα and IL1 cytokines in coal workers' pneumoconiosis. *Exp Toxicol Pathol.* 2011 Jan;63(1-2):175-9. Epub 2009 Dec 11, ISSN: 0940-2993

Benford, DJ.; Hanley, AB.; Bottrill, K.; Oehlschlager, S.; Balls, M.; Branca, F.; Castegnaro, JJ.; Descotes, J.; Hemminiki, K.; Lindsay, D. & Schilter, B. (2000). Biomakers as predictive tools in toxicity testing. The report and recommendations of ECVAM Workshop 40, *ATLA*, pp. 119-131, ISSN: 0261-1929

Beňo, M.; Hurbánková, M.; Černá, S.; Dušinská, M.; Volkovová, M.; Staruchová, M.; Barančoková, M.; Kažimírová, A.; Kováčiková, Z.; Mikulecký, M. & Kyrtopoulos, AS. (2005). Multinucleate cells (MNC) as sensitive semiquantitative biomarkers of the toxic effect after experimental fibrous dust and cigarette smoke inhalation by rats, *Exp Toxicol Pathol.* Vol.57, No.1, pp. 77-87, ISSN: 0940-2993

Bernstein, DM. (2007). Synthetic vitreous fibers: a review toxicology, epidemiology and regulations, *Crit. Rev. Toxicol.*, Vol.37, No.10, pp. 839-86, ISSN: 1547-6898

Boffetta, P.; Saracci, R.; Andersen, A.; Bertazzi, PA.; Chang-Claude, J.; Cherrie, J.; Ferro, G.; Frentzel-Beyme, R.; Hansen, J.; Olsen, JH.; Plato, N.; Teppo, L.; Westerholm, P.; Winter, PD. & Zocchetti, C. (1997) Cancer mortality among man-made vitreous fibre production workers. *Epidemiology*, 8, 259-268, ISSN (printed): 1044-3983. ISSN (electronic): 1531-5487

Boor, P.; Casper, S.; Cele, P.; Hurbánková, M.; Beňo, M.; Heidland, A.; Amann, K. & Šebeková, K. (2009). Renal, vascular and cardiac fibrosis in rats exposed to passive smoking and industrial dust fibre amosite. *J. Cell. Mol. Med.* Vol Vol. 13, No 11-12, pp. 4484-4491, ISSN (printed): 1582-1838. ISSN (electronic): 1582-4934

Bottrill, K. (1998). The use of biomarkers as alternatives to current animal tests on food chemicals, *ATLA*, Vol.26 pp. 421-480, ISSN: 0261-1929

Branche, Ch. (2009). Asbestos fibers and other elongated mineral particles: State of the science and roadmap for research, *NIOSH Current Intelligence Bulletin*, pp. 1-129,

Brüske-Hohlfeld, I. (2009). Environmental and occupational risk factors for lung cancer. *Methods Mol Biol.* 2009;472:3-23, ISSN: 1064-3745

Bunderson-Schelvan, M.; Pfau, JC.; Crouch, R. & Holian, A. (2011). Non-pulmonary outcomes of asbestos exposure. *J Toxicol Environ Health B Crit Rev* 14:122–152, ISSN (printed): 1093-7404. ISSN (electronic): 1521-6950

Burchiel, SW.; Mitchell, LA.; Lauer, FT.; Sun, X.; McDonald, JD.; Hudson, LG. & Liu, KJ. (2009). Immunotoxicity and biodistribution analysis of arsenic trioxide in C57B1/6 mice following a two-week inhalation exposure. *Toxicol Appl Pharmacol.* 2009 December 15; 241(3): 253-259, ISSN (printed): 0041-008X. ISSN (electronic): 1096-0333

Carbonari, D.; Campopiano, A.; Ramires, D.; Strafella, E.; Staffolani, S.; Tomasetti, M.; Curini, R.; Valentino, M.; Santarelli, L. & Amati, M. (2011). Angiogenic effect induced by mineral fibres, *Toxicology*, Vol.288 No.1-3, pp. 34-42, ISSN: 0300-483X

Ciebiada, M.; Gorska-Ciebiada, M. & Gorski, P. (2011). sICAM and TNF-α in asthma and rhinitis: relationship with the presence of atopy. *J. Asthma*, Vol.48, No.7, pp. 660-666, ISSN 0022-1899

Černá, S.; Beňo, M.; Hurbánková, M.; Kováčiková, Z.; Bobek, P. & Kyrtopoulos, SA. (2004). Evaluation of Bronchoalveolar lavage fluid cytotoxic parameters after inhalation exposure to amosite and wollastonite fibrous dusts combined with cigarette smoke, *Cent Eur J Health*. 12 Suppl.: pp. 20-23, ISSN: 1210-7778.

Chauhan, V.; Howland, M.; Kutzner, B.; McNamee, JP.; Bellier, PV. & Wilkins, RC. (2011). Biological effects of alpha particle radiation exposure on human monocytic cells. *Int J Hyg Environ Health*. 2011 Dec 6. Epub ahead of print, ISSN: 1438-4639

Cho, WS.; Duffn, R.; Poland, CA.; Howie, SAM.; MacNee, W.; Bradley, M.; Megson, JL. & Ken Donaldson, K. (2010). Metal Oxide Nanoparticles Induce Unique Infammatory Footprints in the Lung: Important Implications for Nanoparticle Testing, *Environmental Health Perspectives*, 118, 12, December 2010, Epub 2008 Sep 17, ISSN: 0091-6765

Cho, WS.; Duffin, R.; Bradley, M.; Megson, IL.; Macnee, W.; Howie, SE. & Donaldson, K. (2011a). NiO and Co3O4 Nanoparticles Induce Lung DTH-Like Responses and Alveolar Lipoproteinosis. *Eur Respir J*. 2011 Aug 4. Epub ahead of print, ISSN (printed): 0903-1936. ISSN (electronic): 1399-3003

Cho, WS.; Duffin, R.; Howie, SEM.; Scotton, ChJ.; Wallace, WAH.; MacNee, W.; Bradley, M.; Megson, IL. & Donaldson, K. (2011b). Progressive severe lung injury by zinc oxide nanoparticles; the role of Zn2+ dissolution inside lysosomes, *Particle and Fibre Toxicology* 2011, 8:27, ISSN: 1743-8977

Committee for Proprietary Medicinal Products (2000) http://www.emea.eu.int/pdfs/human/swp/104299en.pdf

Corsini, E.; Luster, MI.; Mahler, J.; Craig, WA.; Blazka, ME. & Rosenthal, GJ. (1994). A protective role for T lymphocytes in asbestos-induced pulmonary inflammation and collagen deposition. *Am J Respir Cell Mol Biol*. 1994 Nov;11(5):531-9, ISSN: 1044-1549.

Costantini, LM.; Gilberti, RM. & Knecht, DA. (2011). The phagocytosis and toxicity of amorphous silica. *PLoS One*. 2011 Feb 2;6(2):e14647, ISSN: 1932-6203

D'Amato, G.; Liccardi, G.; D'Amato, M. & Holgate, S. (2005). Environmental risk factors and allergic bronchial asthma. *Clin Exp Allergy*. 2005 Sep;35(9):1113-24, ISSN: 0954-7894 (Print) 1365-2222 (Electronic) 0954-7894 (Linking)

Das, KK. & Buchner, V. (2007). Effect of nickel exposure on peripheral tissues: role of oxidative stress in toxicity and possible protection by ascorbic acid. *Rev Environ Health*. 2007 Apr-Jun;22(2):157-73. ISSN (printed): 0048-7554. ISSN (electronic): 2191-0308

De Rosa, CT.; Smith, LS.; Hicks, H.; Nickle, R. & Williams-Johnson M. (2002). The impact of toxicology on public health policy and service. In: Impact of Hazardous Chemicals on Public Health, Policy and Service, 556pp. De Rosa, CT; Holler, JS & Mehlman,

MA.(eds). In: *Advances in modern environmental toxicology*, vol. XXVI International
Toxicology Books, Inc Princeton, New Jersey, ISSN:0748-2337 vol:19 issue:2

Descotes, J.; Choquet-Kastylevsky, G.; Van Ganse, E.; & Vial, T. (2000). Responses of the
Immune System to Injury, *Toxicol. Pathol.*, Vol.28, pp. 479-481, ISSN (printed): 0192-
6233; ISSN (electronic): 1533- 1601.

Descotes J. (2005). Immunotoxicology: role in the safety assessment of drugs. *Drug Saf.*,
Vol.28, No.2, pp. 127-36, ISSN: 0114-5916

De Jong, W.H. & Van Loveren, H. (2007). Screening of xenobiotics for direct immunotoxicity
in an animal study, *Methods*, Vol.41, Issue 1, pp. 3-8, ISSN (printed): 1046-2023.
ISSN (electronic): 1095-9130

De Vuyst, P.; Dumortier, P.; Swaen, G.M.H.; Pairon, J.C. & Brochard, P. (1995). Respiratory
health effects of man-made vitreous (mineral) fibres, *Eur Respir J*, Vol.8, pp. 2149–
2173, ISSN 0903 - 1936

Dietert, RR. & Holsapple, MP. (2007). Methodologies for developmental immunotoxicity
(DIT) testing. *Methods* 41:123-131, ISSN: 1046-2023

Di Giampaolo, L.; Quecchia, C.; Schiavone, C.; Cavallucci, E.; Renzetti, A.; Braga, M. & Di
Gioacchino, M. (2011) Environmental pollution and asthma. *Int J Immunopathol
Pharmacol*. 2011 Jan-Mar;24(1 Suppl):31S-38S. Review, ISSN: 0394-6320 (Print) 0394-
6320 (Linking)

Doll, NJ.; Diem, JE.; Jones, RN.; Rodriguez, M.; Bozelka, BE.; Stankus, RP.; Weill, H. &
Salvaggio JE. (1983). Humoral immunological abnormalities in workers exposed to
asbestos cement dust, *J Allergy Clin Immunol*, Vol.72, pp. 509-512, ISSN: 0091- 6749

Donald, E.; & Gardner, I. (2006). Toxicology of the Lung., Taylor & Francis Group, USA,
2006: 681 s., ISBN 0-8493-2835-7

Donaldson, K & Tran, L. (2004). An introduction to the short-term toxicology of respirable
industrial fibres, *Mutation Research/Fundamental and Molecular Mechanisms of
Mutagenesis*, Volume 553, Issues 1-2, 3 September 2004, Pages 5-9, ISSN 1386-1964

Duramad, P. & Holland, N.T. (2011). Biomarkers of Immunotoxicity for Environmental and
Public Health Research, *Int. J. Environ. Res. Public Health*, Vol.8, pp. 1388-1401, ISSN
1660-4601

Dusinska, M.; Collins, A.; Kazimírová, A.; Barancoková, M.; Harrington, V.; Volkovová, K,.;
Staruchová, M.; Horská, A.; Wsólová, L.; Kocan, A.; Petrík, J.; Machata, M.;
Ratcliffe, B. & Kyrtopoulos, S. (2004). Genotoxic effects of asbestos in humans.
Mutat Res. 2004 Sep 3;553(1-2):91-102, ISSN: 0027-5107

Dziedzic, D.; Wheeler, C.S. & Gross, K.B., (1993). Bronchoalveolar lavage: detecting markers
of lung injury, in: *Handbook of Hazardous Materials*. New York: Academic Press. pp.
99-111, ISBN: 012189410X 9780121894108

Elder, AC.; Gelein, R.; Azadniv, M.; Frampton, M.; Finkelstein, J. & Oberdorster G. (2004)
Systemic effects of inhaled ultrafine particles in two compromised, aged rat strains.
Inhal Toxicol. 16, 461-71, ISSN: 8750-7587

Food and Drug Administration, Washington, USA (2004).
http://www.fda.gov/cder/guidance/6636dft.htm

Froom, P.; Lahat, N.; Kristal-Boneh, E.; Cohen, C.; Lerman, Y. & Ribak, J. (2000). Circulating
natural killer cells in retired asbestos cement workers, *J. Occup. Environ. Med.*, Vol.2,
No.1, pp. 19-24, ISSN 1076-2752

Fujita, K.; Morimoto, Y.; Ogami, A.; Myojyo, T.; Tanaka, I.; Shimada, M.; Wang, WN.; Endoh, S.; Uchida, K.; Nakazato, T.; Yamamoto, K.; Fukui, H.; Horie, M.; Yoshida, Y.; Iwahashi, H. & Nakanishi, J. (2009). Gene expression profiles in rat lung after inhalation exposure to C60 fullerene particles. *Toxicology.* 2009 Apr 5;258(1):47-55. Epub 2009 Jan 9, ISSN: 0300-483X (Print), 1879-3185 (Electronic)

Gillissen, A.; Gessner, C.; Hammerschmidt, S.; Hoheisel, G & Wirtz, H. (2006). [Health significance of inhaled particles] *Dtsch Med Wochenschr.* 2006 Mar 24;131(12):639-44, ISSN: 0012-0472

Garcia-Garcia, E. (2005). Diversity in PhagocyticSignaling: A Story of Greed, Sharing and Exploitation, In book: *Molecular mechanisms of phagocytosis*, pp.1-154, Springer, ISBN: 1423724070 9781423724070

Garcia-Garcia, E. & Rosales, C. (2005). Adding Complexity to Phagocytic Signaling: Phagocytosis-Associated Cell Response and Phagocytic Efficiency, In book: *Molecular mechanisms of phagocytosis*, pp.1-154, Springer, ISBN:1423724070 9781423724070,

Gaumer, HR.; Doll, NJ.; Kaima, J.; Schuyler, M. & Salvaggio, JE. (1981). Diminished suppressor cell function in patients with asbestosis. *Clin. Exp. Immunol.,* Vol.44, No.1, pp. 108-116, ISSN 0009-9104

Gopinath, C. (1996). Pathology of toxic effects on the immune system. *Inflamm Res* 45(suppl 2): S74-S78, ISSN: 1023-3830

Governa, M.; Amati, M.; Valentino, M.; Visona, I.; Fubini, B ; Botta, GC. ; Volpe, AR. & Carmignani, M. (2000). *In vitro* cleavage by asbestos fibers of the fifth component of human complement through free-radical generation and kallikrein activation, *J. Toxicol. Environ. Health A.,* Vol.59, No.7, pp. 539-52, ISSN:1528-7394

Greim, H.; Borm, P.; Schins, R.; Donaldson, K.; Driscoll, K.; Hartwig, A.; Kuempel, E.; Oberdorster, G. & Speit, G. (2001). Toxicity of fibers and particles. Report of the workshop held in Munich, Germany, 26–27 October, 2000. *Inhal Toxicol* 2001;13:737–54, ISSN: 0895-8378 print

Haley, PJ.; Shopp, GM.; Benson, JM.; Cheng, YS.; Bice, DE.; Luster, MI.; Dunnick, JK. & Hobbs, CH. (1990). The immunotoxicity of three nickel compounds following 13-week inhalation exposure in the mouse. *Fundam Appl Toxicol.* 1990 Oct;15(3):476-87, ISSN: 0272-0590

Haley, P.; Perry, R.; Ennulat, D.; Frame, S.; Johnson, C.; Lapointe, J.M.; Nyska, A.; Snyder, P.W.; Walker, D. & Walter, G. (2005). *Toxicol. Pathol.,* Vol.33, pp. 404-407, ISSN: 0192-6233 print

Hazenbos, WLW. & Brown, EJ. (2006). Phagocytosis: receptors and biology, in book Phagocytosis of Bacteria and Bacterial Pathogenicity, *Ernst JD. & Stendahl O., (September 2006), Cambridge University Press, New York,* ISBN 9780511242977

He, X.; Young, SH.; Schwegler-Berry, D.; Chisholm, WP.; Fernback, JE. & Ma, Q. (2011). Multiwalled Carbon Nanotubes Induce a Fibrogenic Response by Stimulating Reactive Oxygen Species Production, Activating NF-κB Signaling, and Promoting Fibroblast-to-Myofibroblast Transformation. *Chem Res Toxicol.* 2011 Nov 22. Epub ahead of print, ISSN (printed): 0893-228X. ISSN (electronic): 1520-5010

Hess, E.V. (2002). Environmental chemicals and autoimmune disease: cause and effect, *Toxicology* Vol.181–182, pp. 65–70, ISSN: 0300-483X.

Hoet, P.H.M.; Lewis, C.P.L.; Demedts, M. & Nemery, B. (1994). Putrescine and paraquast uptake in human slices and isolated type II pneumocytes, *Biochem. Pharmacol.*, Vol.48, pp. 517-524, ISSN 0006-2952

Horie, M.; Nishio, K.; Fujita, K.; Kato, H.; Nakamura, A.; Kinugasa, S.; Endoh, S.; Miyauchi, A.; Yamamoto, K.; Murayama, H.; Niki, E.; Iwahashi, H.; Yoshida, Y. & Nakanishi, J. (2009). Ultrafine NiO particles induce cytotoxicity *in vitro* by cellular uptake and subsequent Ni(II) release. *Chem Res Toxicol.* 2009 Aug;22(8):1415-26, ISSN (printed): 0893-228X. ISSN (electronic): 1520-5010

Horie, M.; Fukui, H.; Nishio, K.; Endoh, S.; Kato, H.; Fujita, K.; Miyauchi, A.; Nakamura, A.; Shichiri, M.; Ishida, N.; Kinugasa, S.; Morimoto, Y.; Niki, E.; Yoshida, Y. & Iwahashi, H. (2011). Evaluation of acute oxidative stress induced by NiO nanoparticles *in vivo* and *in vitro*. *J Occup Health.* 2011;53(2):64-74. Epub 2011 Jan 11, ISSN: 1341-0725

Horská, A.; Kazimírová, A.; Barancoková, M.; Wsólová.; L, Tulinská, J. & Dusinská, M. (2006). Genetic predisposition and health effect of occupational exposure to asbestos. *Neuro Endocrinol Lett.* 2006 Dec;27 Suppl 2:100-3, ISSN: 1478-4491

Huaux, F. (2007). New developments in the understanding of immunology in silicosis. *Curr Opin Allergy Clin Immunol.* 2007 Apr;7(2):168-73, ISSN (printed): 1528-4050. ISSN (electronic): 1473-6322

Hurbánková, M. & Kaiglová, A. (1999). Compared effects of asbestos and wollastonite fibrous dusts on various biological parameters measured in bronchoalveolar lavage fluid, *J Trace Microprobe Techn.*, 17, pp. 233-43, ISSN: 0272-9172

Hurbánková, M.; Cerná, S.; Gergelová, P. & Wimmerová, S. (2005). Influence of refractory ceramic fibres - asbestos substitute - on the selected parameters of bronchoalveolar lavage 6 months after intratracheal instillation to W-rats, *Biomed Pap Med Fac, Univ Palacky Olomouc Czech Repub.*, Vol.149, No.2, pp. 367-71, ISSN: 2005-6745

Hurbánková, M.; Cerna, S.; Beno, M.; Tatrai, E.; Wimmerova, S. & Kovacikova, Z. (2010). The combined effect of refractory ceramic fibers and smoking in terms of selected inflammatory and cytotoxic parameters of bronchoalveolar lavage and histological findings in the experiment [Kombinovaný účinok keramických vlákien a fajčenia z hľadiska vybraných zápalových a cytotoxických parametrov bronchoalveolárnej laváže a histologických nálezov v experimente]. *Pracovní Lékařství.*, Vol. 62, 2010, No. 3, p. 102–108. ISSN: 0032-6291

IARC. (2002). Man-made Vitreous Fibres, Summary of Data Reported and Evaluation; *IARC Monographs on the Evaluation of Carcinogenic Risks to Humans*, WHO, Lyon, France, Vol.81: pp. 403, ISBN 92-832-1281-9,
http://monographs.iarc.fr/ENG/Monographs/vol81/volume81.pdf

IARC. (2004). Tobacco Smoke and Involuntary Smoking. *IARC Monographs on the Evaluation of Carcinogenic Risks to Humans*, WHO, Lyon, France, Vol.83: pp. 1452, ISBN 92-832-1283-5, http://monographs.iarc.fr/ENG/Monographs/vol83/mono83.pdf

ICICIS (1998). *Toxicology*, Vol.125, pp. 183–201. ISSN: 0300-483X.

Ilavska, S.; Jahnova, E.; Tulinska, J.; Horvathova, M.; Dusinska, M.; Wsolova, L.; Kyrtopoulos, S.A. & Fuortes, L. (2005). Immunological monitoring in workers occupationally exposed to asbestos, *Toxicol.*, Vol.206, pp. 299-308, ISSN: 0300-483X

Inoue, KI. & Takano, H. (2011). Aggravating Impact of Nanoparticles on Immune-Mediated Pulmonary Inflammation, *TheScientificWorldJOURNAL* (2011) 11, 382–390 Special Issue: Nanoparticles and Inflammation, ISSN: 1537-744X

IPCS/WHO, 1999 IPCS/WHO, Environmental health criteria, No. 210. Principles for the Assessment of Risks to Human Health from Exposure to Chemicals, (1999), pp. 7–10, ISSN 0250-863X

Ishihara, Y.; Nagai, A. & Kagawa, J. (1997). Comparison of the effect of exposure to filter cigarette and nonfilter cigarette smoke in rat bronchoalveolar lavage fluid and blood: the antioxidant balance and protease-antiprotease balance *in vivo*, *Inhal Toxicol*. Vol.9, pp. 273-86, ISSN (printed): 0895-8378.

Jacobsen, NR.; Møller, P.; Jensen, KA.; Vogel, U.; Ladefoged, O.; Loft, S. & Wallin, H. (2009). Lung inflammation and genotoxicity following pulmonary exposure to nanoparticles in ApoE-/- mice. *Part Fibre Toxicol*. 2009 Jan 12;6:2, 1-17, ISSN: 1743-8977

Jaurand, M.C. (1997). Mechanisms of fiber-induced genotoxicity, *Environmental Health Perspectives*, Vol.105, suppl. 5, pp. 1073–1084, ISSN: 1082-6076

Johansson, A.; Lundborg, M.; Sköld, C.M.; Lundahl, J.; Tornling, G.; Eklund, A. & Camner, P. (1997). Functional, morphological, and phenotypical differences between rat alveolar and interstitial macrophages, *Am. J. Respir. Cell Mol. Biol.*, Vol.16, pp. 582-588, Print ISSN: 0741-5400; Online ISSN: 1938-3673.

Kagan, E.; Solomon, A.; Cochrane, JC.; Kuba, P.; Rocks, PH. & Webster, I. (1977). Immunological studies of patients with asbestosis. II. Studies of circulating lymphoid cell numbers and humoral immunity. Clin. Exp. Immunol., Vol.28, No.2, pp. 268-275 ISSN 0271-9142

Kaminski, NE.; Kaplan, BLFK. & Holsapple, MP. (2008). Toxic response of the immune system, pp.485-555, In: Klaassen, CD. *Casarett and Doull's Toxicology - The Basic Science of Poisons* (7th Edition). 2008 McGraw-Hill, USA, ISBN-13: 978-0-07-147051-3, ISBN-10: 0-07-147051-4

Kohyama, N.; Tanaka, I.; Tomita, M.; Kudo, M. & Shinohara, Y. (1997). Preparation and characteristics of standard reference samples of fibrous minerals for biological experiments. *Ind Health* 35, 415–32, ISSN: 0895-8378 print 11091-7691

Kristovich, R.; Knight, DA.; Long, JF.; Williams, MV.; Dutta, PK. & Waldman WJ. (2004). Macrophage-Mediated Endothelial Inflammatory Responses to Airborne Particulates: Impact of Particulate Physicochemical Properties, *Chem. Res. Toxicol.*, Vol.17, No.10, pp. 1303-1312, ISSN: 0893-228X (Print) 1520-5010 (Electronic) 0893-228X (Linking)

Kumagai-Takei, N.; Maeda, M.; Chen, Y.; Matsuzaki, H.; Lee, S.; Nishimura, Y.; Hiratsuka, J. & Otsuki, T. (2011). Asbestos Induces Reduction of Tumor Immunity, *Clinical and Developmental Immunology*, Volume 2011, Article ID 481439, 9 pages, doi:10.1155/2011/481439, ISSN: 17402522

Kuper, C.F.; De Heer, E.; Van Loveren, H.; Vos, J.G.; Haschek, W.; Rousseaux, C.G. & Wallig, M.A. (2002). Editors Handbook of Toxicologic Pathology, vol. 2 (2nd ed.), *Academic Press*, San Diego pp. 585–646. ISSN: 0192-6233

Lankveld, DP.; Van Loveren, H.; Baken, KA. & Vandebriel, RJ. (2010). *In vitro* testing for direct immunotoxicity: state of the art. *Methods Mol Biol.* 2010;598:401-23, ISSN: 0022-3042

Lightfoot, NE.; Pacey, MA. & Darling, S. (2010). Gold, nickel and copper mining and processing. *Chronic Dis Can.* 2010;29(Suppl 2):101-24, ISSN: 0228-8699 (Print), 1481-8523 (Electronic)

Liu, F.; Liu, L.; Weng, D.; Chen, Y.; Song, L.; He, Q. & Chen, J. (2010). CD4+CD25+Foxp3+ Regulatory T Cells Depletion May Attenuate the Development of Silica-Induced Lung Fibrosis in Mice, *PLoS One.* 2010; 5(11): e15404, Published online 2010 November 3, ISSN: 1932-6203

Lovik, M.; Hogseth, AK.; Gaarder, PI.; Hagemann, R. & Eide, I. (2003). Diesel exhaust particles and carbon black have adjuvant activity on the local lymph node response and systemic IgE production to ovalbumin. *Eur Respir J* Suppl. 46, 5s-13s, ISSN 1529-7322

Lucarelli, M.; Gatti, A.M.; Savarino, G.; Quattroni, P.; Martinelli, L.; Monari, E. & Boraschi, D. (2004). Innate defence functions of macrophages can be biased by nano-sized ceramic and metallic particles. *Eur Cytokine Netw.,* Vol.15, No. 4,pp. 339-46, ISBN 10 : 2-89631-027-4, ISSN : 0820-8395

Luster,M.; Ackermann, M.F.; Germolec, D.R. & Rosenthal G.J. (1989). Perturbations of the Immune System by Xenobiotics, Environmental Health Perspectives, Vol.81, pp. 157-162, ISSN: 0091-6765.

Manning, CB.; Vallyathan, V. & Mossman, BT. (2002). Diseases caused by asbestos: mechanisms of injury and disease development. *Int. Immunopharmacol*, Vol.2, No.2-3, 191-200, ISSN: 1567-5769.

Marsh, GM.; Buchanich, JM. & Youk, AO. (2001). Historical cohort study of US man-made vitreous fiber production workers: VI. Respiratory system cancer standardized mortality ratios adjusted for the confounding effect of cigarette smoking. *J Occup Environ Med.* 2001 Sep;43(9):803-8, ISSN: 1076-2752

Martin, AK.; Mack, DG.; Falta, MT.; Mroz, MM.; Newman, LS.; Maier, LA. & Fontenot, AP. (2011). Beryllium-specific CD4+ T cells in blood as a biomarker of disease progression. *J Allergy Clin Immunol.* 2011 Nov;128(5):1100-6.e1-5. Epub 2011 Sep 23, ISSN (printed): 0091-6749. ISSN (electronic): 1097-6825

Mascagni, P.; Corsini, E;. Pettazzoni, M.; Baj, A.; Feltrin, G.; Ferraioli, E. & Toffoletto, F. (2003). [Determination of interleukin-8 in induced sputum of workers exposed to low concentrations of asbestos]. *G Ital Med Lav Ergon.* 2003 Jul-Sep;25 Suppl(3):137, ISSN 0022-3166

Matthews, JB.; Green, TR.; Stone, MH.; Wroblewski, BM.; Fisher, J. & Inghani E. (2000). Comparison of the response of primary human peripheral blood mononuclear phagocytes from different donors to challenge with model polyethylene particles of known size and dose. *Biomaterials,* Vol.21, pp. 2033-44, ISSN: 0142-9612.

Mikulski, MA.; Leonard, SA.; Sanderson, WT.; Hartley, PG.; Sprince, NL. & Fuortes, LJ. (2011). Risk of beryllium sensitization in a low-exposed former nuclear weapons cohort from the Cold War era. *Am J Ind Med.* 2011 Mar;54(3):194-204. Epub 2010 Oct 28, ISSN (printed): 0271-3586. ISSN (electronic): 1097-0274

Mitschik, S.; Schierl, R.; Nowak, D. & Jörres, RA. (2008).Effects of particulate matter on cytokine production *in vitro*: a comparative analysis of published studies. Inhal. Toxicol., Vol.20, No.4, pp. 399- 414, ISSN (printed): 0895-8378

Montero, MA.; de Gracia, J. & Morell, F. (2010). Hard Metal Interstitial Lung Disease, *Arch Bronconeumol*. 2010;46(9):489-491, ISSN: 0300-2896 (Print), 1579-2129 (Electronic)

Morimoto, Y. & Tanaka, I. (2001). *In vivo* studies of man-made mineral fibers -fibrosis-related factors, *Ind Health.*, Vol.39, pp. 106-13, ISSN (printed): 0019-8366.

Morimoto, Y.; Ogami, A.; Todoroki, M.; Yamamoto, M.; Murakami, M.; Hirohashi, M.; Oyabu, T.; Myojo, T.; Nishi, K.; Kadoya, C, Yamasaki, S, Nagatomo, H, Fujita, K, Endoh, S, Uchida, K, Yamamoto, K, Kobayashi, N, Nakanishi, J. & Tanaka, I. (2010). Expression of inflammation-related cytokines following intratracheal instillation of nickel oxide nanoparticles. *Nanotoxicology*. 2010 Jun;4(2):161-76, ISSN (printed): 1743-5390. ISSN (electronic): 1743-5404

Morimoto, Y.; Oyabu, T.; Ogami, A.; Myojo, T.; Kuroda, E.; Hirohashi, M.; Shimada, M.; Lenggoro, W.; Okuyama, K. & Tanaka, I. (2011). Investigation of gene expression of MMP-2 and TIMP-2 mRNA in rat lung in inhaled nickel oxide and titanium dioxide nanoparticles. *Ind Health*. 2011;49(3):344-52, Epub 2011 Mar 1, ISSN (printed): 0019-8366. ISSN (electronic): 1880-8026

Mossman, BT.; Kamp, DW. & Weitzman, SA. (1996). Mechanisms of carcinogenesis and clinical features of asbestos-associated cancers, *Cancer Investigation*, Vol.14, No.5, pp. 466–480, ISSN (printed): 0735-7907.

Mossman, BT. & Churg, A. (1998). Mechanisms in the pathogenesis of asbetosis and silicosis. *Am. J. Respir. Crit. Care Med.*, Vol.157, pp. 1666–1680, ISSN (printed): 1073-449X

Mossman, BT.; Lippmann, M.; Hesterberg, TW.; Kelsey, KT.; Barchowsky, A. & Bonner, JC. (2011). Pulmonary endpoints (lung carcinomas and asbestosis) following inhalation exposure to asbestos. *J Toxicol Environ Health B Crit Rev* 14:76–121, ISSN (printed): 1093-7404. ISSN (electronic): 1521-6950

Moulin, JJ.; Mur, JM.; Wild, P.; Perreaux, JP. & Pham, QT. (1986) Oral cavity and laryngeal cancers among man-made mineral fiber production workers. *Scand. J. Work Environ. Health*, 12, 27–31, ISSN: 0355-3140

National Research Council. (1992) Subcommittee on Immunotoxicology, Committee on Biologic Markers, Board on Environmental Studies and Toxicology, National Research Council, Biologic Markers in Immunotoxicology, NATIONAL ACADEMY PRESS, Washington, D.C., 1992, ISBN-13: 978-0-309-04389-2

National Toxicology Program. (2009). Final report on carcinogens background document for glass wool fibers. *Rep Carcinog Backgr Doc*. 2009 Sep;(9-5980):i-280, ISSN: 2151-7746 (Print); 2151-3805 (Electronic); 2151-3805 (Linking)

Nelson, HH. & Kelsey, KT. (2002). The molecular epidemiology of asbestos and tobacco in lung cancer, *Oncogene*, Vol.21, 48, pp. 7284-7288, ISSN: 0950-9232.

Nishi, K.; Morimoto, Y.; Ogami, A.; Murakami, M.; Myojo, T.; Oyabu, T.; Kadoya, C.; Yamamoto, M.; Todoroki, M.; Hirohashi, M.; Yamasaki, S.; Fujita, K.; Endo, S.; Uchida, K.; Yamamoto, K.; Nakanishi, J. & Tanaka, I. (2009). Expression of cytokine-induced neutrophil chemoattractant in rat lungs by intratracheal instillation of nickel oxide nanoparticles. *Inhal Toxicol*. 2009 Oct;21(12):1030-9, ISSN (printed): 0895-8378, ISSN (electronic): 1091-7691

Nkamgueu, EM.; Adnet, JJ.; Bernard, J.; Zierold, K.; Kilian, L.; Jallot, E.; Benhayoune, H.;
    Bonhomme, P. (2000). *In vitro* effects of zirconia and alumina particles on human
    blood monocyte-derived macrophages: X-ray microanalysis and flow cytometric
    studies. *J Biomed Mater Res*. 2000 Dec 15;52(4):587-94, ISSN (printed): 0021-9304.
Nymark, P.; Wikman, H.; Hienonen-Kempas, T. & Anttila, S. (2008). Molecular and genetic
    changes in asbestos-related lung cancer, *Cancer Letters*, Vol. 265, No. 1, pp. 1–15,
    ISSN: 0304-3835.
Oberdorster, G. (1994). Macrophage-associated responses to chrysotile, *Ann Occup Hyg*.,
    Vol.38, No.4, pp. 601-15, 421-2, ISSN (printed): 0003-4878.
Ogami, A.; Morimoto, Y.; Myojo, T.; Oyabu, T.; Murakami, M.; Todoroki, M.; Nishi, K.;
    Kadoya, C.; Yamamoto, M. & Tanaka I. (2009). Pathological features of different
    sizes of nickel oxide following intratracheal instillation in rats. *Inhal Toxicol*. 2009
    Aug;21(10):812-8, ISSN (printed): 0895-8378.
Oostingh, GJ.; Casals, E.; Italiani, P.; Colognato, R.; Stritzinger, R.; Ponti, J.; Pfaller, T.; Kohl,
    Y.; Ooms, D.; Favilli, F.; Leppens, H.; Lucchesi, D.; Rossi, F.; Nelissen, I.; Thielecke,
    H.; Puntes, VF.; Dusch A. & Boraschi, D. (2011). Problems and challenges in the
    development and validation of human cell-based assays to determine nanoparticle-
    induced immunomodulatory effects. *Particle and Fibre Toxicology* (9 February 2011),
    8:8, pp. 1-21, ISSN:1743-8977
Osinubi, OYO.; Gochfeld, M. & Kipen, HM., (2000). Health effects of asbestos and
    nonasbestos fibers. *Environ Health Perspect*, Vol.108, (Supp.4), pp. 665-674, ISSN:
    1078-0475.
Otsuki, T.; Maeda, M.; Murakami, S.; Hayashi, H.; Miura, Y.; Kusaka, M.; Nakano,T.;
    Fukuoka,K ; Kishimoto, T.; Hyodoh, F.; Ueki, A. & Nishimura, Y. (2007).
    Immunological effects of silica and asbestos. *Cell. Mol. Immunology*, Vol.4, No.4, pp.
    261-268, ISSN: 1672-7681.
Oudijk, EJ.; Lammers, JW. & Koenderman, L. (2003). Systemic inflammation in chronic
    obstructive pulmonary disease. *Eur Respir J Suppl*. 46, 5s-13s, ISSN: 0904-1850.
Ozesmi, M.; Hillerdal, G.; Karlsson-parra, A. & Forsum, U. (1988). Phenotypes of peripheral
    blood lymphoid cells in patients with asbestos-related pleural lesions. *Eur. Respir J*.,
    Vol.1, No.10, pp. 938-942, ISSN (printed): 0903-1936.
Panizza, C.; Bai, E.; Oddone, E.; Scaburri, A.; Massari, S.; Modonesi, C.; Contiero, P.;
    Marinaccio, A. & Crosignani, P. (2011). Lung cancer risk in the electroplating
    industry in Lombardy, Italy, using the Italian occupational cancer monitoring
    (OCCAM) information system. *Am J Ind Med*. 2011 Sep 14. doi: 10.1002/ajim.21004.
    [Epub ahead of print], ISSN (printed): 0271-3586. ISSN (electronic): 1097-0274
Pietruska, JR.; Liu, X.; Smith, A.; McNeil, K.; Weston, P.; Zhitkovich, A.; Hurt, R. & Kane,
    AB. (2011). Bioavailability, intracellular mobilization of nickel, and HIF-1α
    activation in human lung epithelial cells exposed to metallic nickel and nickel oxide
    nanoparticles. *Toxicol Sci*. 2011 Nov;124(1):138-48. Epub 2011 Aug 9, ISSN:1096-6080
    (Print)1096-0929 (Electronic)
Rabinovitch, M. (1995). Professional and non-professional phagocytes: an introduction,
    Trends in Cell Biology, 5, 85-87, ISSN: 0962-8924

Richards, RJ.; Davies, N.; Atkins, J. & Oreffo, VIC. (1987). Isolation, biochemical characterization and culture of lung epithelial cell of the rat. *Lung,* Vol.165, pp. 143-158, ISSN (printed): 0341-2040.

Rom, WN.; Weiden, M.; Garcia, R.; Yie, TA.; Vathesatogkit, P.; Tse, DB.; McGuinness, G.; Roggli, V. & Prezant, D. (2002). Acute eosinophilic pneumonia in a New York City firefighter exposed to World Trade Center dust. *Am. J. Respir. Crit. Care Med.,* Vol.166, No.6, pp. 797-800, ISSN (printed): 1073-449X.

Rosenthal, GJ.; Corsini, E. & Simeonova, E. (1998). Selected New Developments in Asbestos Immunotoxicity, *Environ Health Perspect,* Vol.106 (Suppl 1), pp. 159-169, Available from
http://ehpnetl.niehs.nih.gov/docs/1998/Suppl-1/159-169rosenthal/abstract.html
ISSN: 1078-0475.

Rosenthal, G.J.; Simeonova, P. & Corsini, E. (1999) Asbestos toxicity: An immunologic perspective, *Rev. Environ. Health,* Vol.14, No.1, pp. 11-20, ISSN (printed): 0048-7554.

Ruehl-Fehlert, C.; Bradley, A.; George, C.; Germann, P.G.; Bolliger, A.P. & Schulte, A. (2005). Harmonization of immunotoxicity guidelines in the ICH process--pathology considerations from the guideline Committee of the European Society of Toxicological Pathology (ESTP) . *Exp. Toxicol. Pathol.,* Vol.57, pp. 1-5, ISSN: 0940-2993.

Sabo-Attwood, T.; Ramos-Nino, M.; Bond, J.; Butnor, KJ.; Heintz, N.; Gruber, AD.; Steele, C.; Taatjes, DJ.; Vacek, P. & Mossman, BT. (2005). Gene expression profiles reveal increased mClca3 (Gob5) expression and mucin production in a murine model of asbestos-induced fibrogenesis. *Am. J. Pathol.,* Vol.167, No.5, pp. 1243-56, ISSN (printed): 0002-9440.

Schenker, MB; Pinkerton, KE.; Mitchell, D.; Vallyathan, V.; Elvine-Kreis, B. & Green, FHY. (2009). Pneumoconiosis from Agricultural Dust Exposure among Young California Farmworkers. *Environmental Health Perspectives* 117, 6, June 2009, ISSN: 0091-6765

Shannon, H.; Muir, A.; Haines, T. & Verma, D. (2005). Mortality and cancer incidence in Ontario glass fiber workers. *Occup Med (Lond).* 2005 Oct;55(7):528-34, ISSN (printed): 0962-7480. ISSN (electronic): 1471-8405

Shukla, A.; Lounsbury, KM.; Barrett, TF.; Gell, J.; Rincon, M.; Butnor, KJ.; Taatjes, DJ.; Davis, GS.; Vacek, P.; Nakayama, KI.; Nakayama, K.; Steele, C. & Mossman, BT. (2007). Asbestos-induced peribronchiolar cell proliferation and cytokine production are attenuated -oslabene-in lungs of protein kinase C-delta knockout mice. *Am. J. Pathol.,* Vol.170, No.1, pp. 140-51, ISSN (printed): 0002-9440.

Schuurman, HJ; Kuper CF. & Vos JG. (1994). Histopathology of the immune system as a tool to assess immunotoxicity. *Toxicology* 86:187-212, ISSN: 0300-483X.

Simeonova, PP. & Luster, MI. (1996). Asbestos induction of nuclear transcription factors and interleukin 8 gene regulation. *Am. J. Respir. Cell. Mol. Biol.* Vol.15, No.6, pp. 787-795, ISSN: 1044-1549.

Sjörstrand, M.; Rylander, R. & Bergström, R. (1989). Lung cell reactions in guinea pigs after inhalation of asbestos (amosite), *Toxicology,* Vol.57. pp. 1-14, ISSN: 0300-483X.

Song, Y. & Tang, S. (2011). Nanoexposure, Unusual Diseases, and New Health and Safety Concerns, *TheScientificWorldJOURNAL* (2011) 11, 1821-1828, ISSN: 1537-744X

Immune System and Environmental Xenobiotics - The Effect of Selected Mineral Fibers and
Particles on the Immune Response

93

Sood, A. (2009). Current Treatment of Chronic Beryllium Disease, *J Occup Environ Hyg.* 2009 December ; 6(12): 762–765, ISSN (printed): 1545-9624. ISSN (electronic): 1545-9632

Spiegelberg, T.; Kördel, W. & Hochrainer, D. (1984). Effects of NiO inhalation on alveolar macrophages and the humoral immune systems of rats. *Ecotoxicol Environ Saf.* 1984 Dec;8(6):516-25, ISSN: 0147-6513

Staruchova, M.; Collins, AR.; Volkovova, K.; Mislanová, C.; Kovacikova, Z.; Tulinska, J.; Kocan.; A, Staruch, L.; Wsolova, L. & Dusinska, M. (2008). Occupational exposure to mineral fibres. Biomarkers of oxidative damage and antioxidant defence and associations with DNA damage and repair. *Mutagenesis.* 2008 Jul;23(4):249-60, Epub 2008 Feb 14, ISSN (printed): 0267-8357

Tátrai, E.; Ungváry, G. & Adamis, Z. (1994). On the structural differences in the membranes between ciliated bronchial and non-ciliated lymphoepithelium in rats. *Eur. J. Histochem.* Vol.38, pp. 59-64, ISSN (printed): 1121-760X.

Tátrai, E.; Kováčiková, Z.; Brózik, M. & Six, E. (2004). Pulomary toxicity of wollastonite *in vivo* and *in vitro*. *J. Appl. Toxicol.*, Vol.24, pp. 147-154, ISSN: 1099-1263

Tátrai, E.; Brózik, M.; Drahos, A.; Kováčiková, Z.; Six, E.; Csík, M. & Dam, A. (2006a). The effect of stone-wool on rat lungs and on the primary culture of rat alveolar macrophages and type II pneumocytes. *J. Appl. Toxicol.* Vol.26, pp. 16-24, ISSN: 1099-1263

Tátrai, E.; Kováčiková, Z.; Brózik, M.; Six, E.; Csík, M.; Drahos, A. & Dam, A. (2006b). The influence of refractory ceramic fibres on pulmonary morphology, redox and immune system in rats, *J. Appl. Toxicol,* Vol.26, pp. 500-508, ISSN: 1099-1263

Topinka, J.; Loli, P.; Georgiadis, P.; Dusinská, M.; Hurbánková, M.; Kováciková, Z.; Volkovová, K.; Kazimírová, A.; Barancoková, M.; Tatrai, E.; Oesterle, D.; Wolff, T. & Kyrtopoulos, SA. (2004). Mutagenesis by asbestos in the lung of lambda-lacI transgenic rats. *Mutat Res.* 2004 Sep 3;553(1-2):67-78, ISSN: 1383-5718

Topinka, J.; Loli, P.; Dusinská, M.; Hurbánková, M.; Kováciková, Z.; Volkovová, K.; Kazimírová, A.; Barancoková, M.; Tatrai, E.; Wolff, T.; Oesterle, D.; Kyrtopoulos, SA. & Georgiadis, P. (2006). Mutagenesis by man-made mineral fibres in the lung of rats. *Mutat Res.* 2006 Mar 20;595(1-2):174-83, ISSN: 1383-5718

Toyokuni, S. (2009a). Mechanisms of asbestos-induced carcinogenesis, *Nagoya Journal of Medical Science,* Vol.71, No.1-2, pp. 1– 10. ISSN: 0027-7622.

Toyokuni, S. (2009b). Role of iron in carcinogenesis: cancer as a ferrotoxic disease, *Cancer Science,* Vol.100, No.1, pp. 9–16, ISSN (printed): 1347-9032.

Tsuda, T.; Morimoto, Y.; Yamato, H.; Nakamura, H.; Hori, H.; Nagata, N.; Kido, M.; Higashi, T. & Tanaka, I. (1997). Effects of Mineral Fibers on the Expression of Genes Whose Product May Play a Role in Fiber Pathogenesis, *Environ Health Perspect,* Vol.105(Suppl 5), pp.1173-1178, ISSN: 1078-0475.

Tsang, PH.; Chu, FN.; Fischbein, A. & Bekesi, JG. (1988). Impairments in functional subsets of T-suppressor (CD8) lymphocytes, monocytes, and natural killer cells among asbestos-exposed workers. *Clin. Immunol. Immunopathol.,* Vol.47. No.3, pp. 323-32, ISSN: 0090-1229.

Tulinska, J.; Jahnova, E.; Dusinska, M.; Kuricova, M.; Liskova, A.; Ilavska, S.; Horvathova, M.; Wsolova, L.; Kyrtopoulos, S.A.; Collins, A.; Harrington, V. & Fuortes, L. (2004).

Immunomodulatory effects of mineral fibres in occupationally exposed workers. *Mutat. Res.*, Vol.553, No.1-2, pp. 111-24, ISSN: 1383-5718

Tulinska, J.; Kuricova, M.; Liskova, A.; Kovacikova, Z. Tatrai E, (2005). The effect of ceramic fibres on the immune system, *Biomed Pap Med Fac Univ Palacky Olomouc Czech Repub.* 2005, 149(2):397-9, ISSN:1213-8118

Urso, C. & Caimi, G. (2011). Oxidative stress and endothelial dysfunction, *Minerva Med.*, Vol.102, No.1, pp. 59-77, ISSN: 0026-4806

van Eeden, SF. & Hogg, JC. (2002). Systemic inflammatory response induced by particulate matter air pollution: the importance of bone-marrow stimulation. *J Toxicol Environ Health* A. 65, 1597-613, ISSN (printed): 1528-7394.

van Helden, YG.; Keijer, J.; Knaapen, AM.; Heil, SG.; Briede, JJ.; van Schooten, FJ. & Godschalk, RW. (2009). Bete-carotene metabolites enhance inflammation-induced oxidative DNA damage in lung epithelial cells. *Free Radic. Biol. Med.*, Vol.46, No.2, pp. 299-304, ISSN: 0891-5849.

Van Loveren, H.; Vos, J.G.; Germolec, D.; Simeonova, P.P.; Eijkemanns, G. & McMichael, A.J. (2001). Meeting report. Epidemiologic associations between occupational and environmental exposures and autoimmune disease: Report of a meeting to explore current evidence and identify research needs, *Int. J. Hyg. Environ. Health*, Vol.203, pp. 483-495, ISSN: 1438-4639.

Venarske, D. & deShazo, RD. (2003). Molecular mechanisms of allergic disease, *South Med. J.*, Vol.96, No.11, pp. 1049–1054, ISSN: 0038-4348.

Vial, T. & Descotes, J. (1996). Drugs affecting the immune system. In: *Meyler's Side-Effects of Drugs*, 13th ed, Dukes MNG (ed). Elsevier, Amsterdam, pp 1090-1165, ISBN: 0 85369 460 5.

Wu, J.; Liu, W.; Koenig, K.; Idell, S. & Broaddus, VC. (2000). Vitronectin adsorption to chrysotile asbestos increases fiber phagocytosis and toxicity for mesothelial cells. *Am. J. Physiol. Lung Cell. Mol. Physiol.*, Vol.279. No. 5, pp. 916-23, ISSN:1040-0605.

Yamato, H.; Morimoto, Y.; Tsuda, T.; Ohgami, A.; Kohyama, S. & Tanaka, I (1998) Fiber numbers per unit weight of JFM standard reference samples determined with scanning electron microscope. *Ind Health* 36, 384–7, ISSN: 1549-3199.

Yagil-Kelmer, E.; Kazmier, P.; Rahaman, MN.; Bal, BS.; Tessman, RK.; Estes, DM. (2004). Comparison of the response of primary human blood monocytes and the U937 human monocytic cell line to two different sizes of alumina ceramic particles, *Journal of Orthopaedic Research* 22 (2004) pp.832-838, ISSN: 1554-527X

Zhao, J.; Shi, X.; Castranova, V. & Ding M. (2009). Occupational toxicology of nickel and nickel compounds, *J Environ Pathol Toxicol Oncol.* 2009;28(3):177-208, ISSN: 0731-8898

3

Development of the Immune System - Early Nutrition and Consequences for Later Life

JoAnn Kerperien[1], Bastiaan Schouten[2], Günther Boehm[2,3],
Linette E.M. Willemsen[1], Johan Garssen[1,2],
Léon M.J. Knippels[1,2] and Belinda van't Land[2,4]
[1]*Pharmacology, Utrecht Institute for Pharmaceutical Sciences (UIPS),
University of Utrecht,*
[2]*Danone Research – Centre for Specialised Nutrition, Wageningen,
The Netherlands and Friedrichsdorf,*
[3]*Sophia Children's Hospital, Erasmus University Rotterdam,*
[4]*Wilhelmina Children's Hospital, University Medical Center, Utrecht,
The Netherlands*

1. Introduction

The immunological interaction between mother and fetus during pregnancy causes the fetal immune system to avoid excessive and destructive immunological reactions. This particular physiologic situation coexists with an immature immune system, which makes the infant very vulnerable for infections and susceptible to the development of immune system related disorders. At birth, the immune system of the infant is particularly characterized by a not fully developed non-specific immune system. In addition, a suppressed capacity of antigen-specific T cells, a deletion of activated T cells, and the presence of high amounts of regulatory T cells (Treg) hamper proper immune responsiveness. During the first months of life the antigen-specific immune response has to be developed in parallel to the maintenance of immune tolerance against compounds commonly found in the environment of mother and infant. There is evidence that disturbances of these complex developmental processes will have impact on the function of the immune system during lifetime causing immunological disorders such as allergy and autoimmunity.

Human milk contains several immunological active compounds which protect the infant from infection. Many of them such as antibodies are individually adapted to the maternal environment which is similar to the environment of the infant thus providing individual protection to the infant. Apart from this protection activated immediately after birth, human milk modulates also the described developmental processes. Although the mechanisms of this modulation are not fully understood there is evidence that human milk can transfer "immunological memory of the mother" to the infant. This concept of the role of human milk underlines the importance of quality of nutrition during first months of life for total development of the immune system. Individual human milk analyses will provide insight in components that are important modulators. Immunologic active peptides, long chain polyunsaturated fatty acids, several glycolipids and non-digestible oligosaccharides have already been identified as such modulators. The interaction of these active components with different parts of the immune system is very complex allowing a graduate and balanced development of the immune system.

One problem of studies in animals and humans is the fact that no single biomarker exists which describes completely the developmental status of the immune system. Although the question which biomarkers are of relevance is still a matter of intensive research there is evidence that many "classical" biomarkers are not useful. Many of these "classical" biomarkers are only sensitive in case the immune system is out of balance but not during a normal development. Consequently, research to identify relevant biomarkers characterizing healthy development is strongly required. There are many questions still open. However, first results are promising indicating that the quality of nutrition early in life might support development of the immune system for lifetime. Acceptance of such a concept might provide opportunities for new ways of primary prevention of immune related diseases later in life.

This chapter will summarise the newest and some specific insights of the mechanisms and impact of nutrition on the development of the immune system early in life.

2. Influences prior life

The nutritional status in early life has an important influence on human immune development, for example, a positive association is clearly observed between birth weight and antibody response to certain vaccines later in life (McDade, Beck et al. 2001). The precise relationship however between nutritional exposures during critical periods of development and later immune function warrants further investigation. The early postnatal environment is a vital determinant of adult health. An environmental exposure, like nutritional modulation of the evolving intestine during early infancy makes an impact on the development and function. A concept like this (as illustrated in *Figure 1*) will provide opportunities for primary prevention from immune related diseases later in life.

In order to understand the impact of nutrition on immune development early in life it is of key importance to know which steps in immune development are subjective to change and depend on specific nutrition. During embryogenesis, stem cells start to differentiate into specific progenitor stem cells, creating a pool of more specific and less totipotent stem cells. Hematopoietic stem cells (HSC) are the progenitor cells for our whole immune system (*Figure 2*). Identification of the first HSC is still difficult, because these regions don't contain many HSC and unique markers are lacking (Medvinsky, Rybtsov et al. 2011). After these few first HSC have colonized the human fetal liver, these cells expand and will relocate under influence of adhesion molecules and chemo-attractants to thymus, spleen and bone marrow (Mazo, Massberg et al. 2011). The bone marrow will start to produce immune cells from the hematopoietic lineage at four to five months of gestation in human pregnancy. Upon stimulation with 'early acting cytokines' a HSC will proliferate and differentiate into a myeloid or a lymphoid precursor cell depending on their surroundings (Grassinger, Haylock et al. 2010).

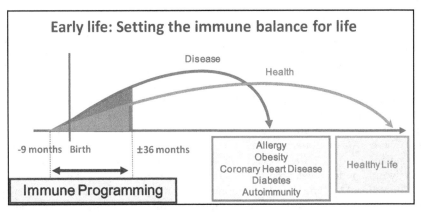

Fig. 1. Disturbances of immune developmental processes will have impact on the function of the immune system during life causing immunological disorders such as allergic disorders and autoimmunity. Although there are many questions still open first results are promising indicating that feeding early in life might support the development of the immune system for lifetime.

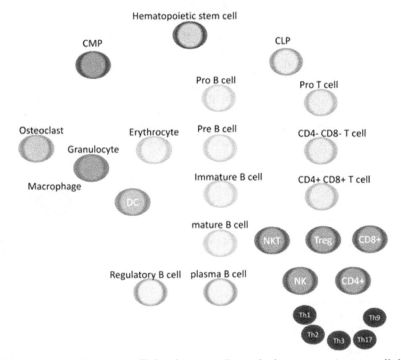

Fig. 2. Hematopoiesis/ immune cell development; From the hematopoetic stem cell the different immune cells develop, including; CMP, common myeloid precursor; CLP, common lymphoid precursor; DC, dendritic cell; NKT, natural killer T cell; NK, natural killer cell; Treg, regulatory T cell; CD8+, cytotoxic T cell; CD4+ Th, T helper cell.

2.1 Lymph node formation

Recent investigation showed that during lymph node development retinyl hydrogenase (RALDH) 2 is one of the enzymes essential in initial cross talk between different cell types (van de Pavert and Mebius 2010). RALDH-2 converts retinaldehyde to retinoic acid (RA). In absence of this enzyme proper lymphoid follicles are not developed. Retinoic acid is the active form of vitamin A and is important during embryogenesis, when axial patterning and organ formation take place (Campo-Paysaa, Marletaz et al. 2008). RA is involved in nerve development and expression of RALDH is found in nerve fibers near the lymph node anlagen, where RA can influence stromal cells to produce specific chemokines. Because RA is produced and used for different developmental processes, other factors should be present to direct lymph node development. One of these factors is CXC chemokine ligand 13 (CXCL13) produced by lymph node surrounding stromal cells. After a small cluster of pre-T- and -B cells is formed, more cells are attracted to this specific site for example via CC chemokine receptor (CCR) 7 and CC chemokine ligand (CCL) 19 and CCL21. When there are enough cells in the cluster, differentiation into lymph nodes occurs. Lymph nodes in the intestine are essential for priming of the whole immune system; therefore detailed development of the intestinal tract and intestinal immune tissues are described in *Box 1*. Peyers patches (PP) are the local small intestinal lymph nodes and mesenteric lymph nodes (MLN) are the collecting lymph nodes for small and large intestine. In essence these lymph structures develop very similar but there are some differences. For the development of PP the CD11c+ cells are required. In addition there are differences in essential transcription factors which are necessary to develop lymph nodes or PP, like interleukin (IL) 7 and RANK (Chappaz, Gartner et al. 2010). Using mice deficient for IL7 or Kit or both they showed that IL7 is important for lymph node anlagen but not for PP development whereas both Kit and Il7 are important for MLN anlagen (Chappaz, Gartner et al. 2010). But growth factors needed for lymph node development still remain poorly understood. The influence of vitamin A on the development of lymphoid structures is already a strong indication that nutritional components are of key importance at the base of infant's immune system.

A human embryo consists two weeks after fertilisation of three layers, called ectoderm, endoderm and mesoderm. Ectoderm forms the nervous system and the exterior, endoderm forms among others the gastrointestinal tract and the mesoderm forms for example connective tissue and the cells of the immune system. In the fourth week of embryogenesis the flat tissue folds lateral and folds from head to toe, via which the endoderm is enclosed by the ectoderm and a foregut, midgut and a hindgut are being formed, surrounded by mesoderm. At the end of the fourth week the liver is also beginning to form. From one of the pouches in the forgut, thymus will be formed, between 3rd and fourth month during pregnancy.

The loop of the midgut remains in contact with the yolk sac via the vitalline duct. In the same period that the definitive duodenum is formed, the midgut elongates and the hindgut becomes enlarged. When these changes in the pre-intestinal tract occur, the midgut migrates to the umbilical cord and returns in the embryo before the 4th month. During retraction the gut rotates to its final position. Throughout the whole gut enlargement of the surface is initiated via formation of crypts, villi and microvilli. The villi and microvilli start to develop after 9 to 10 weeks and at a later stage the colon loses it's villi. After birth the intestine needs approximately one week to organize it's lymph nodes with specific T- and B-cell regions and six months to acquire a tight epithelial barrier.

Box 1.

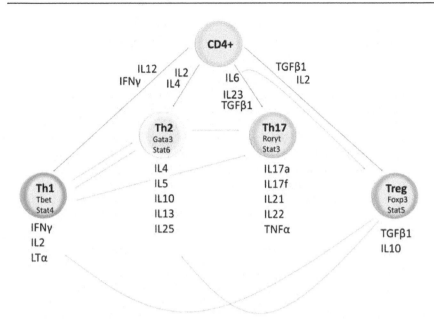

Fig. 3. Immune cell plasticity; Upon antigen encounter and T cell activation, naïve CD4+ T cells mature into several subsets. Several factors including cytokines, as described above determine the type of immune response, including Th1, Th2, Th17 and regulatory T cells. For example Th1 cell differentiation Interleukin (IL)12 and interferon gamma (IFNγ) is needed (blue arrow indicates stimulation). These cytokines help up regulate specific transcription factors like Tbet and Signal transducer and activator of transcription 4 (Stat4). These transcription factors activate certain genes to produce other cytokines like, IL2, LTα and IFNγ. When these cytokines are produced they help inhibit the differentiation of other Th-cells (red arrows indicate inhibition).

2.2 Immune cell development

The fetal common lymphoid progenitor cells (CLP) differ from the adult CLPs. The fetal CLPs have the ability not only to differentiate into all lymphoid cell types but also into macrophages. It is currently not known whether adult CLP are restricted to the division in myeloid and lymphoid progenitors or whether it is a gradual loss in lineage commitment (Chi, Bell et al. 2009). Via complex processes involving, a positive and negative selection, a lineage specific development in the thymus occurs. Only naïve T cells, intermediately recognizing the Major Histocompatibility Complex (MHC)-self-peptide and expressing CD4 or CD8, are allowed to migrate to their target organ (Singer, Adoro et al. 2008). CD4+ T cells form a subset of T cells called T helper (Th) cells and these cell types help to activate the B cells and CD8+ T cells. Th cells need binding of CD4 and CD28 to become activated Th cells and dependent on a specific set of cytokines, CD4+ T cells mature into different kinds of effector T cells, memory T cells or regulatory T (Treg) cells [Box 2]. Many factors are important for the development of both B and T cells, IL7 is of uttermost importance for both lymphocyte lineages (Kang, Der, et al. 2004). Recently it was shown that IL7 helps establish B cells, producing IgM, in the marginal zone of the spleen (Willems, Li, et al. 2011). Directly after birth maternal IL7 increases T cell production in the thymus and supports survival of T cells in other lymphoid structures in offspring, underlines the importance of IL7 during lymphogenesis (Aspinall, Prentice, et al. 2011).

The thymus is critically sensitive to malnutrition, with protein nutrition deficiency causing atrophy of the thymus (Savino and Dardenne 2010). This suggests that the thymus is a putative target for early-life programming effects. Most immune defence mechanisms are impaired in malnutrition, even in moderate nutritional deficiency. Protein-energy malnutrition is accompanied by deficiencies of micronutrients such as vitamin A, vitamin E, vitamin B6, vitamin C, folate, zinc, iron, copper, and selenium. Rapid proliferating T cells are especially affected by the lack of essential nutrients. Severe and chronic malnutrition may even lead to thymus atrophy affecting the basis of our immune system. The potential of adding certain nutrients, like vitamin C, D, or E, at levels above recommended dietary allowances (RDA) to the diet may improve immune function, is subject to increasing research.

Naïve CD4+ T cells are activated upon encountering an antigen presenting cell expressing MHC class II and the co-stimulatory signal CD28. They mature into effector, memory- of Treg dependent on which cytokines are produced by their APC. Already in 1986 two subsets were discovered by Mosmann and Cofmann (Zhu and Paul 2008) and now many more are well characterized. For Th1 Tbet and Signal transducer and Activator of transcription (Stat)1 are the initiating transcription factors , producing IFNγ, then Stat4 is amplifying the Th1 response. Th2 differentiation is activated by IL4, which induces Stat6. Stat6 in turn will activate the transcription factor Gata3. For Th17 RORγt is crucial, it is induced by transforming growth factor (TGF) β with IL6, then Stat3 and IRF4 are expressed. The transcription factors Foxp3 and Stat5 are needed, but without RA Tregs aren't formed. After the infection is cleared most cells die by apoptosis and some cells become memory cells to establish a faster response upon another infection (Zhu and Paul 2008; Zhu, Yamane et al. 2011).

Box 2.

The B cell lineage develops from HSC at the same sites as T cell development occurs. A major difference in lymphocyte development is that B cell development starts earlier, already in the pre-aorta gonad mesonephros region, which is also the most potent site for B cell development in the fetus (Dorshkind and Montecino-Rodriguez 2007). The HSC that migrate into the bone marrow are post natal responsible for B cell production. When B cells are activated they start to produce immunoglobulins, soluble and cell surface products to neutralize pathogens. Follicular B2 cells respond to microbial infections, they will present processed bacterial peptide to their CD4+ T cell partner. Because of this interaction B cells will undergo isotype switching and mature into plasma cells secreting antibodies to clear the infection. Some of these mature cells become memory B cells in peripheral lymphoid organs. Marginal B cells respond to bacterial polysaccharides without T cell stimulation. Recently it has been found that regulatory B cells can negatively influence the immune response via IL10 and transforming growth factor (TGF)β secretion (Vaughan, Roghanian et al. 2010). There are T cell independent B cell activators as mentioned above, but there is also T cell dependent B cell activation. Th1 type of CD4+ T cells are capable of helping B cells redirect to IgG2a in mice and IgG2 in humans. Th2 type of environment can induce switching towards IgE and IgG1 in mice and IgE and IgG4 in humans. At first the B cells will start with producing IgM and IgD. Upon stimulation they can switch towards an IgA,

IgE or IgG, depending on their surroundings and seem to be influenced by dietary components as discussed later. Neonatal B cells are capable of switching to IgG1 and IgG3 during the first 2 years of life, but the switch to IgG2 and IgG3 is inadequate during this period. To compensate the lack of protection in fetus and newborn, microbe-specific maternal IgG antibodies move across the placental barrier to provide some vital protection. During the last trimester of pregnancy IgGs are transferred intrauterine to the infant, because new-borns memory T cells capable of generating IgG and isotype switching aren't present yet. IgG1 and IgG4 are most effectively transported across the placenta compared to IgG3 and IgG2. Transfer of maternal antigen-specific IgG regulates the development of allergic airway inflammation early in life in a neonatal Fc region (FcRn)-dependent manner (Nakata, Kobayashi et al. 2010). This active transfer of IgGs from mother to child starts at week 17 and continues until birth. Moreover, just before birth, IgG levels of prenatal infants are even higher than levels present in the mother. The transfer and amount of pathogen specific IgGs is dependent on vaccinations and diseases the mother acquired during life. Many factors influence the IgG transportation processes which are described in a review by (Chucri, Monteiro et al. 2010). IgA IgD, IgM are the only known antibodies acquired after birth via breast feeding, covering the lack time during increasing antibody productions of infant's immune system itself. When the infant can produce the different B-cell antibodies, the activation, isotype switching and survival of B cells is for example under influence of B – cell activating factor (BAFF), TGFß1, IL-6, -7 and -10 produced by PP stromal cells (Finke, 2009). Not much is known about the involvement of Ig free light chains (IgfLC) in humoral immune response early in life. However the release of antigen specific IgfLC by B-cells/plasma cells like for example IgE may have implications for the health status of the newborn (Redegeld Nat Med 2003, Schouten JACI 2010). Furthermore compromised immune status may result in enhanced production and secretion of IgfLC at the cost of other immunoglobulins (van Esch CEA 2010).

Whereas T and B cell lineage experienced an in dept research into their origin, the origin and differentiation of dendritic cells (DC) is in its initial phase. One problem is to define specific precursor DC types (Liu and Nussenzweig 2010). Microbial exposure is one of the key developing factors for DCs (Plantinga, van Maren et al. 2011). The lamina propria (LP) contains mostly fractalkine positive DCs which sample the gut lumen with protrusions across the epithelial barrier, and are able to induce a Th17 response. Furthermore, in addition to the non-migrating DC population in PP there is a majority of DCs which will migrate to specific sites after encountering an antigen. For example the intestinal LP derived CD103+ DC subtype will migrate towards the MLN and is known for its capability to elicit a regulatory response, in the presence of RA and TGFβ. However if other factors are present a Th1 of a Th2 response can be induced. The activated T cell in the MLNs will migrate to the site of inflammation for instance in the intestine to initiate a proper immune response (*Figure 4*). Intestinal development is already influenced during pregnancy by the amniotic fluid as intestinal epithelial cells of the fetus can react to components in the amniotic fluid by different receptor expression (Drozdowski, Clandinin et al. 2010). So during gestation the gut can readily react to its micro-environment, but still much is unknown about the influence of maternal status on infantile gut development.

An increasing number of studies have identified interesting links between early nutrition, epigenetic processes and disease development later life (Boehm and Moro 2008). As the plasticity of growing and developing tissues shapes, the base of the responses to later

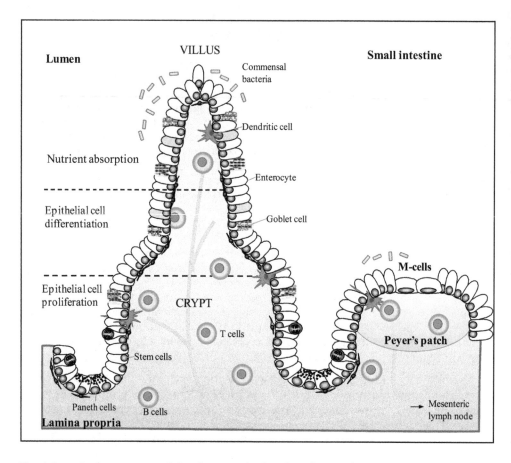

Fig. 4. Intestinal structure and development is already influenced during pregnancy and reacts to its micro-environment. The complex structure includes a variety of cross talk between different cells including epithelial cells, dendritic cells and lymphocytes. The lamina propria contains mostly dendritic cells which sample the lumen with protrusions across the epithelial barrier; in addition, the CD103+ DC subtype will migrate towards the mesenteric lymph nodes (MLN), after which the activated T cell in the MLNs will migrate back to the site of inflammation to initiate a proper immune response.

challenges is established, therefore the exposures during early life may be critical. Folate deficiency during pregnancy is associated with increased risk for aberrant reprogramming of DNA methylation inducing neural tube defects. Dietary folate intake can restore these deficiencies and neural tube defects. Folate is however not the only determinant of DNA methylation. Other methyl donor nutrients like betaine, vitamins B2, B6 and B12, and methionine, and choline, can also change DNA methylation status and therefore have an impact on development early in life (Niculescu and Lupu 2010).

3. Postnatal immune development in the gut

After birth a newborn changes from a sterile environment of the uterus into a world of constant challenges. In the first months of life newborns are more dependent on their innate immunity and immunoglobulins derived from the mother as described before. IgG is already acquired intrauterine but IgM and IgA are ingested via human milk to have an early defence against pathogens. Triggering the innate immunity repeatedly to microbial challenges after birth helps establishing a normal Th1 response postnatal. But the immune response is still less adequate compared to the adult response, possibly due to a general lower number of immune cells present. To build up an effective and balanced immune system interaction with germs and bacteria is needed (van't Land, Schijf et al. 2011). It is important that the immune balance is restored properly because a deregulation early in life could trigger an adverse reaction leading to an allergic reaction. The gut is the main processing site of food and, here immune tolerance against new food particles is established. But an improper chemical barrier and weak mucosal barrier integrity will complicate acquiring immune tolerance. There are some factors positively influencing development of the gut and immune system during pregnancy and after birth, of which only few of them will be discussed in detail below.

3.1 Influence of vitamins during and after pregnancy

Vitamin A has been recognized for its importance in lymphoid structure formation during embryogenesis. Sources of vitamin A are carrots, liver, sweet potatoes and butter. For example vitamin A supplementation before, during and after pregnancy using restricted dosages, results in long term positive effects on lung function which could be measured nine to thirteen years later.(Checkley, West et al. 2010). Shortly after the recognition of vitamin A essence during pregnancy, the teratogenic effect of excess vitamin A was shown. Malformations of the central nervous system, the eye and the thymus were found due to excessive use of vitamin A (Gutierrez-Mazariegos, Theodosiou et al. 2011). The teratogenic danger of vitamin A can also be induced via extra prolonged ingestion of this vitamin because it is stored in fat cells in the liver. It was already mentioned that RA could increase the progression from HSC into myeloid cell lineage. When RA is lacking from the diet CD4+ and CD8+ T cells and IgA+ B cells aren't found in the LP of the intestine, whereas CD4+ T cells were still present in lung tissue (Iwata 2009). Recently it was shown that stromal cells and DCs in the MLN induce high levels of RALDH expression postnatally, dependent on vitamin A and not on toll like receptor (TLR) signalling (Molenaar, Knippenberg et al. 2011). They compared MLN with other lymph nodes at different postnatal weeks and found an increased expression of RALDH only in the MLN residing DC, almost exclusively in CD103+ MHC-II+ CD11c+ DC cells. Vitamin A deficiency reduces this RALDH expression significantly. In addition, RA skews DC towards tolerance induction via instruction of Foxp3 Treg in the mother during pregnancy and in the infant just after birth (Coombes, Siddiqui et al. 2007; Duriancik, Lackey et al. 2010). Also vitamin A is necessary for the intestinal homing properties of activated T cells, Treg and certain B cells. *In vitro* it was shown that naïve CD4+ cells induce gut homing receptors when they are activated by CD3 and CD28 together with RA, this combination simultaneously down regulates skin homing receptors (Iwata 2009). In *vitro* DC from the gut associated lymphoid tissue could also induce activated IgA secreting B cells more effectively when RA was present in the medium, however the intracellular mechanism needs to be determined (Mora and von Andrian 2009). Not only RA is important for IgA secreting B cells, IL5 is essential for IgA production and TGFβ increases IgA secretion *in vitro*. There is also a positive feedback loop, IL6 stimulates IgA induction by DC and IL6 is induced by RA. Synergistic effect on IgA induction could be obtained by the aforementioned cytokines and therefore immune protection of the infant could be achieved (Mora and von Andrian 2009; Duriancik, Lackey et al. 2010). This indicates that also during early infancy the level of vitamin A is of importance for proper immune functioning, which may have profound consequences later in life.

An additional vitamin of interest for immune development is vitamin D. Worldwide there is no consensus on the healthy levels of vitamin D intake before and during pregnancy. Already during the first trimester of pregnancy vitamin D could be of importance for the development of the fetus. The 25-hydroxy vitamin D-1α-hydrolase CYP27B1), which converts vitamin D into its more active metabolite 1,25 $(OH)_2D$, can be detected in the placenta. There is some speculation about vitamin D deficiency and reduced fertility, this fertility problem may be caused by a reduced down regulation of the Th1 response by high levels of vitamin D as well as circumstantial evidence pointing at a relation between gestational diabetes and preeclampsia in correlation to circulating vitamin D levels (Dror and Allen 2010). In addition, vitamin D is important for the clearance of certain infections (Hoyer-Hansen, Nordbrandt et al. 2010).

Vitamin D is linked to monocyte activation via activation of TLR2 and TLR1(Lagishetty, Liu et al. 2011). Recently it was shown that IL4 and IFNγ are involved in the regulation of vitamin D expression (Edfeldt, Liu et al. 2010). IL4 promotes expression of CYP24A1, which down regulates active vitamin D, and IFNγ positively influences the expression of CYP24B1 in monocytes. Then it is suggested that vitamin D could skew the balance between Th1 and Th2 towards a Th2 phenotype directly or indirectly via monocyte activation, which however may be much more complex *in vivo* (Adams and Hewison 2008). Low vitamin D levels during pregnancy are suggested to be related in the development of food allergy (Nwaru, Ahonen et al. 2010). It was recently shown that active vitamin D can suppress DC maturation and inhibit T cell proliferation. Mature DC have high levels of vitamin D converting enzymes, suggesting that upon Vitamin D addition, mature DC can inhibit the development of immature DC. Suppression of DC maturation could then via vitamin D promote tolerance. Research with vitamin D receptor (VDR) and CYP27B1 knockout mice showed abnormal lymph node development due to the presence of more mature DC and increased DC trafficking (Hewison 2011).

There is still debate about the healthy amount of vitamin D intake during pregnancy (West, Videky et al. 2010). Indeed some studies show that vitamin D intake is associated with diminished wheeze, asthma and eczema in offspring (West, Videky et al. 2010). For vitamin D it is clear that lymphocytes are influenced, but to what extent this affects function later in life remains to be established. Increasing evidence from observational studies in infants at older ages, indicate that vitamin D insufficiency and deficiency might increase the risk of chronic diseases such as type 1 diabetes and multiple sclerosis. However, clear randomized trials on this association need to be conducted to confirm these findings. In the last decades, observations accumulate that vitamin D deficiency leads to more often and more serious respiratory infections than in individuals with sufficient vitamin D plasma levels. This illustrates the importance of the nutritional status early in life, to set the proper immune balance (Karatekin, Kaya et al. 2009).

3.2 Human milk

It is well established that breastfeeding reduces the incidence of gastrointestinal and non-enteric infections in infants, due to its antimicrobial activity against several viruses, bacteria, and protozoa (Chirico, Marzollo et al. 2008). In addition, it was shown that infants, breastfed for more than 4 months experienced significant reduced incidences of respiratory tract infection requiring hospitalization, as compared to infants who were not breastfed (Bachrach, Schwarz et al. 2003). Moreover, other studies showed that breastfeeding provides protection against urinary tract infections and otitis media and it reduces the development of inflammatory conditions like allergy (Fiocchi, Martelli et al. 2003), Crohn's disease and ulcerative colitis (Hanson 2007). This, moreover, emphasizes the diversity of activity and active components present in human breast milk. Although it is clear that allergy development is influenced by breast milk as well as atopy related disorders, still some controversy exists regarding the beneficial length of breastfeeding (van Odijk, Kull et al. 2003). These protective effects of human breast milk seem to persist at least during the first decade of life.

Fortunately prenatally the infant is supplied with maternal immunoglobulins, for the first protection against infections. It takes at least one year before an infant can produce about 60% of its IgG levels on its own. After birth the child can be supplied with essential IgG, IgM and IgA via human milk. For example, IgA is necessary as the first line of defence against microorganisms. This immunoglobulin also controls commensal (also called beneficial) bacteria all without activation of an inflammatory response. Because infants do not have an optimized Treg response and no memory cells, B cells cannot be directed to produce the right amount of Ig antibodies quickly as a first defence. IgM helps to eliminate the pathogen before IgGs are produced. As earlier mentioned IgM is normally produced by naive B cells before isotype switching occurs. The B cell response needs time after birth to be fully functional, so acquiring this component via human milk strengthens the first line of defence. Not only antibodies are factors present in human milk, other immune modulating components are present, including cytokines, non digestible oligosaccharides and poly unsaturated fatty acids (PUFA), which are discussed in more detail below.

3.3 Cytokines

TGFβ and IL10 are held responsible for the induction of oral tolerance in the intestine (du Pre and Samsom 2010). They educate the immune system locally not to respond to harmless antigens. In human milk TGFβ2 is the predominant isoform of the three existing mammalian isoforms. Addition of TGFβ2 to infant formula, can skew the Th2 allergic effector response towards Th1 in rat pups exposed to β-lactoglobulin, a cow's milk allergy protein (Penttila 2009). Not TGFβ2 but TGFβ1 is the major player to establish immune tolerance to food in the adult system. To guarantee the uptake of TGFβ, TGFβ receptors are abundantly expressed in the neonatal intestine, even the soluble TGFβ2 receptor is present in breast milk. But in addition it was found that TGFβ is not essential for tolerance induction when milk born-IgG antigen immune complexes are present (Verhasselt, Milcent et al. 2008). Moreover it is known that high levels of TGFβ together with RA skew the immune system towards a regulatory suppressive function, a low dose of TGFβ combined with IL6 or IL21 or IL23 will result in inflammatory Th17 activation instead of Treg upregulation (Konkel and Chen 2011). Recently Hering et al (2009) showed that *in vitro* TGFβ probably helps forming the intestinal epithelial barrier via exerting its effect on the reinforcement between the epithelial cells (van't Land, Meijer et al. 2002; Hering and Schulzke 2009). The production of IgA is also positively influenced by TGFβ (Cazac and Roes 2000; Borsutzky, Cazac et al. 2004). This indicates that the immune modulating components have their function alone, but this needs to be further investigated in combination.

3.4 Nondigestible oligosaccharides

There are different types of soluble dietary fibres e.g. (hemi)cellulose, lignin, β-glucans, pectins, gums, inulin and oligofructose. In addition different non-digestible oligosaccharides with specific properties are obtained or manufactured from natural sources (Calder, Krauss-Etschmann et al. 2006). Human milk contains approximately 7-12 g/L oligosaccharides (Hoppu, Kalliomaki et al. 2001). At least 130 different oligosaccharides have been isolated from human milk and the two main categories are neutral and acidic oligosaccharides (Lara-Villoslada, Olivares et al. 2007; Greer, Sicherer et al. 2008). These oligosaccharides are non-digestible carbohydrates that have many different properties and are believed to act on the microbiota in the gut (Host, Koletzko et al. 1999; Halken, Hansen et al. 2000; Hill, Murch et al. 2007; Niggemann and Beyer 2007). Due to physicochemical properties of non-digestible carbohydrates the absorption of minerals and fecal consistency improves. Some of these have specific properties and can be used as prebiotics as a dietary supplement. Prebiotics are defined as "a selectively fermented ingredient that allows specific changes, both in the composition and/or activity in the gastrointestinal microflora that confers benefits upon host wellbeing and health" (Host and Halken 2004). Prebiotics enhance defense mechanisms of the host by stimulation of growth of Bifidobacteria and Lactobacilli. As the intestinal microbiota plays a critical role in the establishment and maintenance of healthy immune responses, the delayed colonisation of the infant gut with commensal bacteria are suggested to be a risk factor for the development of immune mediated chronic disorders such as allergic and autoimmune diseases. Short-chain fatty acids, released by these bacteria upon fermentation of prebiotics, are essential nutrients for intestinal epithelial cells and support gut function (Gibson and Roberfroid 1995; Nakhla, Fu et al. 1999; Boehm and Stahl 2007). *In vivo* and *in vitro* studies have shown beneficial effects of prebiotics on the innate as well as the adaptive immune system (Boehm, Fanaro et al. 2003). Short-chain galacto-oligosaccharides (scGOS), long-chain fructo-oligosaccharides (lcFOS) and pectin-derived acidic oligosaccharides (pAOS) are some examples of non-digestible oligosaccharides that mimic the functionality and molecular size distribution of human milk oligosaccharides.

The effects of scGOS and lcFOS (9:1)(Immunofortis®) have been studied in a murine vaccination model (Vos, Haarman et al. 2006), in an allergic asthma model (Vos, van Esch et al. 2007) and a cow's milk allergy model (Schouten, van Esch et al. 2009). The response to vaccination of mice fed the scGOS/lcFOS diet was significant enhanced, as well as the fecal Bifidobacteria and Lactobacilli proportions. pAOS enhanced the murine vaccination response and the combination (scGOS/lcFOS/pAOS) was even more effective (Vos, Haarman et al. 2007). To stimulate the entire microbiota a great variation in the oligosaccharide structures will exert this effect, as human milk oligosaccharides comprise of many different oligosaccharides. The pAOS are not only another group of oligosaccharides, they act very specifically to their acidity. Based on this they are able to interact with surfaces and might prevent the adhesion of pathogens on the intestinal epithelium. In infants pAOS showed no difference in stool characteristics, pH, growth, crying, vomiting and regurgitation patterns as compared to control formula. In addition pAOS alone did not affect intestinal microecology (Fanaro, Jelinek et al. 2005). Furthermore, systemic Th1 dependent immune responses were enhanced using the prebiotics without inducing autoimmunity, as Th1 is low in newborn infants. In addition, in a murine model for cow's milk allergy dietary intervention with scGOS/lcFOS showed significant decrease of the allergic response and increased specific IgG2a levels (Meyer 2004; Schouten, van Esch et al. 2009).

Recently it was found in mice that dietary intervention with scGOS/lcFOS/pAOS reduces the development of an acute allergic response upon antigen challenge, although specific immunoglobulins levels remain high. *Ex vivo* depletion of CD25$^+$ Treg abrogated the diminished acute allergic response, combined with adoptive transfer studies, imply crucial involvement of antigen specific CD25$^+$ Treg cells in the suppression of the allergic effector response (Schouten, van Esch et al. 2010; van't Land, Schijf et al. 2010; Schouten, van Esch et al. 2011). Furthermore, clinical trials have been performed with the scGOS/lcFOS mixture in children at high risk for allergies. A reduction in the incidence of atopic dermatitis (AD) (Moro, Arslanoglu et al. 2006) and the incidence of allergic manifestations during the first 6 months of life (Arslanoglu, Moro et al. 2007) was observed, furthermore this reduction lasted at least until 2 years of age (Arslanoglu, Moro et al. 2008).

Recently, it was also shown, in a multicenter trial, that the scGOS/lcFOS/pAOS mixture could reduce the incidence of AD in healthy not at risk children (Gruber, van Stuijvenberg et al.). In another clinical study, using the scGOS/lcFOS mixture, fecal secretory IgA was increased in healthy infants (Bakker-Zierikzee, Tol et al. 2006). Also in healthy infants there is cumulative evidence that prebiotic mixtures might beneficially affect the host in both Th1 as well as Th2 prone settings as it might prevent food allergy (Th2) and enhances the vaccination response (Th1). Although it is believed that prebiotics exert their effect via stimulation of growth of selective bacterial species that beneficially improve host health, there is debate about this mechanism and there are potentially microbiota-independent mechanisms as well (Boehm, Fanaro et al. 2003; Vos, M'Rabet et al. 2007). As it was shown that epithelial cells can transport scGOS, lcFOS and pAOS across from apical to the basolateral side (Eiwegger, Stahl et al. 2010), this illustrates that besides a prebiotic immune modulating effect the oligosaccharides also come in direct contact with immune cells themselves, making it possible to act directly on the immune cells.

3.5 Poly unsaturated fatty acids

Omega-3 and omega-6 poly unsaturated fatty acids (PUFA) are essential for humans and have to be provided via the diet especially found in seafood. PUFA are incorporated into the cellular membrane and are eicosanoid precursors hereby affecting the immune response. In this regard in particular n-3 long chain (LC)-PUFA eicosapentaenoic acid (EPA) and docosahexaenoic acid (DHA) are regarded to be anti-inflammatory while n-6 LCPUFA, like linoleic and arachidonic acid, are able to boost inflammatory responses. Arachidonic acid, for example can be converted into 2 series prostaglandins, these are able to increase IL4 and decrease IFNγ, and 4 series of leukotrines, which are able to induce endothelial permeability and production of inflammatory cytokines (Moreno 2009).

In westernized countries the n-3 fatty acid ingestion is no longer favoured over n-6 PUFA which may have implications for immune homeostasis. It has been stated that the original diet of the human race had an n-6 : n-3 ratio of approximately 1:1 and that this has changed over the past decades to a ratio of at least 15:1 (Simopoulos 2008). This shift is suggested to be explanatory for the increased incidence of cardiovascular diseases, chronic inflammatory diseases, obesity and also allergic diseases. Therefore pre-clinical as well as clinical trials are performed in order to investigate this hypothesis. It has been reviewed that n-3 LCPUFA intake reduces the incidence of allergic disorders, e.g. AD, less sensitization to egg in the clinical trials (Blumer, Pfefferle et al. 2007). Two studies by Dunstan *et al.* show reduced sensitization to egg and less AD in offspring when pregnant woman were supplemented with fish oil, which contains EPA and DHA (Dunstan, Mori et al. 2003; Dunstan, Roper et al. 2004). They found a positive influence of n-3 LCPUFA on TGFβ mRNA levels in maternal peripheral blood and cord blood. This could imply a regulatory function of n-3 LCPUFA, but mRNA still needs to be processed towards an active component. Recently, it was shown that maternal n-3 LCPUFA intake decreased the risk of food allergy and IgE-associated eczema in children at risk for allergy (Furuhjelm, Warstedt et al. 2009). This shift in the decrease of allergy can be explained since n-3 LCPUFA is incorporated in the membrane of immune cells at the cost of n-6 LCPUFA as arachidonic acid, skewing towards a less inflammatory cytokine surrounding. In contrast, in a clinical study by Almqvist et al., (Almqvist, Garden et al. 2007) it is shown that supplementation of n-3 PUFA, starting at a maximum of six months of age, did not prevent children with a family history of asthma from developing atopy, eczema nor asthma at the age of 5 years. Hence discrepancy on effects of n-3 PUFA in prevention of allergic disease exists. There are also discrepancies between studies in the preparation of fish oil, influencing EPA and DHA content (Prescott and Calder 2004). Of concern is the dosage in human studies, this is often much lower than used in animal studies, which makes it difficult to extrapolate the outcome and could explain differences observed. However interventions using dietary factors like LCPUFAs are under-explored and that there is a need for additional research. One of the strategies that are proposed is the use of selected LCPUFA in the formula feeding of young children at high risk for allergies (Vanderhoof 2008). Another strategy could be to supplement a novel LCPUFA during pregnancy; LCPUFA maybe has its largest positive effect on an infant health status when primary immune responses are still developing. In addition novel synthetic LCPUFA may reveal to be potent in the reduction of the allergic burden (Prescott and Calder 2004).

4. Consequences later in life conclusion

During the different phases of life, several nutritional factors influence our immune system and immune responsiveness in collaboration with endogenous immune modulating mediators like humoral factors, lipids and oligosaccharides. A vast amount of literature is available on the role that nutrients and human milk (as reviewed in this article), have on the development of the immune system; a lot less is known about the exact requirements in the phases thereafter, in toddlers, during adolescence, and in the later stages of life. Moreover, as no single biomarker exists able to determine a proper functioning immune system, it is almost impossible to describe completely the developmental status of the immune system and the important influences of nutrition. Although it is clear that each phase in life puts specific requirements on nutrition, no clear statement can be made based on literature as to what the exact dietary requirements are in order to fully support the immune system during these stages in life. But food as a beneficial dietary component is currently under very active scientific investigation, so more information about nutrition will be available soon.

5. References

Adams, J. S. and M. Hewison (2008). "Unexpected actions of vitamin D: new perspectives on the regulation of innate and adaptive immunity." *Nat Clin Pract Endocrinol Metab* 4(2): 80-90.

Almqvist, C., F. Garden, et al. (2007). "Omega-3 and omega-6 fatty acid exposure from early life does not affect atopy and asthma at age 5 years." *J Allergy Clin Immunol* 119(6): 1438-44.

Arslanoglu, S., G. E. Moro, et al. (2007). "Early supplementation of prebiotic oligosaccharides protects formula-fed infants against infections during the first 6 months of life." *J Nutr* 137(11): 2420-4.

Arslanoglu, S., G. E. Moro, et al. (2008). "Early dietary intervention with a mixture of prebiotic oligosaccharides reduces the incidence of allergic manifestations and infections during the first two years of life." *J Nutr* 138(6): 1091-5.

Aspinall, R., Prentice, A.M., Ngom, P.T. Interleukin 7 from maternal milk crosses the intestinal barrier and modulates T-cell development in offspring. PloS One, 2011;6(6) e20812

Bachrach, V. R., E. Schwarz, et al. (2003). "Breastfeeding and the risk of hospitalization for respiratory disease in infancy: a meta-analysis." *Arch Pediatr Adolesc Med* 157(3): 237-43.

Bakker-Zierikzee, A. M., E. A. Tol, et al. (2006). "Faecal SIgA secretion in infants fed on pre- or probiotic infant formula." *Pediatr Allergy Immunol* 17(2): 134-40.

Blumer, N., P. I. Pfefferle, et al. (2007). "Development of mucosal immune function in the intrauterine and early postnatal environment." *Curr Opin Gastroenterol* 23(6): 655-60.

Boehm, G., S. Fanaro, et al. (2003). "Prebiotic concept for infant nutrition." *Acta Paediatr Suppl* 91(441): 64-7.

Boehm, G. and G. Moro (2008). "Structural and functional aspects of prebiotics used in infant nutrition." *J Nutr* 138(9): 1818S-1828S.

Boehm, G. and B. Stahl (2007). "Oligosaccharides from milk." *J Nutr* 137(3 Suppl 2): 847S-9S.

Borsutzky, S., B. B. Cazac, et al. (2004). "TGF-beta receptor signaling is critical for mucosal IgA responses." *J Immunol* 173(5): 3305-9.

Calder, P. C., S. Krauss-Etschmann, et al. (2006). "Early nutrition and immunity - progress and perspectives." *Br J Nutr* 96(4): 774-90.

Campo-Paysaa, F., F. Marletaz, et al. (2008). "Retinoic acid signaling in development: tissue-specific functions and evolutionary origins." *Genesis* 46(11): 640-56.

Cazac, B. B. and J. Roes (2000). "TGF-beta receptor controls B cell responsiveness and induction of IgA in vivo." *Immunity* 13(4): 443-51.

Chappaz, S., C. Gartner, et al. (2010). "Kit ligand and Il7 differentially regulate Peyer's patch and lymph node development." *J Immunol* 185(6): 3514-9.

Checkley, W., K. P. West, Jr., et al. (2010). "Maternal vitamin A supplementation and lung function in offspring." *N Engl J Med* 362(19): 1784-94.

Chi, A. W., J. J. Bell, et al. (2009). "Untangling the T branch of the hematopoiesis tree." *Curr Opin Immunol* 21(2): 121-6.

Chirico, G., R. Marzollo, et al. (2008). "Antiinfective properties of human milk." *J Nutr* 138(9): 1801S-1806S.

Chucri, T. M., J. M. Monteiro, et al. (2010). "A review of immune transfer by the placenta." *J Reprod Immunol* 87(1-2): 14-20.

Coombes, J. L., K. R. Siddiqui, et al. (2007). "A functionally specialized population of mucosal CD103+ DCs induces Foxp3+ regulatory T cells via a TGF-beta and retinoic acid-dependent mechanism." *J Exp Med* 204(8): 1757-64.

Dorshkind, K. and E. Montecino-Rodriguez (2007). "Fetal B-cell lymphopoiesis and the emergence of B-1-cell potential." *Nat Rev Immunol* 7(3): 213-9.

Dror, D. K. and L. H. Allen (2010). "Vitamin D inadequacy in pregnancy: biology, outcomes, and interventions." *Nutr Rev* 68(8): 465-77.

Drozdowski, L. A., T. Clandinin, et al. (2010). "Ontogeny, growth and development of the small intestine: Understanding pediatric gastroenterology." *World J Gastroenterol* 16(7): 787-99.

du Pre, M. F. and J. N. Samsom (2010). "Adaptive T-cell responses regulating oral tolerance to protein antigen." *Allergy* 66(4): 478-90.

Dunstan, J. A., T. A. Mori, et al. (2003). "Fish oil supplementation in pregnancy modifies neonatal allergen-specific immune responses and clinical outcomes in infants at high risk of atopy: a randomized, controlled trial." *J Allergy Clin Immunol* 112(6): 1178-84.

Dunstan, J. A., J. Roper, et al. (2004). "The effect of supplementation with fish oil during pregnancy on breast milk immunoglobulin A, soluble CD14, cytokine levels and fatty acid composition." *Clin Exp Allergy* 34(8): 1237-42.

Duriancik, D. M., D. E. Lackey, et al. (2010). "Vitamin A as a regulator of antigen presenting cells." *J Nutr* 140(8): 1395-9.

Edfeldt, K., P. T. Liu, et al. (2010). "T-cell cytokines differentially control human monocyte antimicrobial responses by regulating vitamin D metabolism." *Proc Natl Acad Sci U S A* 107(52): 22593-8.

Eiwegger, T., B. Stahl, et al. (2010). "Prebiotic oligosaccharides: in vitro evidence for gastrointestinal epithelial transfer and immunomodulatory properties." *Pediatr Allergy Immunol* 21(8): 1179-88.

Fanaro, S., J. Jelinek, et al. (2005). "Acidic oligosaccharides from pectin hydrolysate as new component for infant formulae: effect on intestinal flora, stool characteristics, and pH." *J Pediatr Gastroenterol Nutr* 41(2): 186-90.

Finke, D. Induction of intestinal lymphoid tissue formation by intrinsic and extrinsic signals. Semi. Immunopathol. 2009, july; 31(2) 151-169

Fiocchi, A., A. Martelli, et al. (2003). "Primary dietary prevention of food allergy." *Ann Allergy Asthma Immunol* 91(1): 3-12; quiz 12-5, 91.

Furuhjelm, C., K. Warstedt, et al. (2009). "Fish oil supplementation in pregnancy and lactation may decrease the risk of infant allergy." *Acta Paediatr* 98(9): 1461-7.

Gibson, G. R. and M. B. Roberfroid (1995). "Dietary modulation of the human colonic microbiota: introducing the concept of prebiotics." *J Nutr* 125(6): 1401-12.

Grassinger, J., D. N. Haylock, et al. (2010). "Phenotypically identical hemopoietic stem cells isolated from different regions of bone marrow have different biologic potential." *Blood* 116(17): 3185-96.

Greer, F. R., S. H. Sicherer, et al. (2008). "Effects of early nutritional interventions on the development of atopic disease in infants and children: the role of maternal dietary restriction, breastfeeding, timing of introduction of complementary foods, and hydrolyzed formulas." *Pediatrics* 121(1): 183-91.

Gruber, C., M. van Stuijvenberg, et al. "Reduced occurrence of early atopic dermatitis because of immunoactive prebiotics among low-atopy-risk infants." *J Allergy Clin Immunol* 126(4): 791-7.

Gutierrez-Mazariegos, J., M. Theodosiou, et al. (2011). "Vitamin A: A multifunctional tool for development." *Semin Cell Dev Biol* 22(6): 603-10.

Halken, S., K. S. Hansen, et al. (2000). "Comparison of a partially hydrolyzed infant formula with two extensively hydrolyzed formulas for allergy prevention: a prospective, randomized study." *Pediatr Allergy Immunol* 11(3): 149-61.

Hanson, L. A. (2007). "Session 1: Feeding and infant development breast-feeding and immune function." *Proc Nutr Soc* 66(3): 384-96.

Hering, N. A. and J. D. Schulzke (2009). "Therapeutic options to modulate barrier defects in inflammatory bowel disease." *Dig Dis* 27(4): 450-4.

Hewison, M. (2011). "Vitamin D and innate and adaptive immunity." *Vitam Horm* 86: 23-62.

Hill, D. J., S. H. Murch, et al. (2007). "The efficacy of amino acid-based formulas in relieving the symptoms of cow's milk allergy: a systematic review." *Clin Exp Allergy* 37(6): 808-22.

Hoppu, U., M. Kalliomaki, et al. (2001). "Breast milk--immunomodulatory signals against allergic diseases." *Allergy* 56 Suppl 67: 23-6.

Host, A. and S. Halken (2004). "Hypoallergenic formulas--when, to whom and how long: after more than 15 years we know the right indication!" *Allergy* 59 Suppl 78: 45-52.

Host, A., B. Koletzko, et al. (1999). "Dietary products used in infants for treatment and prevention of food allergy. Joint Statement of the European Society for Paediatric Allergology and Clinical Immunology (ESPACI) Committee on Hypoallergenic Formulas and the European Society for Paediatric Gastroenterology, Hepatology and Nutrition (ESPGHAN) Committee on Nutrition." *Arch Dis Child* 81(1): 80-4.

Hoyer-Hansen, M., S. P. Nordbrandt, et al. (2010). "Autophagy as a basis for the health-promoting effects of vitamin D." *Trends Mol Med* 16(7): 295-302.

Iwata, M. (2009). "Retinoic acid production by intestinal dendritic cells and its role in T-cell trafficking." *Semin Immunol* 21(1): 8-13.

Kang, J., Der, S.D. Cytokine functions in the formative stages of a lymphocyte's life. Current opinion in Immunology, April 2004, Vol. 16, issue 2, 180-190

Karatekin, G., A. Kaya, et al. (2009). "Association of subclinical vitamin D deficiency in newborns with acute lower respiratory infection and their mothers." *Eur J Clin Nutr* 63(4): 473-7.

Konkel, J. E. and W. Chen (2011). "Balancing acts: the role of TGF-beta in the mucosal immune system." *Trends Mol Med* 17(11): 668-76.

Lagishetty, V., N. Q. Liu, et al. (2011). "Vitamin D metabolism and innate immunity." *Mol Cell Endocrinol* 347(1-2): 97-105.

Lara-Villoslada, F., M. Olivares, et al. (2007). "Beneficial effects of probiotic bacteria isolated from breast milk." *Br J Nutr* 98 Suppl 1: S96-100.

Liu, K. and M. C. Nussenzweig (2010). "Development and homeostasis of dendritic cells." *Eur J Immunol* 40(8): 2099-102.

Mazo, I. B., S. Massberg, et al. (2011). "Hematopoietic stem and progenitor cell trafficking." *Trends Immunol* 32(10): 493-503.

McDade, T. W., M. A. Beck, et al. (2001). "Prenatal undernutrition, postnatal environments, and antibody response to vaccination in adolescence." *Am J Clin Nutr* 74(4): 543-8.

Medvinsky, A., S. Rybtsov, et al. (2011). "Embryonic origin of the adult hematopoietic system: advances and questions." *Development* 138(6): 1017-31.

Meyer, P. D. (2004). "Nondigestible oligosaccharides as dietary fiber." *J AOAC Int* 87(3): 718-26.

Molenaar, R., M. Knippenberg, et al. (2011). "Expression of retinaldehyde dehydrogenase enzymes in mucosal dendritic cells and gut-draining lymph node stromal cells is controlled by dietary vitamin A." *J Immunol* 186(4): 1934-42.

Mora, J. R. and U. H. von Andrian (2009). "Role of retinoic acid in the imprinting of gut-homing IgA-secreting cells." *Semin Immunol* 21(1): 28-35.

Moreno, J. J. (2009). "Differential effects of arachidonic and eicosapentaenoic Acid-derived eicosanoids on polymorphonuclear transmigration across endothelial cell cultures." *J Pharmacol Exp Ther* 331(3): 1111-7.

Moro, G., S. Arslanoglu, et al. (2006). "A mixture of prebiotic oligosaccharides reduces the incidence of atopic dermatitis during the first six months of age." *Arch Dis Child* 91(10): 814-9.

Nakata, K., K. Kobayashi, et al. (2010). "The transfer of maternal antigen-specific IgG regulates the development of allergic airway inflammation early in life in an FcRn-dependent manner." *Biochem Biophys Res Commun* 395(2): 238-43.

Nakhla, T., D. Fu, et al. (1999). "Neutral oligosaccharide content of preterm human milk." *Br J Nutr* 82(5): 361-7.

Niculescu, M. D. and D. S. Lupu (2010). "Nutritional influence on epigenetics and effects on longevity." *Curr Opin Clin Nutr Metab Care* 14(1): 35-40.

Niggemann, B. and K. Beyer (2007). "Diagnosis of food allergy in children: toward a standardization of food challenge." *J Pediatr Gastroenterol Nutr* 45(4): 399-404.

Nwaru, B. I., S. Ahonen, et al. (2010). "Maternal diet during pregnancy and allergic sensitization in the offspring by 5 yrs of age: a prospective cohort study." *Pediatr Allergy Immunol* 21(1 Pt 1): 29-37.

Penttila, I. A. (2009). "Milk-derived transforming growth factor-beta and the infant immune response." *J Pediatr* 156(2 Suppl): S21-5.

Plantinga, T. S., W. W. van Maren, et al. (2011). "Differential Toll-like receptor recognition and induction of cytokine profile by Bifidobacterium breve and Lactobacillus strains of probiotics." *Clin Vaccine Immunol* 18(4): 621-8.

Prescott, S. L. and P. C. Calder (2004). "N-3 polyunsaturated fatty acids and allergic disease." *Curr Opin Clin Nutr Metab Care* 7(2): 123-9.

Savino, W. and M. Dardenne (2010). "Nutritional imbalances and infections affect the thymus: consequences on T-cell-mediated immune responses." *Proc Nutr Soc* 69(4): 636-43.

Schouten, B., B. C. van Esch, et al. (2010). "Oligosaccharide-induced whey-specific CD25(+) regulatory T-cells are involved in the suppression of cow milk allergy in mice." *J Nutr* 140(4): 835-41.

Schouten, B., B. C. van Esch, et al. (2011). "A potential role for CD25+ regulatory T-cells in the protection against casein allergy by dietary non-digestible carbohydrates." *Br J Nutr*: 1-10.

Schouten, B., B. C. van Esch, et al. (2009). "Cow milk allergy symptoms are reduced in mice fed dietary synbiotics during oral sensitization with whey." *J Nutr* 139(7): 1398-403.

Simopoulos, A. P. (2008). "The importance of the omega-6/omega-3 fatty acid ratio in cardiovascular disease and other chronic diseases." *Exp Biol Med (Maywood)* 233(6): 674-88.

Singer, A., S. Adoro, et al. (2008). "Lineage fate and intense debate: myths, models and mechanisms of CD4- versus CD8-lineage choice." *Nat Rev Immunol* 8(10): 788-801.

van't Land, B., H. P. Meijer, et al. (2002). "Transforming Growth Factor-beta2 protects the small intestine during methotrexate treatment in rats possibly by reducing stem cell cycling." *Br J Cancer* 87(1): 113-8.

van't Land, B., M. Schijf, et al. (2010). "Regulatory T-cells have a prominent role in the immune modulated vaccine response by specific oligosaccharides." *Vaccine* 28(35): 5711-7.

van't Land, B., M. A. Schijf, et al. (2011). "Influencing mucosal homeostasis and immune responsiveness: The impact of nutrition and pharmaceuticals." *Eur J Pharmacol* 668 Suppl 1: S101-7.

van de Pavert, S. A. and R. E. Mebius (2010). "New insights into the development of lymphoid tissues." *Nat Rev Immunol* 10(9): 664-74.

van Odijk, J., I. Kull, et al. (2003). "Breastfeeding and allergic disease: a multidisciplinary review of the literature (1966-2001) on the mode of early feeding in infancy and its impact on later atopic manifestations." *Allergy* 58(9): 833-43.

Vanderhoof, J. A. (2008). "Hypoallergenicity and effects on growth and tolerance of a new amino acid-based formula with DHA and ARA." *J Pediatr Gastroenterol Nutr* 47 Suppl 2: S60-1.

Vaughan, A. T., A. Roghanian, et al. (2010). "B cells--masters of the immunoverse." *Int J Biochem Cell Biol* 43(3): 280-5.

Verhasselt, V., V. Milcent, et al. (2008). "Breast milk-mediated transfer of an antigen induces tolerance and protection from allergic asthma." *Nat Med* 14(2): 170-5.

Vos, A. P., M. Haarman, et al. (2006). "A specific prebiotic oligosaccharide mixture stimulates delayed-type hypersensitivity in a murine influenza vaccination model." *Int Immunopharmacol* 6(8): 1277-86.

Vos, A. P., M. Haarman, et al. (2007). "Dietary supplementation of neutral and acidic oligosaccharides enhances Th1-dependent vaccination responses in mice." *Pediatr Allergy Immunol* 18(4): 304-12.

Vos, A. P., L. M'Rabet, et al. (2007). "Immune-modulatory effects and potential working mechanisms of orally applied nondigestible carbohydrates." *Crit Rev Immunol* 27(2): 97-140.

Vos, A. P., B. C. van Esch, et al. (2007). "Dietary supplementation with specific oligosaccharide mixtures decreases parameters of allergic asthma in mice." *Int Immunopharmacol* 7(12): 1582-7.

West, C. E., D. J. Videky, et al. (2010). "Role of diet in the development of immune tolerance in the context of allergic disease." *Curr Opin Pediatr* 22(5): 635-41.

Willems, L., Li, S., Rutgeerts, O., Lenaerts, C., Waer, M., Billiau, A.D. IL-7 is required for the development of the intrinsic function of marginal zone B cells and the marginal zone microenvirnment. J. Immunol., October 2011; 187 (7); 3587-3594

Zhu, J. and W. E. Paul (2008). "CD4 T cells: fates, functions, and faults." *Blood* 112(5): 1557-69.

Zhu, J., H. Yamane, et al. (2011). "Differentiation of effector CD4 T cell populations (*)." *Annu Rev Immunol* 28: 445-89.

Section 2

Basic of Immunology and Parasite Immunology

4

Toll Like Receptors in Dual Role:
Good Cop and Bad Cop

Saba Tufail*, Ravikant Rajpoot* and Mohammad Owais
Aligarh Muslim University
India

1. Introduction

Every living organism tends to protect itself from harmful effects of pathogens or molecules of pathogenic origin that can disturb its well-being state. The first line of defence that comes into action upon encounter with the pathogen is referred to as innate immune defence mechanism. It had been a matter of great inquisitiveness how innate immune defence mechanism is able to render the body protected against such a diverse variety of pathogens. But with the discovery of germ line encoded pattern recognition receptors (PRRs) that can sense the pathogen associated molecular patterns (PAMPs), it is to an extent possible to answer the query, how innate immune system copes to recognise such a wide variety of micro-organisms and harmful microbial elements. PAMPs are usually of pathogenic origin and absent from the cells of host origin. PRRs can be transmembrane receptors like Toll like receptors (TLRs) (Beutler & Rietschel, 2003; Janeway & Medzhitov, 2002), C-type lectin receptors (CLRs) or these can be cytosolic receptors like Nod like receptors (NLRs) and Rig like helicases (RLRs). Every PRR is capable of recognising specific conserved molecular patterns on the micro-organism and later can start a downstream signalling process upon proper interaction of PAMP and PRR that leads to synthesis of effector molecules like antimicrobial peptides and pro-inflammatory cytokines that prevent the body from otherwise harmful microbes.

In the late 90's a protein was discovered in *Drosophila* named as Toll. Toll is a transmembrane receptor that is required for the establishment of proper dorso-ventral polarity during embryo formation in *Drosophila* (Hashimoto et al., 1988). Mutation in Toll gene results in a weird phenotype of the fruitflies. Later it was found that signalling pathways of *Drosophila* Toll and mammalian IL-1 receptor showed marked resemblance leading to the assumption that Toll may be involved in the regulation of immune responses. Now, it is well established that Toll signalling is required for the defence against Gram-positive, Gram-negative bacterial and fungal infections. Toll is responsible for the production of Drosomycin, antifungal peptide (Lemaitre et al., 1996). Mutants lacking in components of Toll mediated signalling pathway (Toll, Spatzle, Tube, Pelle) are highly susceptible to fungal infections. A year succeeding the discovery of Toll in *Drosophila*, through database searches, Toll homologues in mammals as well were revealed known as

---

* Saba Tufail and Ravikant Rajpoot contributed equally to this work

Toll like receptors (TLRs). TLRs recognise PAMPs of diverse origin from bacteria, virus, fungi, protozoa and others. TLRs can also sense the molecules that are generated within the host cells alarming a sort of danger signal like heat shock proteins (Hsp60, Hsp70, Hsp90), fibrinogen, surfactant protein A, heparin sulphate and others. Thirteen TLRs are reported so far, out of which TLR1 to TLR9 are conserved between human and mice. TLR10 is only functional in human while TLR11 is found to be functional only in mice. Upon interaction with their cognate ligands, TLRs either homodimerise or heterodimerise to further proceed the downstream signalling.

2. Structure of TLRs

Toll like receptors are type-I transmembrane receptors having an extracellular domain containing multiple leucine rich repeats (LRRs). There are about 19-25 tandem repeats of LRR motif each having 20-29 residue sequence motif LXXLXLXXNXLXXLXXXXXXXLXX where X is any amino acid (Bell et al., 2003). LRR motifs are responsible for interacting and recognising specific ligands and thereby initiating downstream signal transduction. LRRs are varied among different TLRs enabling them to sense a wide variety of PAMPs. Interaction of the pathogen with the LRR motif is supposed to take place at the concave side of the horse shoe shaped LRR motif. Mammalian TLRs are found to have homology with IL-1 receptor in cytoplasmic domain known as Toll/IL-1R or TIR domain while extracellular regions are devoid of any homology having three immunoglobulin domains in IL-1R and LRR motifs in TLRs. TIR domain consists of about 200 amino acids (Slack et al., 2000) and is composed of five β strands (βA, βB, βC, βD and βE) alternated with five α helices (αA, αB, αC, αD and αE) (Xu et al., 2000) connected via 8 loops. Box1, Box2 and Box3 are three highly conserved regions found to be present in TIR domain. BB loop is formed when Box2 forms a loop connecting the second β strand and α helix. This BB loop is of primary importance in further downstream signalling because any single amino acid residue substitution in this loop can lead to the complete impairment of its function. In C3H/HeJ mice, a point mutation in BB loop replacing conserved proline leads to hypo-responsiveness to the LPS resulting in loss of function of BB loop (Poltorak et al., 1998).

3. Distribution of TLRs

TLRs are generally expressed on the cells of innate immune system like dendritic cells, monocytes and macrophages (Beutler & Rehli, 2002) that are likely to have interacted with the pathogen earlier. TLR expression is found to be highest on the phagocytic cells like tissue macrophages, neutrophils and dendritic cells. Macrophages express all TLRs except TLR3. However, not all TLRs are expressed by all cell types i.e. TLR expression is tissue specific eg. TLR5 is shown to be exclusively expressed on the intestinal epithelial cells' basolateral surface. Also TLR expression may vary with the maturation stage of the cell, eg. TLR1, 2, 4 and 5 are shown to be expressed on the immature dendritic cells but there expression decreases as the cells undergo maturation. TLR3 is shown to be expressed only on mature dendritic cells. Yet tissue specific demarcation of TLR expression is not clear, it is observed that most of the tissues express atleast one type of TLR. Also TLR expression is found to be different in the two subsets of blood dendritic cells i.e. Myeloid dendritic cells express TLR1, 2, 4, 5 and 8 while plasmacytoid dendritic cell express TLR7 and TLR9 exclusively. TLR2 and 4 are highly expressed on the surface of macrophages but are also reported to be expressed on the endothelial cells, smooth muscle cells, intestinal cells and

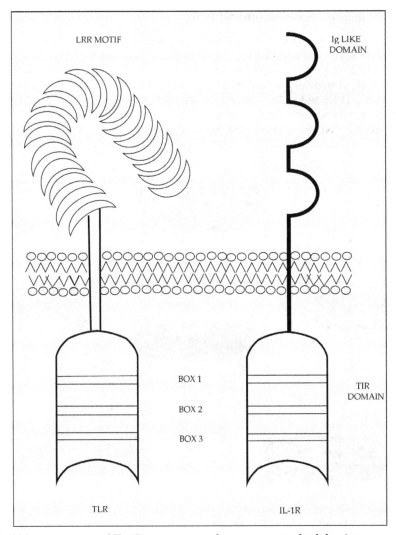

Fig. 1. Toll like receptors and IL-1R are transmembrane receptors both having a conserved region of about 200 amino acids in their cytoplasmic domain known as TIR domain. Three highly conserved regions in TIR domain are referred to as Box1, Box2 and Box3. TLRs and IL-1R though similar in their cytoplasmic domains are markedly different in their extracellular components; TLRs have LRR motif and IL-1R has Ig like domain extracellularly.

others. Studies also indicate subcellular location of TLRs. TLR1, TLR2, TLR4, TLR5 and TLR6 have been found to be expressed on the cell surface, as demonstrated by positive staining of the cell surface by specific antibodies and these recognize bacterial products while TLR3, TLR7, TLR8 and TLR9 have been shown to be expressed in intracellular compartments such as endosomes and recognize microbial nucleic acids (Takeda & Akira, 2005).

4. Phylogenetic relationship among TLRs

A sequence similarity search of different human TLRs revealed that TLRs can be subdivided into five subfamilies i.e. TLR2, TLR3, TLR4, TLR5 and TLR9 subfamilies. While the TLR3, TLR4 and TLR5 are the only respective members of their subfamily, TLR2 subfamily comprises of four members viz. TLR1, TLR2, TLR6 and TLR10; TLR9 family has three members TLR7, TLR8 and TLR9. Members within a subfamily exhibit high ratio of similar sequences than members of other subfamily eg. TLR1 and TLR6 show about 70% similarity in their amino acid sequence, identity approaches about 90% in their TIR domains.

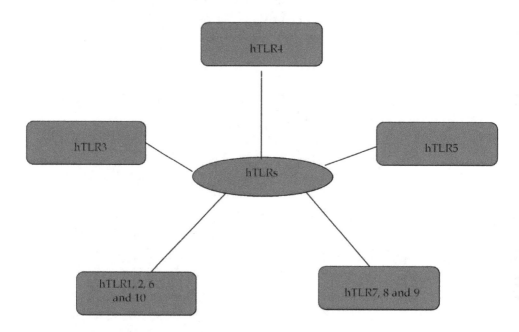

Fig. 2. Human TLRs can be divided into five subfamilies- TLR2, TLR3, TLR4, TLR5 and TLR9. Division is based on the amino acid sequence similarity.

5. Ligands of TLRs

TLRs are able to recognise a wide variety of pathogens and thereafter signal transduction commences that leads to mounting of desirable immune response against the pathogen like expression of inflammatory cytokines, chemokines, antibacterial peptides, enhanced expression of co-stimulatory molecules etc. Generally every TLR recognises more than one type of PAMP e.g. TLR4 (first TLR to be discovered in mammals) has the ability to recognise a variety of PAMPs diverse in nature, for instance it can recognise LPS from bacteria, taxol from plant, different proteins of viral origin, Hsp 60 and 70 from the host cell itself etc. Like TLR4 other TLRs are also able to recognise a wide variety of pathogens which is briefly summarised in Table 1.

TLR	LIGANDS
TLR1	Tri-acyl lipopeptides (bacteria, mycobacteria)
	Soluble factors (Neisseria meningitides)
TLR2	Lipoprotein/lipopeptides (a variety of pathogens)
	Peptidoglycan (Gram-positive bacteria)
	Lipoteichoic acid (Gram-positive bacteria)
	Lipoarabinomannan (mycobacteria)
	A phenol-soluble modulin (Staphylococcus epidermidis)
	Glycoinositolphospholipids (Trypanosoma Cruzi)
	Glycolipids (Treponema maltophilum)
	Porins (Neisseria)
	Zymosan (fungi)
	Atypical LPS (Leptospira interrogans)
	Atypical LPS (Porphyromonas gingivalis)
	HSP70 (host)
TLR3	Double-stranded RNA (virus)
TLR4	LPS (Gram-negative bacteria)
	Taxol (plant)
	Fusion protein (RSV)
	Envelope proteins (MMTV)
	HSP60 (Chlamydia pneumoniae)
	HSP60 (host)
	HSP70 (host)
	Type III repeat extra domain A of fibronectin (host)
	Oligosaccharides of hyaluronic acid (host)
	Polysaccharide fragments of heparan sulfate (host)
	Fibrinogen (host)
TLR5	Flagellin (bacteria)
TLR6	Di-acyl lipopeptides (mycoplasma)
TLR7/8	Imidazoquinoline (synthetic compounds)
	Loxoribine (synthetic compounds)
	Bropirimine (synthetic compounds)
TLR9	CpG DNA (bacteria)
	Hemozoin (protozoa)
TLR10	?
TLR11	Component of uropathogenic bacteria (bacteria)
	Profilin like molecule (protozoa *Toxoplasma gondii*)

Table 1. TLRs and their corresponding ligands.

6. TLRs bridge innate and adaptive immunity

TLRs serve as a link between innate and adaptive immunity by induction of dendritic cell (DC) maturation and directing T helper responses (Parker et al., 2006). It has been reported that stimulation of specific TLRs leads to induction of either IL-10 or IL-12 that results in a response biased towards either Th1 or Th2 cytokines. TLR2 mediated response preferentially leads to release of Th2 cytokines while TLR4 induces Th1 cytokine release. DCs have been reported to express TLRs on their surfaces which respond to different microbial antigens differently. Immature DCs have high phagocytic activity but low T cell activation potential and these are capable of detecting, capturing and phagocytosing pathogens that ultimately leads to activation of TLRs and cytokine release. A signalling cascade commences after TLR activation (as described later) which serves as a complex differentiation programme for DCs, collectively termed DC maturation. This DC maturation is characterised by up-regulation of co-stimulatory molecules such as CD40, CD80, and CD86. CD80 and CD86 are the two requisite signals for naïve T cell activation (Banchereau & Steiman, 1998; Parker et al., 2006).

Also, when TLRs on many cell types are stimulated by TLR agonists, bacteria and viruses, it leads to the production of type I interferon (IFN-α/β) (Parker et al., 2006). This response is popularly attributed to be part of first line of defence against infection and a central modulator of adaptive immunity. Proliferation of memory T cells, inhibition of T cell apoptosis, enhanced IFN-γ secretion, B-cell isotype switching and differentiation into plasma cells and NK cell activation are some of the attributes of IFNs owing to their diverse functions in the development of adaptive immunity.

In addition to up-regulation of CD80/CD86 molecules on DCs and production of type I interferon (IFN-α/β) to control T cell activation, another mechanism of T cell activation exists in which T cell responses are regulated by $CD4^+$ $CD25^+$ suppressor or regulatory T cells (Treg cells). The Treg cells function to induce tolerance in peripheral T cells (both self-reactive and non-self-reactive T cells), a malfunctioning of these cells leads to autoimmune diseases. It has been reported that DCs produce IL-6 in response to TLR activation that is critical for T cell activation as it relieves suppression of effector T cells (non-self-reactive T cells) by Treg cells (Pasare & Metzitov, 2003). Pasare & Metzitov also report that T cell activation occurs even in the absence of IL-6 when Treg cells are removed. This suggests that induction of co-stimulatory molecules on DCs is enough for T cell activation in the absence of Treg cells.

7. TLR signalling

Toll like receptors after recognising PAMPs initiate intracellular signalling that leads to the activation of NF-κB (Nuclear factor kappa B) or IRF3 (Interferon regulating factor 3) and subsequently expression of genes under their control takes place. To induce intracellular signal transduction, TLRs either homodimerise or heterodimerise upon interaction with PAMPs. Probably there are two pathways regarding TLR signal transduction, MyD88 (Myeloid Differentiation Factor 88) dependent and MyD88 independent.

MyD88 dependent signalling pathway is found to be central to all TLRs except TLR3. TIRAP (TIR domain containing adaptor protein) is essential for MyD88 dependent signalling through TLR2 and 4 as revealed by the studies with TIRAP deficient mice.

MyD88 dependent signalling involves a number of molecules which are briefly described below.

MyD88

It is encoded by MyD88 gene (Muzio et al., 1997; Wesche et al., 1997; Burns et al., 1998). This protein is utilised by all TLRs except TLR3 as an adaptor to transmit the signal inside the cell resulting in activation of transcription factor NF-κB. Data indicates that another protein TIRAP also known as MAL (MyD88 adaptor like protein) is required by MyD88 to be recruited to TLR2 and TLR4. MyD88 protein has two domains- N terminal death domain (DD domain) and C terminal TIR domain. It interacts with the TIR domain of TLR via its C terminal TIR domain. MyD88 is also reported to interact with IL-1R, IRAK1, IRAK2, RAC1 (Ras mediated C3 botulinum toxin1) and many other proteins.

IRAK

IRAKs (IL-1R associated protein kinases) are protein kinases that act downstream of MyD88. Four IRAKs are identified in mammals- IRAK1, 2, 4 and M (Janssens & Beyaert, 2003). While IRAK1 and 4 are expressed in all cell types, IRAK2 shows narrower distribution and IRAK M is reported to be only expressed in cells of myeloid origin. IRAKs have an N terminal death domain but lack a TIR domain. But a central serine threonine kinase domain is present. IRAK1 and 4 have intrinsic kinase activity while IRAK2 and M are with no kinase activity.

TRAF

TRAFs (TNF receptor associated factors) are proteins having an N terminal coiled coil domain known as TRAF-N and a conserved C terminal domain known as TRAF- C (Bradley & Pober, 2001). There are six members in the mammalian TRAF family (TRAF1, TRAF2, TRAF3, TRAF4, TRAF5 and TRAF6). Binding of TRAF to its interacting proteins require that proteins should contain TRAF binding motif of which consensus sequence is identified and found to be as Pro-X-Glu-X-X-(aromatic/acidic residue) (Ye et al., 2002). This motif is found to present in CD40, IRAK1, IRAK2, IRAK4, TRANCER (TNF related activation induced cytokine receptor).

TAK1 and TABs

Activation of IKK complex (Inhibitor of NF-KB kinase complex) by TRAF6 requires two factors TRIKA1 (TRAF6 regulated IKK activator1) and TRIKA2 (TRAF6 regulated IKK activator2). Further studies revealed that TRIKA1 is composed of Ubc13 (Ubiquitin conjugating enzyme 13) and Uev1A (Ubiquitin conjugating enzyme variant1) which act as ubiquitin conjugating enzyme complex. Polyubiquitination of TRAF6 is done by TRIKA1 complex with lysine 63 (K63) of ubiquitin. This polyubiquitination directly activates the TAK1 in a proteasome independent manner. TRIKA2 is composed of TAK1, TAB1 and TAB2. TAK1 (TGF-β activated kinase) belongs to a MAPKKK family of protein kinases (Yamaguchi et al., 1995). TABs are TAK1 binding proteins (Shibuya et al., 1996; Takaesu et al., 2000). TAB1 acts as co-activator of TAK1 enhancing its kinase activity while TAB2 has an adaptor function linking TAK1 to TRAF6.

NF-κB

NF-κB (Nuclear factor kappa B) is a transcription factor that controls the expression of genes involved in inflammation, immunity and apoptosis. It was discovered as a transcription factor for the K chains in immunoglobulins. About 100 genes are under the transcriptional control of NF-κB. It belongs to rel family of proteins. NF-κB is an evolutionary conserved protein having five members in mammals- p50, p52, RelA/p65, RelB and RelC. All these function either as homodimer or heterodimer for e.g. p50 homodimer and p50/p65 heterodimer. Their ability to regulate and control transcription also differs markedly, for instance p65 and Rel-C are most potent transcriptional activators while p50 homodimers seem to repress transcription. NF-κB is composed of two subunits p50 and p65. It is bound to an inhibitory protein IκB via non-covalent interaction which hampers its activity. Studies indicate that p50 and p65 dimerise around a 10 base pair region referred to as κB sites. Sequence of this site is 5'GGGRNNYYCC3' where R, Y and N refer to purine, pyrimidine and any base respectively.

7.1 MyD88 dependent signalling pathway

MyD88 is an adaptor protein that is recruited to the TIR domain of TLR upon its activation via C terminal TIR domain. MyD88 also has a death domain at its N terminal end spaced with a short linker sequence from its C terminal. MyD88 then recruits IRAK4 (IL-1R associated protein kinase 4) at its death domain via its N terminal. IRAK4 has N terminal death domain and a central serine/threonine kinase domain that is essentially required for its kinase activity and downstream signalling. This recruitment of IRAK4 to MyD88 induces conformational changes in IRAK4 that allows the interaction of IRAK1 with it and then IRAK4 acts on IRAK1 to phosphorylate it. Also upon activation, IRAK1 starts auto-phosphorylating itself (Takeda & Akira, 2005). To this assembly, TRAF6 (TNF receptor associated factor 6) further associates via phosphorylated IRAK1. TRAF6 acts as a signalling mediator for both IL-1R/TLR superfamily and TNF receptor superfamily. Association of TRAF6 with phosphorylated IRAK1 leads to the dissociation of both these mediators from the assembly and binding to TAK1 (Transforming growth factor β activated kinase), TAB1(TAK1 binding protein 1) and TAB2 (TAK1 binding protein 2). TAK1 belongs to MAPKKK (Mitogen activated protein kinase kinase kinase) family. TAB1 acts as an activator of TAK1 while TAB2 functions as an adaptor molecule linking TAK1 to TRAF6. Recently, another TAK1 binding protein, TAB3 came into being and might function similar to TAB2. This causes phosphorylation of TAB2 & TAK1 and degradation of IRAK1. This remaining complex i.e. TAK1, TAB1, TAB2 and TRAF6 now gets associated with ubiquitin ligase UBC13 (Ubiquitin conjugating enzyme 13) and UEV 1A (Ubiquitin conjugating enzyme E2 variant 1). This leads to activation of TRAF6 which in turn activates TAK1. TAK1 activation takes place through linkage of a lysine63 linked polyubiquitin chain via TRAF6-UBC13 complex where TRAF6 acts as an E3 Ubiquitin ligase (Wang et al., 2001). Activated TAK1 is responsible for the phosphorylation of MAPK and IKK complex (Inhibitor of NF-κB (IκB) kinase complex). IKK has three subunits, IKK1 or IKKα, IKK2 or IKKβ and IKKγ or NEMO (NF-κB essential modulator) (Karin & Ben-Neriah, 2000). This kinase complex phosphorylates IκB at conserved serine residues in N terminal which mark it for ubiquitination and its subsequent degradation via proteasome. Removal of inhibitor from NF-κB leads to its activation and translocation from cytosol to nucleus where it binds to NF-κB binding regions (present in the genes under the control of NF-κB transcriptional activation) and induce the transcription of genes responsible for synthesis of effector molecules that act against the invading pathogen or PAMPs and lead to their destruction.

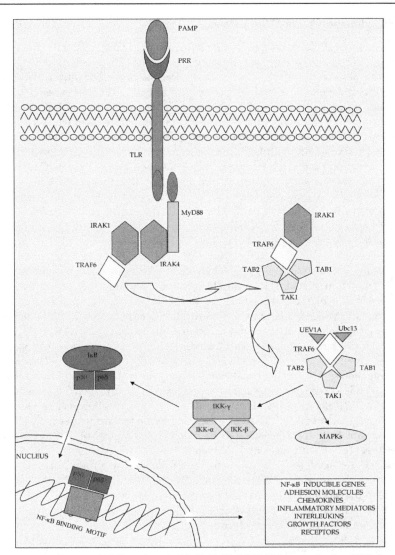

Fig. 3. Upon stimulation of TLR with suitable PAMP, MyD88 is recruited to TIR domain of TLR. IRAK4 then associates with MyD88. This causes IRAK1 to attach with IRAK4 which causes its phosphorylation. TRAF6 then joins this complex and thereafter causes IRAK1 to dissociate from IRAK4 along with it. Later TRAF6 and IRAK1 bind to TAK1, TAB1 and TAB2. Later IRAK1 is degraded and remaining complex joins Ubc13 and Uev1A which causes polyubiquitination of TRAF6 and activates TAK1 in a proteasome independent manner. Activated TAK1 phosphorylates both MAPK and IKK complex. IKK complex phosphorylates IκB that leads to its ubiquitination and then degradation in proteasome. Release of IκB from NF-κB activates it which then translocates into the nucleus and causes the expression of genes which are under its transcriptional control including genes involved in apoptosis, inflammation and immunity.

7.2 MyD88 independent signalling pathway

Studies have revealed that upon stimulation with LPS in MyD88 deficient cells, there is still production of NF-κB, although the production is delayed. This leads to the fact that TLR signalling can also occur in the absence of MyD88 i.e. independently of MyD88. TLR3 utilizes MyD88 independent signalling pathway to activate IRF3 that is responsible for the up-regulation of interferon (IFN) inducible genes and the production of IFN-β. This MyD88 independent signalling pathway utilizes another adaptor molecule known as TRIF/TICAM1 (TIR domain containing adaptor protein inducing IFN-β/ TIR domain containing molecule 1). TRIF has TRAF6 binding motifs (T6BM) in its N terminal and a TIR domain and RHIM (Receptor interacting protein 1 homotypic interaction motif) domain at its C terminal. TRIF is the only molecule meant to be involved in signalling through TLR3. Studies with TRIF deficient mice showed impaired response in activation of IRF3 and expression of IFN inducible genes only with ligands of TLR3 and TLR4 (Hoebe et al.,2003). IRF3, 5 and 7 play important roles in expression of IFN inducible genes during viral infection. IRF3 is typically required for the expression of genes encoding IFN-β and genes under the control of other interferons (Yoneyema et al., 1998). Upon activation of TLR3 with its ligand, TRIF is recruited to the TIR domain of TLR3. Then TRIF associates at its N terminus via two molecules- TRAF6 and TBK1 (TRAF family member associated NF- κB activator (TANK) binding kinase 1). TBK1 is responsible for phosphorylating the IRF3 at its C terminal regulatory domain which leads to their dimerization (Sharma et al., 2003). Dimers are then able to translocate into the nucleus and associate with co-activators p300 and CBP(cAMP responsive element binding protein).This then causes the expression of genes encoding IFN-β and other TypeI interferons (Taniguchi & Takaoka, 2002). These TypeI interferons via JAK-STAT signalling pathway are capable of inducing the expression of IFN inducible genes like GARG16 (Glucocorticoid attenuated responsive gene 16), IPG1(Immunoresponsive gene1) and CXCL10 etc. Also, IRF7 is produced later in viral infections via interferons whose expression is regulated by IRF3. TRAF6, another molecule that associates with TRIF at its N terminal is meant to activate NF-κB. TRAF6 binds to N terminal of TRIF via its TRAF-C. TRIF has three T6BM with consensus sequence Pro-X-Glu-X-X-(aromatic/acidic residue). Also, to the C terminal of TRIF, RIP1 (Receptor interacting protein 1) binds which is discovered recently and also found to activate NF- κB (Meylan et al., 2004). Activated NF-κB then is able to translocate and causes the expression of genes under its control. It has been found that transcriptional activation of IFN-β encoding gene needs both NF-κB and IRF3. However, inflammatory cytokine production still remains impaired.

Search for adaptors containing TIR domain led to the discovery of a new adaptor molecule known as TRAM/TICAM2 (TRIF related adaptor molecule/TIR domain containing molecule2) (Bin et al., 2003). Studies with TRAM deficient mice revealed that TRAM is involved in signalling through TLR4 in a MyD88 independent/TRIF dependent manner (Yamamoto et al., 2003). TRAM has a TIR domain in the C terminal and it acts upstream of TRIF while mediating TLR4 signalling exclusively. Studies showed that siRNA mediated inhibition of TRAM expression causes impairment of IRF3 activation and expression of IFN inducible genes only in response to TLR4 ligand, eg. LPS. However, TRAM knockout mice shows normal activation of IRF3 and expression of IFN inducible genes in response to TLR3 activation. Hence, TRAM is only involved in signalling through TLR4 but not TLR3. MyD88 deficient macrophages when stimulated with LPS show activation of IRF3 and also production of NF-κB, although production is delayed. Also, the production of inflammatory cytokines is impaired in these cells. Studies with TRIF and TRAM deficient mice showed that for the production of inflammatory cytokines via TLR4, activation of both the signalling pathways is required i.e. MyD88 dependent and independent, although the mechanism is not clear. However, the production is not affected via MyD88 dependent pathway in response to ligands of TLR2, 7 and 9. Another adaptor that is involved in signalling via TLR4 is TIRAP/MAL (TIR domain containing adaptor protein/MyD88 adaptor like protein) (Horngs et al., 2001). TIRAP deficient mice show impaired production of inflammatory cytokines in response to TLR2 and 4 ligands but not to TLR3, 5, 7 and 9 ligands. This confirms its role in signalling through TLR2 and 4. TIRAP deficient mice also show IRF3 activation and production of late phase NF-κB as seen in the studies with MyD88 deficient mice. TIRAP has a C terminal TIR domain but it lacks a death domain that is present in MyD88. It acts upstream of MyD88.

LPS signalling through TLR4 is mediated with the help of several other proteins eg. MD-2 is a novel protein that mediates the TLR4 signalling in response to LPS. MD2 functions to bind LPS and then presents this LPS to TLR4 via physically interacting with it. MD2 is found to attach with TLR4 extracellular domain. Also, another protein CD14 is found to facilitate LPS signalling via TLR4. CD14 along with LBP (LPS binding protein) binds to LPS (Wright et al., 1990) and can initiate signalling via transmembrane receptors like TLR4.

7.2.1 Genes under transcriptional control of NF-κB

NF-κB is crucial for the expression of genes which are involved in immune responses (both innate and adaptive), inflammation, viral infection, stress, cytokine signalling, acute phase responses etc. Genes under the regulation of NF-κB have NF-κB binding sites in their promoter region. Adhesion molecules like ICAM-1, VCAM-1, E-selectins are expressed as a result of NF-κB transcriptional activation. ICAM-1/CD54 (Intercellular adhesion molecule -1) is expressed on endothelial and immune system cells. ICAM-1 expression upon required stimulus is enhanced via NF-κB activity. ICAM-1 binds to LFA1 (Lymphocyte function-associated antigen1), a receptor on leukocytes. Leukocytes adhere and then migrate into the tissues via ICAM-1 and LFA-1 interaction and carry out the required actions. VCAM-1(Vascular cell adhesion protein-1) is present in the endothelial cells and function to adhere lymphocytes, basophils, monocytes etc. to vascular endothelium. E-selectin/CD62E/ELAM-1(Endothelial leukocyte adhesion molecule-1) is expressed on vascular endothelium in response to TNF-α and IL-1β. It binds to carbohydrate moieties on some leukocytes. Genes expressing growth factors are also up-regulated by NF-κB like genes for GM-CSF (Granulocyte macrophage colony stimulating factor), M-CSF/CSF1 (Macrophage colony stimulating factor/ Colony stimulating factor3) and G-CSF(Granulocyte colony stimulating factor/ Colony stimulating factor 3). GM-CSF is a cytokine that stimulates stem cells to differentiate into neutrophils, eosinophils, basophils, granulocytes and monocytes. M-CSF is also a cytokine that stimulates stem cells to differentiate into macrophages and related cell types. G-CSF acts on bone marrow to form more of granulocytes and stem cells. Various chemokine genes also show enhanced expression in response to NF-κB like genes for Eotaxin, RANTES (Regulated upon activation, normal T cell expressed and secreted), MIP 1α (Macrophage inflammatory protein 1 α) etc. Eotaxin is a chemokine that recruits eosinophils while RANTES is a chemoattractor for T cells, K cells, eosinophils, dendritic cells and is also responsible for recruiting leukocytes at inflammatory sites. Several cell surface receptor genes are up-regulated eg. CCR5 (C-C chemokine receptor

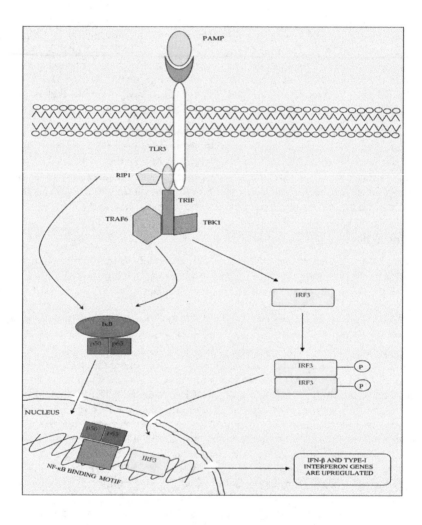

Fig. 4. TLR3 recruits TRIF upon stimulation with its ligand. To N terminal of TRIF, TBK1 associates which carries out later phosphorylation of IRF3. Upon phosphorylation, IRF3 forms dimer and translocates into nucleus and causes the expression of genes of IFN-β and Type I interferons. Also, to the N terminal of TRIF, TRAF6 binds which activates NF-κB which is then able to translocate and causes the transcription of genes under its control. Genes encoding IFN-β require activation of both NF-κB and IRF3.

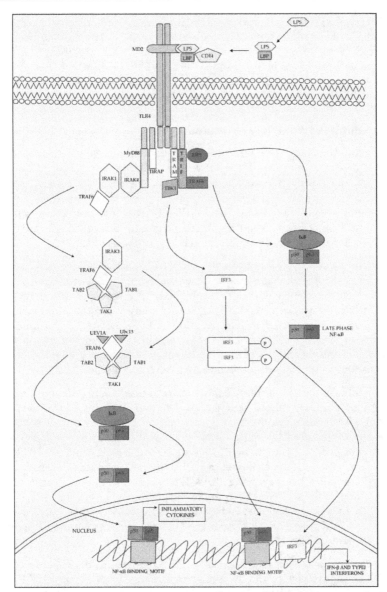

Fig. 5. Response to LPS is mediated through TLR4; LPS binds to LBP, and then forms a complex with CD14. This complex interacts with MD-2 which is able to interact physically with TLR4. Signalling downstream afterwards proceeds either via MyD88 dependant or MyD88 independent pathway. In MyD88 dependant pathway, NFκB is activated which induces transcription of several genes including genes of inflammatory cytokines. On the other hand, in TIRAP and MyD88 knockout mice, activation of IRF3 and late phase NFκB takes place both of which are able to initiate transcription of the genes under their respective control.

type 5), CD86, TCR(T cell receptor), MHC class I & II, PAF(Platelet activating factor) receptor. Enhanced expression of MHC molecules and TCR means to up-regulate T cell activation and hence adaptive immunity. CD80 and CD86 are the major T cell co-stimulatory molecules. CCR5 is the receptor for RANTES, MIP 1α and 1β. Cytokine IL-1β, IL-2, IL-6 and TNFα show enhanced expression after NF-κB activation. NF-κB dependent stimulation of iNOS promoters also takes place.

8. TLR signalling is negatively regulated

Docking of pathogen onto TLRs and their subsequent stimulation induces production of inflammatory cytokines such as TNF-a, IL-6 and IL-12. An uncontrolled and excessive cytokine production can lead to manifestation of serious autoimmune and inflammatory diseases. Hence, to avoid an excessive inflammatory response, organisms have evolved mechanisms which make a balance between TLR activation and inactivation. Several molecules modulating TLR-mediated responses have been unravelled. Negative regulators of TLRs can either be extracellular or intracellular (Arancibia et al., 2007).

Extracellular regulators comprise of soluble form of TLRs. Soluble form of TLR2, sTLR2, is produced by a post-translational modification of the membrane bound TLR2. It is reported that if sTLR2 splice variant expression is inhibited, an augmented response to bacterial lipopeptide is seen (Lebouder et al., 2003). Alternate splice variant of TLR4 (soluble TLR4), sTLR4, is shown to be involved in the inhibition of LPS-mediated TNFα production and NFκB activation, blocking MD-2 (a co-receptor of TLR4) recruitment to the TLR4-CD14 complex. Also, soluble product of TLR5, sTLR5, is seen to be implicated in cellular response of flagellin that induces an increased NF-κB activation by an unknown cellular mechanism.

A variety of intracellular molecules (adaptors and kinases) are found to regulate TLR signalling. An alternatively spliced variant of MyD88 that lacks the intermediary domain of MyD88 (MyD88s) is induced in monocytes upon LPS stimulation. Overexpression of MyD88s results in impaired LPS-induced NF-κB activation through inhibition of IRAK-4-mediated IRAK-1 phosphorylation. IRAK-M is another negative regulator of TLR signalling cascade and it lacks catalytic kinase activity. IRAK-M inhibits expression of pro-inflammatory cytokines by preventing IRAK-1/IRAK-4 dissociation from MyD88, hence causing inhibition of IRAK-1-TRAF6 complex formation. The fact that IRAK-M plays a crucial role in regulating MyD-88 dependant signalling pathway can be established from the information that IRAK-M-/- mice overproduce inflammatory cytokines in response to LPS and CpG DNA (Arancibia et al., 2007).

A protein associated with Toll-Like Receptor 4 (PRAT4A) regulates cell surface expression of TLR4. PRAT4A is associated with the immature form of TLR4 but not with MD-2 (a TLR4 co-receptor) or TLR2. PRAT4A knockdown led to the profound defect in LPS responsiveness in a cell line expressing TLR4/MD-2, probably due to impaired maturation of TLR4, leading to the lack of mature TLR4/MD-2 on the cell surface. PRAT4A is likely to be a component of the machinery facilitating TLR4/MD-2 trafficking to the cell surface. Hence, PRAT4A is another negative regulator of TLR4.

SOCS1 and SOCS3 belong to SOCS (Suppressor of cytokine signaling) family of proteins. These proteins themselves induced by cytokines, negatively regulate TLR4/NFκB signalling pathways (Gingras et al. 2004). In SOCS 1-/- mice defective induction of LPS tolerance was observed as they were found to be hypersensitive to LPS-endotoxin. In the same manner, LPS induced TNF-α production was found to be suppressed in macrophages exposed to IL-10 and IL-6 isolated from SOCS3-/-(Arancibia et al., 2007).

PI3K, implicated in TLR signalling, has been found to suppress both MAPKs and NFκB induced by LPS, thereby decreasing TNF-α production (Arancibia et al., 2007). Tollip (Toll interacting protein) has also been found to play an inhibitory role in TLR signalling. Tollip when in association with TIR domain decreases IRAK-1 phosphorylation upon LPS activation. A plausible role of PI3K in regulating inhibitory effects of Tollip has been proposed. PI3K does that by interacting with 3′ phosphorylated phosphatidylinositides (Arancibia et al., 2007).

SIGIRR (single immunoglobulin IL-1 receptor-related molecule) and T1/ST2, membrane bound proteins adhered to the TIR domain, have also been found to be negative regulators of TLR signalling (Takeda & Akira, 2005). Nucleotide oligomerization domain receptor (NOD2), a mammalian PRR, too seems to be a negative regulator as NOD2-/- macrophages when stimulated by TLR agonists produce significantly higher amount of cytokines but on restoration of NOD phenotype, cytokine expression is lowered (Arancibia et al., 2007).

Activating Transcription Factor-3 (ATF-3) has also been found to negatively regulate TLR-signalling pathways (Whitmore et al., 2007). It has been observed that different TLR ligands (i.e., zymosan for TLR2/3, pIC for TLR3, LPS for TLR4, and CpG-ODN for TLR9) stimulate rapid induction of ATF3 in cultured mouse macrophages. It is reported that primary macrophages of mice lacking atf3 gene (ATF3-knockout (KO)) show enhanced expression of TLR-induced IL-12 and IL-6 when compared to wild type macrophages. In a reporter assay, ectopic expression of ATF3 was found to antagonize TLR-stimulated IL-12p40 activation. Further, CpG oligodeoxynucleotide, a TLR9 agonist when introduced in ATF3-KO mice resulted in enhanced cytokine production from splenocytes. Hence, it can be concluded that atf3 deficiency leads to altered pattern of immunological response and ATF-3 is a negative regulator of TLR pathways.

In addition to these, degradation of TLRs (either ubiquitination mediated or lysosomal) is also proposed as a mechanism for negatively regulating TLR signaling (Takeda & Akira, 2005; Wang et. al., 2007). A RING finger protein, Triad3A, has been found to act as an E3 ubiquitin ligase, ligating ubiquitin molecules onto the TLR4 and TLR9 and enhancing their proteolytic degradation. A recent study by Wang et. al. (Wang et. al., 2007) reveals another mechanism of negative regulation of TLR4 signalling, by lysosomal degradation of TLRs. They propose that Rab7b, a lysosome associated small GTPase negatively regulates NF-κB and IRF3 signalling pathways in macrophages by promoting lysosomal degradation of TLR4 and decreasing the cell surface expression of TLR4. These complex mechanisms of negative regulation of TLRs emphasize that it is important for prevention of uncontrolled immune activation in the host.

9. TLRs in various diseases

9.1 TLRs in nervous system diseases

TLRs have been considered earlier as receptors expressed solely on antigen presenting cells of the immune system i.e. B cells, dendritic cells, monocytes, macrophages etc. and mediate innate immunity. However, with advancement in techniques, it is clear that nearly all cells within the body express TLRs, including different brain cell types such as microglial cells, astrocytes, oligodendrocytes and neurons within the CNS (Central Nervous System). The present section will focus the role of TLRs in these brain cells.

Microglia

Microglial cells are bone marrow-derived macrophage-like cells constituting about 10% of the adult CNS and mediate neuronal immune interactions under both physiological and pathological conditions (Pessac et al., 2001). Microglial cells are the key defence against invading pathogens within the CNS, and it is not surprising, therefore, that activation of these cells either by a single type of ligand or a combination of ligands, leads to secretion of a milieu of cytokines and chemokines. It is now well known that microglial cells express wide receptors of TLRs in addition to their adapter proteins, required for functional downstream TLR signalling. Recent studies showed that TLR1-9 are expressed in microglia (Jack et al., 2005). Upon activation, TLR mRNA and protein expression is increased in microglia. As a result of TLR activation, these cells secrete higher amounts of pro-inflammatory cytokines and hence show pathogen specific responses. TLR signalling in microglia may also have a role in cell death and survival following inflammatory activation which suggests a paradigm in which auto-regulation of the innate immune system exists in the CNS which helps to prevent excessive inflammation during pathogen infection (Jack et al., 2007; Tanaka et al., 2008; Okun et al., 2009).

Astrocytes

Astrocytes are characteristic star-shaped glial cells in the brain and spinal cord and perform many functions, including biochemical support to endothelial cells that form the blood–brain barrier provision of nutrients to the nervous tissue, maintenance of extracellular ion balance, and a role in the repair and scarring process of the brain and spinal cord following traumatic injuries. Similar to microglial cells, astrocytes exhibit a wide expression of TLRs. Astrocytes express robust TLR 3 with low expression of TLR 1, TLR4, TLR5 and TLR9, and with rare expression of TLR2, TLR6, TLR7, TLR8 and TLR10. Several cytokines and chemokines are reportedly produced following TLR activation in astrocytes. TLR 3 signalling induces strongest pro-inflammation polarizing response by secreting increased levels of IL-12, TNF-alpha, IL-6, CXCL-10, IFN-beta and IL-10 (Jack et al., 2005). Both cytokines and TLR agonists induce expression of chemokine ligands i.e. CCL2, CCL3, CCL5, ICAM-1 and vascular cell adhesion molecule-1 (VCAM-1) (Carpentier et al., 2005 ; Okun et al., 2009).

Oligodendrocytes

Oligodendrocytes are a type of neuroglia and function as an insulation of axons in the CNS. As compared to other CNS cell types, very little is known regarding the expression and function of TLRs in oligodendrocytes. The first report on TLRs in these cells has shown the predominant expression of TLR2 and 3 as evidenced by promotion of survival, differentiation, and myelin-like membrane formation and induction of apoptosis by TLR2 agonist, zymosan and TLR3 agonist, poly-I:C respectively (Bsibsi et al., 2002). While the exact role of TLR2 in oligodendrocytes is unknown, *in vivo* evidences suggest that activation of this receptor is involved in CNS repair by enhancing myelination of neurons in the CNS and damage repair after spinal cord injury (Okun et al., 2009).

Neurons

Neurons are the core components of the CNS which processes and transmits information by electrical and chemical signalling. During the past few years, evidence for the neuronal expression of TLRs has increased, suggesting a role for this receptor family in neurons during physiological as well as pathological conditions. The expression of the mRNA for TLRs1-9 as well as protein levels of TLR 2, 3 and 4 has been shown *in vivo* following infection in a parasitic model of neurocysticercosis (Tang et al., 2007). Studies provide evidence that neurons from both the central and peripheral nervous systems express TLR3 and that it is concentrated at the growth cones of neurons. In addition to TLR expression in brain diseases, it is known that neuronal TLR activation plays a role in development. It has been reported recently that treatment of cultured embryonic cortical neurospheres with a TLR3 ligand significantly reduced proliferating (BrdU-labeled) cells and neurosphere formation, whereas neural progenitor cells (NPC) from TLR3-deficient embryos formed greater numbers of neurospheres compared to neurospheres from wild-type embryos (Okun et al., 2009). A distinct difference is apparent between the effects of TLR activation in differentiated neurons and neuronal progenitor cells. Apart from the classical TLR ligands such as LPS (TLR4) or Pam3CSK4 (TLR2), it is considered that neuronal TLRs respond to endogenous ligands but not to pathogen-derived ligands (Okun et al., 2009).

9.1.1 TLRs in neurodegeneration

TLRs generally respond against invading pathogens, however, they can also be activated in the absence of microbial infection and regulate neurogenesis. Studies examining inflammatory markers in normal brain aging have also suggested a dynamic regulation of TLRs and hence, showed its participation in aging and age-related disease. Despite the emerging role of TLRs in stokes, AD (Alzheimer's disease) and MS (Multiple sclerosis), very little is known regarding the function of these receptors in other neurodegenerative disorders. In this context, the role of TLRs in brain diseases such as, Alzheimer's disease, multiple sclerosis and other neurodegenerative conditions is discussed herewith.

9.1.2 TLRs in Alzheimer's disease

Alzheimer's disease (AD) is a progressive neurodegenerative disease characterized by gradual onset and advancement of memory loss and other cognitive deficits. Definitive diagnosis of AD is based on the presence of extracellular amyloid plaques comprised of neurotoxic amyloid β-peptide (Aβ) which is generated by proteolysis of the β-amyloid precursor protein (APP), and intracellular neurofibrillary tangles composed of hyper-phosphorylated insoluble forms of *tau* protein. TLR expression is up-regulated and increased in the AD brain. A screening of TLRs in murine models of AD revealed an up-regulation of TLR2 and TLR7 transcription levels compared to wild-type controls. Further, multiple TLR genes (1-8) are expressed in microglia in post-mortem tissue from AD patients, with varying levels of expression. The increased expression of TLRs in AD positions them as potential players in neurodegenerative mechanisms and disease progression. The TLR4 gene has emerged as a candidate susceptibility gene for AD. A common missense polymorphism occurs at the TLR4 gene locus resulting from an adenine to guanine substitution 896 nucleotides downstream of the transcription start site. This substitution causes the replacement of glycine for aspartic acid at amino acid 299 (Asp299Gly), and alters the structure of the extracellular domain of TLR4. This mutation attenuates TLR4 signalling in response to LPS and diminishes the ability to induce inflammation (Arbour et al, 2000). In AD brain, activated glia expressing high levels of TLR4 and TLR2 surround Aβ plaques. The close association between Aβ plaques and reactive astrocytes and microglia has led to the assertion that these cells contribute to plaque formation (Walter et al., 2007). TLR4 expression increases during exposure to Aβ and the lipid peroxidation product 4-hydroxy-nonenal (HNE). Further, c-Jun N-terminal kinases (JNK) and caspase-3 activity levels are augmented in neurons exposed to Aβ and HNE. Selective elimination of TLR4 function significantly suppresses the abilities of Aβ and HNE to induce activation of JNK and caspase-3 (Tang et al., 2007) suggesting that TLR4 expression increases neuronal vulnerability to Aβ-induced damage (Okun et al., 2009). Neurons expressing TLR4 have increased sensitivity to Aβ and are vulnerable to degeneration in AD. In addition to epidemiological studies that suggest mutations in TLR4 lead to decreased susceptibility to neurodegeneration, several data indicate that activation of TLR4 is required for clearance of Aβ in AD. In addition to TLR4, activation of other TLRs may also contribute to Aβ clearance. Whereas TLRs are activated by exogenous pathogens, mounting evidence indicates that Aβ itself activates TLRs and mediates microglial activation. At present, it still remains to be determined if the activation of TLRs by Aβ contributes to and/or inhibits AD progression. Contrasting data exist on the precise role of TLRs in Aβ deposition. Therefore, there may be a balance of TLR activation in which mild activation is beneficial, promoting Aβ uptake and breakdown. However, excessive activation of TLRs on microglia may lead to the accumulation of cytotoxic compounds such as reactive oxygen species, cytokines, complements and proteases causing damage and eventual neuronal loss. TLR signalling pathways are a potential therapeutic target in AD; however more work remains to delineate the complex interaction of TLRs in Aβ deposition and clearance and its precise role in AD development (Okun et al., 2009; Akiyama et al., 2000).

9.1.3 TLRs in Multiple Sclerosis

Multiple Sclerosis (MS) is a chronic inflammatory and demyelinating disease of the CNS and characterized by recurrent neurological dysfunction. It is believed to be an immune-mediated disease in which auto-reactive T cells enter the CNS and drive a pro-inflammatory reaction resulting in tissue injury after infection. There is a marked increase in TLR expression in multiple sclerosis lesions. Microglial cells from MS patients express TLRs 1-8, while, healthy white matter from patients does not contain TLRs. Examination of TLR3 and TLR4 localization revealed that early active MS lesions are associated with vesicular localization of TLR3 and TLR4 within microglia, located near blood vessels at the outer edges of lesions. In contrast, late active lesions also contain astrocytes bearing surface TLR3 and TLR4. This suggests that early lesions are characterized by microglia infiltration, while astrocytes are also active in later MS lesions. Researchers showed that TLR expression is up-regulated in the brain and spinal cord in animal models of MS. The exact role and mechanism of TLRs and its activation in these lesions is still unclear. One hypothesis asserts that in response to pro-inflammatory cytokines, microglial cells are capable of serving as antigen-presenting cells which can activate CD4+ T cells and facilitate neuroinflammation. Therefore, TLR activation may be an essential step in converting microglia to antigen presenting cells and facilitate T cell infiltration of MS lesions. Alternatively, TLRs may induce production of pro-inflammatory cytokines and thereby inflict damage. It can also happen that endogenous ligands like ganglioside and sialic acid containing glycosphingolipids released from apoptotic neurons may bind to TLR4 present on microglia and activate it resulting in either neurodegeneration by releasing pro-inflammatory molecules or provide neuroprotection by attracting oligodendrocyte progenitor cells to lesion sites in MS to promote remyelination. Although TLRs often recognize pathogen-associated molecular patterns and protect the body from invasion of microbial pathogens, the expression of TLRs within multiple sclerosis suggests novel roles for these receptors in mediating neurological disease and hence can be used as a biomarker of the neurodegenerative disorders (Okun et al., 2009). Moreover, it is important to determine the precise role of distinct TLRs in Aβ recognition and clearance, and the activation of glial cells. This may open a window of hope (Arroyo et al, 2011).

9.1.4 Therapeutic approaches

TLRs are not only activated in response to microbial infection, but are critically involved in mediating neurological dysfunction. The extensive involvement of TLRs in neurodegenerative disorders provides wide opportunity for promoting and inhibiting their signalling to intervene the progression of the disease. However, it may be difficult to achieve the correct balance and appropriate timing of such interventions. There is huge variation in the TLR expression and hence the modifications will be varied across different disorders and there may exist variability within patients of the same disease. Proper TLR targeting will require extensive understanding of the pathways, mechanism activated, cell-specific responses and the course of disease progression. Both human and animal studies implicating TLRs in neural degeneration suggest direct modulation of TLR signalling as an ideal therapy. Specific strategies are necessary to circumvent this barrier and allow administration of TLR treatments to the CNS. Targeting TLRs in neurological disease will not be without difficulties. One potential obstacle to targeting TLR signalling in disease is that virtually all cells in the body express TLRs. If chronic administration of TLR agonists is necessary, it may result in overstimulation of the immune system, which limits dosage capability as well as frequency of application. CNS- specific isoforms of TLR agonists which possess high selectivity could prevent such overstimulation of peripheral immune responses. In addition, partial agonists may be useful in preventing overstimulation of TLRs in the same tissues. Another potential hurdle to TLR- directed therapeutics is cross-talk between receptor subtypes. Alternatively, specific TLR activation can induce tolerance to stimulation for other TLRs sharing same cascade. Therefore, the consequences of targeted TLR stimulation on similar signalling pathways must be carefully considered while adapting the therapeutic approaches (Okun et al., 2009).

9.2 TLRs in cancer and anti-cancer immunotherapy

Tumour cells in order to survive try to modulate their microenvironment by providing signals for uncontrolled growth, anti-apoptosis, angiogenesis and metastasis. Despite all these efforts tumour cells get noticed by the immune system which treat cancer cells as foreign. The studies have shown that tumour cells have devised sets of strategies to escape the surveillance by immune system. TLRs were earlier thought associated only with immune cells but recent findings have suggested that tumour cells too have TLRs on their surface and may play important role in tumour growth and immune surveillance escape.

The tumour cells are able to escape the immune surveillance probably by inhibitory cytokines, inflammatory factors, proteinases, and other small molecules such as nitric oxide, IL-6 and IL-12. These molecules in conjugation with TLRs may play role in development of cancer by providing resistance to tumour cells to apoptosis and immune surveillance. It has been seen that upon activation of TLR4, level of X-linked inhibitor of apoptosis and phosphorylated Akt (Protein Kinase B, PKB) are increased. Apoptosis inhibition has been seen as the case also in lymphoma and lung cancer cells. Previous studies have given evidence in support of LPS as tumour growth promoter through the NF-κB resulting in up-regulation of iNOS and MMP2 and the β1 integrin subunit (Harmey et al, 2002; Wang et al, 2003). Apart from microbial origin ligands for TLRs, the source of endogenous ligands which may promote tumour growth is not clear. The answer to the endogenous source of ligands may not only provide some insight to tumour growth but may also help to understand autoimmune diseases. It has been proposed that the TLR-4-MyD88 signalling pathway may be a risk factor for developing cancer and may represent a novel target for the development of bio-modulators. Heat shock proteins such as Hsp60, Hsp70 and Hsp90 may induce the production of pro-inflammatory cytokines such as TNF-α, IL-1, IL-6 and IL-12, release of NO and chemokines by monocytes, macrophages and dendritic cells (Neill., 2008; Asea et al., 2000; Kol et al., 2000; Singh-Jasuja et al., 2000) . There are strong possibilities of Hsp60, Hsp70 and Hsp90 being putative endogenous ligands for TLR4. Ulcerative colitis, a chronic inflammatory disease of the colon may put an individual at risk of colorectal carcinoma. Chronic hepatitis and cirrhosis, pose a risk for the development of hepatocellular carcinoma. Research in the past few years have given strong evidence that an inflammatory profile of cytokines and chemokines persisting at a particular site would lead to the development of a chronic disease. The innate immune system may give in to the promotion of tumour growth through inflammation-dependent mechanisms. Recognition of molecules either of viral or bacterial origin bearing molecular signature or pattern by TLRs on immune cells may induce an inflammatory response associated with tumour promotion. It has been observed that bacterial infection post-surgery may promote metastasis of previously dormant tumour, and LPS have implicated in leading to this situation (Hsu et al, 2011). The MyD88-independent TLR signalling involves the activation of the late phase of NF-κB in addition to the activation of IFN regulatory factor 3, which ultimately leads to the production of type I IFN (IFN a/h), IFN-inducible gene products, and an immune regulatory response. Activated TLRs on the surface of tumour cells not only promote their own proliferation but also help to build resistance to apoptosis. Further, rouge TLRs may enhance tumour cell invasion and metastasis by regulating metalloproteinases and integrins. Moreover, the control of TLRs may also lie beyond the traditional boundaries of protein molecules into world of miRNA, and their role is still being uncovered. In fact, the discovery of miRNAs has indeed brought a paradigm shift in our understanding towards the eukaryotic gene regulation. Their uniqueness lies in the fact that these molecules show cell or tissue specific expression. In principle, the miRNAs fine tune the gene expression, and similar to the classical oncogenes and tumour suppressor genes, miRNA may play part in promotion or suppression of malignancies. They act mainly by inhibiting the translation or by promoting the degradation of mRNA. For example, miRNAs like miR-146, which targets two proteins involved in TLR signalling, TRAF6 and IRAK1, negatively regulates mRNAs of both TRAF6 and IRAK1 proteins whereas its own level gets up-regulated in response to LPS. Another miRNA, miR-155 targets Src domain containing inositol 5-phophate 1(SHIP-1) and negatively regulates NF-κB signalling. Owing to their role of fine tuner of gene expression pattern, the administration of single miRNA may affect the expression pattern of the target gene. Despite some apprehensions over the safety and efficacy of miRNA based therapies, a judicial extrapolation to TLR regulated miRNAs may provide some therapeutic solution. Also the role of innate immune system in cancer development is being looked into more seriously.

TLRs, tumour cells and Treg cells have been linked. TLR agonists can induce differentiation, proliferation or activation of Treg cells. Several TLR agonists such as Streptococcal agent OK-432, double stranded RNA and CpG DNA have anti-tumour activity (Chen & Oppenheim, 2009). TLR agonists overcome tolerance to self-antigens or tumour-antigens by directly or indirectly relieving suppression of effector T cells by Treg cells. A TLR2 agonist has been reported to transiently suppress FoxP3 (a member of forkhead/winged helix family of transcription factors and a master regulator of Treg development) expression and render resistance to suppression by Treg cells of CD4+CD25+ effector T cells. Treg cells express TLR4, 5, 7 and 8 in mice. It has been reported that transfer of Treg cells enhanced tumour growth in mice but it was reversed upon stimulation of Treg cells with a TLR8 ligand. Administration of LPS also abrogates Treg activity reveals latent anti-tumour immunity ((Chen & Oppenheim, 2009). The biggest problem in using TLRs as anti-cancer targets lies in the fact that many cancer patients have very low immunity because of anti-cancer therapy side effect, thus it becomes very difficult to get innate immune response. The quest to arrive at a point where innate immune system's stimulatory compounds are used along with anticancer agents may bear some fruit. The TLR3 has been shown to be receptor for viral dsRNA, and also seems to be potentially promising in anti-cancer therapy. Reports have shown that cancer cells themselves express TLR3 *in vivo* and agonist ploy (I:C) is activating the signalling pathway leading to the anticancer effects (Elizabeth et al., 2010; O'Neill et al., 2011). Hence, this complex relationship of tumour cells and TLRs seems to be crucial to determine the balance between beneficial and pathological roles of TLRs.

9.3 TLRs in asthma and allergy

Lungs are continuously exposed to microbial pathogens because of their constant relationship with the surrounding environment. Therefore, innate immune response in lungs to eliminate the pathogen requires expression of TLRs which would be activated upon pathogen exposure and subsequently commencing in signalling cascade. This signalling culminates in the elevated expression of IL-1-β, TNF-α, IL-12, and IFN-γ. The nature and intensity of response is regulated by the display of polarized cytokine profiles, either Th1 or Th2. Th2 cytokines are reported to play a crucial role in initiation and perpetuation of allergy and asthma (Bauer et al., 2007). Exposure to low doses of LPS results in Th2 biased response leading to onset of allergic response. On the contrary, high doses of LPS show protective effect. This is confirmed by the studies revealing an inverse relationship between allergy and asthma and early childhood exposure to rural farm environment. Although the exact mechanistic pathway is yet to be explored, but it becomes quite evident that LPS-TLR4 complex can either protect or aggravate the severity of asthma, depending on the timing of the LPS exposure. This is supported by "hygiene hypothesis" that favours that development of asthma and allergies is executed by the reduction in microbial exposure in early childhood and decrease in naturally occurring infections. Asthma and allergies are found to be less prevalent among individuals brought up in rural farm areas in their childhood (Gehring et al., 2002). Such early exposure to farms and barns or early exposure to microbes and microbial components is attributed to the protection rendered in development of allergies in later life. This might be because of the induction of regulatory T cells that down-regulate the adaptive immune responses.

Apart from the role of TLR4 in allergies, recently it has been reported that TLR2 too modulates the development of allergic disease (Bauer et al., 2007). Studies conducted on children of farmers of Germany who have decreased risk of developing allergies were found to have augmented expression of TLR2 mRNA. The presence of asthma and allergies in the children of farmers was co-related with the genetic variation in TLR2. It was found that asthma and atopy were less prevalent in the children carrying T allele in TLR2/-16934 (Chen et al., 2007).

9.3.1 TLRs, regulatory T cells and allergy

A few studies recently have sparked widespread interest in the regulation of allergy as they claim that control of allergy is not only restricted to Th1/Th2 bias but other mechanisms as well are responsible for controlling inflammatory response and regulatory T cells (Treg cells) play a pivotal role in this regulation (Akbari et al., 2002). TLRs are expressed on Treg cells (Bauer et al., 2007). A study shows that in adults allergic to pollen, a significant reduction in the number of Treg cells and their capacity to restrain allergic response occurs when compared to healthy controls. Another finding supports that Treg cells can block allergic responses by demonstrating that activation of TLR4 expressed on the CD4+CD25+ subset of Treg cells in response to high doses of LPS may prevent activation of pathogenic T effector cells and airway inflammation and hyper-reactivity can be overcome by CD4+CD25+ Treg cell function in IL-10 dependant manner (Chen et al., 2007). Recently, a report elaborates a link between TLR2 and Treg cells as well because in TLR2 mice, CD4+CD25+ Treg cell subset was found to be significantly reduced when compared to wild type mice (Sutmuller et al., 2006).

9.3.2 Therapeutic potential of TLR ligands in allergy

The discovery that TLR signalling culminates in the activation of DCs leading to increased Th1 bias can also be applied in the treatment of allergic diseases. Particularly, TLR9 stimulation by un-methylated CpG-motif that promotes a Th1 response has been explored as potential treatment for atopic diseases like asthma and allergic rhinitis (Horner et al., 2001). In mice sensitized with allergen, CpG administration has been shown to inhibit the development of airway hyper-responsiveness and eosinophilia. It has also been demonstrated that CpG-DNA when conjugated to allergen offer a new anti-allergic strategy in which the complexes so formed show a more promising result by augmenting the immunotherapeutic effect when compared CpG-DNA given alone or CpG-DNA given mixed to allergen (Tighe et al., 2000; Horner et al., 2001). These studies encourage usage of selectively targeted allergen TLR-fusion proteins for manipulating and eliciting specific immune responses and studies are also suggestive that CpG-DNA might be a valuable and potent agent for treatment of allergies. Interestingly, imidazoquinoline resiquimod (R-848), a ligand for TLR8 has the potential to revert Th2 allergic response to Th1 because of its exceptional capability to induce Th1 response

(Hemmi et al., 2002). Hence, ligands like imidazoquinoline resiquimod too can be therapeutic targets for allergic reactions.

9.4 TLRs in autoimmune and inflammatory diseases

9.4.1 Systemic Lupus Erythematosus (SLE)

SLE is an autoimmune disorder in which antibodies are directed against a range of self-antigens. Out of these, autoantibodies to nuclear antigens are of keen importance to the clinical diagnosis of SLE. Nuclear antigens include dsDNA, ssDNA, nucleolar RNA, histone proteins and others. Emerging researches have revealed the involvement of TLRs in the progression of autoimmune diseases like SLE, rheumatoid arthritis, diabetes mellitus etc. TLR7 and TLR9 are of particular interest in the studies of SLE which are located in the endosomal compartments (Anders, 2005; Christensen et al., 2005). It has been seen that unregulated or misregulated activation of TLRs can lead to an autoimmune phenotypic appearance. Nucleic acids which are usually not immunogenic are not able to induce an immune response, but these can become immunogenic via several chemical modifications like hypo-methylation, increased oxidation and high CpG content. Immune complexes having DNA or RNA which are formed as a consequence of necrosis thus are capable of activating TLRs. It has been reported that DNA found in immune complexes has 5-6 times more of CpG content and is hypo-methylated in SLE patients. Release of autoantibodies and inflammatory cytokines which are responsible for chronic inflammation (Christensen et al., 2007; Savarese et al., 2008) can be traced to the improper activation of TLR7. In SLE patients, levels of IFNα and TypeI interferons are excessively high and it is found that higher levels of IFNα are beneficiary to the disease progression. Nowadays, TLR signalling pathways are directed for therapeutic intervention. Various key molecules of TLR7 and TLR9 signalling pathways are targeted to block downstream signalling and hence the effector responses. Molecules targeted are MyD88, TRAF6, IRAK1 & 4. Other approaches are monoclonal antibodies directed against IFNα. Also immunoregulatory DNA sequences (IRS) bind to TLRs and block their activation. Hence, these can be used as effective strategies in reduction of SLE progression molecules. Research for absolute treatment is still in its early stages.

9.4.2 Rheumatoid Arthiritis (RA)

RA is an autoimmune disorder which affects the joints most severely. RA is caused due to generation of autoantibodies against the Fc region of IgG. Usually these autoantibodies are of IgM type and referred to as rheumatoid factors. Recent studies have revealed that TLRs play a significant role in the development of RA. TLR2 & 4 seems to play a crucial role in RA. TLR2 & 4 over expression is found in the blood monocytes, synovial fluid macrophages and fibroblasts in RA (Iwahashi et al., 2004). Patients with RA are found to have presence of TLR ligands in the joints synovial fluid. These ligands can be endogenous (Heat shock proteins, HMGB1, hyaluronan etc) (Huang et al., 2009) or can be exogenous like peptidoglycan. It has been seen that MyD88 and TLR2/4 deficient mice show reduced severity of RA. Currently various approaches are investigated to treat RA effectively. TLR antagonists and various TLR signalling molecules are targeted as a promising agent for treating RA.

9.4.3 Inflammatory Bowel Disease (IBD)

TLR2, TLR4 and TLR5 have been found to play a role in the pathogenesis of IBD. IBD comprises of Crohn's disease (CD) and ulcerative colitis (UC). Elevated expression of TLR4 is seen in the colonic tissue of UC and CD patients (Cairo & Podolsky, 2000), but TLR2 is found to be highly expressed in mouse manifested with colitis (Singh et al., 2005). This shows that IBD may be a consequential result of mutations and dysregulation in TLRs. Another family of PRRs, nucleotide binding oligomerization domain proteins (Nod) have been reported to contribute to IBD pathogenesis in conjunction with TLRs (Chen et al., 2007). Polymorphism in Nod2 is attributed to the development of CD.

9.4.4 Psoriasis

Psoriasis is a dermatological disorder of chronic autoimmune inflammatory nature. Expression of TLR2, TLR5 and TLR1 is altered in psoriatic individuals when compared to normal individuals (Chen et al., 2007). TLR2 is found to be highly expressed in the upper epidermis in contrast to normal skin where TLR2 is expressed in basal keratinocytes. Basal keratinocytes of the lesions also show reduced expression of TLR5 (Baker et al., 2003) and an enhanced and diffused expression of TLR1 when compared to normal skin (Curry et al., 2003). One of the mechanistic explanations of inflammatory response to psoriasis can be that the DNA released from keratinocytes in psoriatic skin binds to antimicrobial peptide cathelicidin LL37 thus mimicking bacterial DNA and triggers TLR expression on surface of immune cell/dendrocytes to activate NF-kB which controls the inflammation.

9.5 TLRs in infectious diseases

Apart from inflammatory and immune diseases associated with TLRs, TLRs are vital players in infectious diseases as well. One of these is *Mycobacterium tuberculosis* infection in which TLR2, TLR4 and TLR9 have been found to play some role. At an early stage of infection TLR2- and TLR4-knockout mice showed an increased susceptibility to the bacteria but it subsided at the later stage of infection (Tjarnlund, 2006). It has also been reported that absence of TLR2 in mice leads to aggravated inflammatory response (Drennan et al., 2004). A study reports that mice double deficient in TLR9 and TLR2 are highly susceptible to mycobacterial infection, however, single knockouts in either TLR2 or TLR9 did not show this phenomenon (Bafica et al., 2005). Another mycobacterial species, *Mycobacterium leprae,* results in various clinical manifestations associated with host immune response (Chen et al., 2007). TLR1 and TLR2 have been found to be highly expressed in patients with tuberculoid lesions whereas lepromatous lesions lack these TLRs indicating their role in the progression of tuberculoid form of the disease (Krutzik et al., 2003).

Altered expression of TLR4, TLR5 and TLR9 has been observed in *Helicobacter pylori* infection (Chen et al., 2007). TLR4 and MD-2 have been found to be expressed at significantly higher levels in gastric mucosa. This indicates the possible role of TLR4/MD-2 complex in host response to *H. pylori* derived LPS (Ishihara et al., 2004). Interestingly, TLR5 and TLR9 are located on both apical surface and basolateral surface but during *H. pylori* infection, these TLRs are not found to be expressed at the apical surface (Schmausser et al., 2005). TLR adaptor protein, MyD88, is found to be crucial in eliciting a protective host innate response against *Cryptococcus neoformans* and *Legionella pneumophila* infections (Archer et al., 2006; Yauch et al., 2004). The response is generated via activation of TLR2. Also *Chlamydia pneumonia* infection is prevented by TLR2 and TLR4 expression (Rodriguez et al., 2006).

Lyme disease, caused by infection by spirochete *Borrelia* is also associated with TLRs. Outer surface protein A lipoprotein (OspA) is an antigen belonging to *Borrelia burgdorferi* that when docks onto TLR2 and TLR6 culminates in the induction of NFκB in human dermal endothelial cells (HMEC) (Bulut et al., 2001). TLR2/1heterodimerization is essential for the macrophages to recognize OspA and initiate desirable immune response against *B. Burgdorferi* (Chen et al., 2007). Absence of chemokine receptor XCR2 results in decreased inflammation which is considered as a novel therapeutic target for lyme disease.

Role of TLRs in viral disease progression is not yet completely elucidated, however, TLR3, TLR7, TLR8 and TLR9 have been associated with viral sensing (Kanwar et al., 2011). TLR3 and TLR9 have been conferred the foremost place in generating viral immunity. TLR3 and TLR9 recognize viral double stranded RNA and non-methylated CpG di-nucleotides (both of viral and bacterial origin) respectively. TLR7 and TLR8 too leave their signature in viral immunity by initiating IFN–α and IFN-β production in DCs and monocytes through IRAK-4 TLR adaptor (Kanwar et al., 2011). Role of TLR3 has been of prime importance in the immune response of lung epithelial cells to Influenza A virus (IAV). Influenza infection causes enhanced pulmonary expression of TLR3 in mice. However, IAV-infected TLR3-/- mice exhibited significantly reduced levels of inflammatory mediators and lower number of CD8+ T lymphocytes in broncho-alveolar space (Le Goffic et al., 2006). Therefore, it can be concluded that TLR3-IAV interaction renders the body protected against debilitating host inflammatory response.

10. TLRs as adjuvant vaccines and their role in immune stimulation

Adjuvant is an agent that may stimulate the immune system and increase the response to an antigen or a vaccine without showing any antigenic property of its own. Adjuvants are used to augment the effect of a particular vaccine by putting in action the innate and then adaptive immune system in action so that the response to a vaccine is more vigorous. Adjuvants mimic molecules of bacterial or viral origin which are conserved and bear molecular signatures called PAMPs or pattern in terms of conservation. These pattern bearing molecules act as a ligand for toll like receptors (TLRs). When TLRs come in contact with their appropriate ligands, the receptor-ligand complex gives rise to innate immune response which in turn activates adaptive immune system. Since the distribution of TLRs is not limited to the innate cells such as DCs, macrophages, natural killer cells, but are also found on B cells, T cells, and other non-immune cells such as epithelial, endothelial and fibroblast, the importance of giving adjuvant based vaccines can be gauged from the fact that ligands will be able to elicit strong immune response from innate to adaptive immunity. The adjuvant simply mimics natural infection, which in turn first puts the innate then adaptive immune system on, subsequently the purpose of generation of memory cells against the desired target is achieved (Kaisho & Akira, 2002).

The role of TLRs as adjuvant receptors may be exploited to control the TLR signalling using immunity modulating reagents which may be used against the pathogens, autoimmune diseases, inflammation and cancers. Since TLRs are crucial in recognition of viral and bacterial pathogens, current treatment aims at activating these receptors, generation of pro-inflammatory response and finally destruction of these pathogens. Ribavarin in combination with IFNα and resiquimod are currently being used as antiviral drugs. But these molecules have their own sets of limitations in terms of side effects. Agonist molecules like ANA773 and IMO-2125 have shown promising results with their respective receptors TLR7 and TLR9. TLR agonists have also been supplemented to boost immune responses to cancer vaccines. TLR7 imidazoquinoline ligand 3M-019 has been found to be a potent adjuvant for pure protein prototype vaccines (Johnston et al., 2007). TLR2 agonist SMP-105 has been approved for the bladder cancer treatment. The compound has shown strong adjuvant and antitumor activities. In experimental model, SM-105 has shown anti-tumour property. Thus TLRs as adjuvant receptors may open up new avenues of medical treatments. MPL has been approved in Europe as adjuvant vaccine. This molecule is a component of the hepatitis B vaccine and papillomavirus virus vaccine. It act as a ligand to TLR4 and activates the TRAM/TRIF pathway leading to the induction of IFNβ and regulation of CD80/86. MGN-1703 and MGN-1706 are double stem loop, non-coding DNA based adjuvants which ligate with TLR9 are being developed as anticancer agents. Another vaccine adjuvant, VAX-102, which acts as TLR5 agonist is also under trial to treat the viral infections (Elizabeth., 2010). This adjuvant vaccine if successful will provide protection from all strains of seasonal and pandemic influenza. Synthetic TLR agonists poorly reproduce the essential 'pattern' component of the larger natural ligands. To overcome this, an agonist PolyMAP, has been generated in which individual ligand is presented in a more natural linear pattern along the length of a biocompatible polymer. PolyMAP agonists can boost the immune response up to 200 times higher on a per molecule basis. PolyMAP has three key properties that contribute to the enhanced adjuvant activity and safety: (1) increased receptor avidity through cooperative, multi-valent interactions, (2) clustering of receptors through cross-linking and (3) improved solubility of TLR ligands that are otherwise difficult to use in their free form. Recently, Kasturi et al. (Kasturi et al., 2011) have reported synthetic nanoparticle adjuvant that stimulates TLR4 and TLR7, ensuing in enhanced generation of antigen-specific antibodies by synergistic action. Hence, conferring protection to lethal viral challenges in mice and inducing robust immunity against the pandemic H1N1 influenza strain in *Rhesus macaques*. Researchers developed poly(d,l-lactic-co-glycolic acid) (PGLA), a biodegradable polymer based nanoparticle to administer the TLR4 and TLR7 ligands, it was found that in comparison to the stimulation of either TLR4 or TLR7 alone, the double TLR stimulation significantly enhanced antibody response and was found to be evident even after secondary immunization.

Overall it can be concluded that adjuvants mimicking the natural molecules of viral or bacterial origin may be used to modulate the immune system resulting in the treatment of autoimmune diseases, cancers, other diseases, and when combined with vaccines, they may help in the generation of memory cells against a particular invader. The potential of adjuvant alone or as an adjuvant vaccine is yet to be fully exploited.

11. TLRs in transplantation

Transplantation is a surgical procedure by which cells, tissues or organs can be moved from one part of body to another or from one individual to another. Despite the advancement in surgical and medical sciences, the immune system remains the biggest barrier to transplantation. Till recently, the rejection of a transplant was taken as an adaptive immune response mediated by killer T cells capable of inducing apoptosis as well as antibody secreting B cells with only small and finishing role of innate immune system like phagocytosis and complement activation. However, the emerging results have shown the importance of innate immune system in the transplant rejection via TLRs. Although direct role of TLRs are yet to be found but the activation of adaptive immune system because of TLRs may be the reason. As we know that TLRs need specific ligands to activate the signalling pathway and it is quite possible that during transplantation there is release of putative endogenous ligands such as heat shock proteins (Hsp), uric acid, hyaluronan, fibrinogen and chromatin (Goldstein, 2006). Some of these putative ligands have been seen to work with the TLRs. At the same time the role of exogenous ligands cannot be ruled out completely, which may be because of infection contracted while surgery. LPS from gram negative bacteria has been shown to activate the TLR mediated signalling pathway and create complications in graft or transplant acceptance. The recognition of alloantigen by adaptive immune system, in principle, made active because of TLRs may show increased level of complications on the development of cross reactivity with alloantigen and viral molecules. Previous studies have shown that lung, intestine and skin are more prone than kidney, heart and pancreas to acute rejection after transplantation (Wang et al., 2010). This observation may be explained that these organs which are less likely to be accepted as graft have commensals or pathogens, which in turn may activate innate immune system through TLRs leading finally to the activation of adaptive immunity. The identification of endogenous and control of exogenous TLR ligands may pave way for longer period of acceptance of transplants.

12. TLRs in trophoblast

During pregnancy the placenta is not only exposed to the maternal immune system, but also to microorganisms. It has been shown recently that in first trimester trophoblastic cells have TLR2 and TLR4 on their surface by which they can recognize and respond to invading pathogens. Interestingly, both of these TLRs show divergent response. TLR4 activation results in a more classical response, characterized by the induction of cytokine production whereas activation of TLR2 results in the induction of apoptosis. This induction of apoptosis by TLR2 may provide a mechanism by which pathogens may give rise to complicated pregnancies in the first trimester, although a clear picture remains elusive. It has been seen that in several complicated pregnancies the case of intrauterine infection was found to be the leading cause. It has been seen that during first trimester TLR2 assisted trophoblastic cell apoptosis level rises. In turn this may give rise to several medical conditions like preterm labour, IUGR, and preeclampsia. Usually, the uterine infection takes place before the implantation of trophoblast. The pathogen gets the recognition only when it is able to penetrate the placental wall and is able to reach the layer where trophoblastic cells are expressing TLRs. The TLR expression is not limited to the cell surface but has been seen also in cytoplasm may be to facilitate emergency call on infection or to face the intracellular infections, if any. The TLR4 when comes in contact with its ligand, LPS, triggers classical response whereas TLR2 induces apoptosis by coming in contact with Gram positive bacterial peptidoglycan or lipoteichoic acid, but at the same time it has been reported that recognition of these bacterial products by TLR2 requires recruitment of TLR6 or TLR1. Further studies have shown that TLR6 may show increased effect but is not essential for TLR2 mediated response and response may be executed through

TLR2 homodimer or TLR1/TLR2 heterodimer. The TLR2 induces apoptotic effect through the activation of caspases. The TLR4 interaction with LPS does not give rise to pro-apoptotic signals during first trimester because the anti-apoptotic signals generated may outweigh the pro-apoptotic signals leading to the survival of trophoblastic cells. There is also a possibility of indirect induction of apoptosis due to the high level of cytokine production such as TNF and IFN to which placenta cells are sensitive (Vikki et al., 2006).

13. Conclusion

Earlier confusion of innate immunity being nonspecific as compared to adaptive immunity got cleared with the discovery of Toll like Receptors (TLRs) which ligate with the molecules having either exogenous origin like viral or bacterial or endogenous origin like Hsp. These ligands bear molecular patterns or signatures which make them unique for their receptors. The induction by these molecules may have either positive or negative effect on the body depending on the type of ligand and TLR. It has been seen that though ligands get recognised because of molecular pattern by a specific receptor, occasionally the same receptor may ligate with two to three different molecules with each having its own signature or pattern. This may be possibly due to assistance by some co-receptors. Further study is needed to arrive at some conclusion about this enigma. The protein-ligand complex crystal structures may provide insight into the still unclear picture of TLR signalling. The TLRs have been implicated in the development of cancers, autoimmune diseases, nervous system disorders and other inflammatory diseases. TLRs agonist or antagonist may help to get the desired result. Also their role as receptor for adjuvant alone or adjuvant vaccine is being explored much vigorously than before. Role of TLRs from premature birth, complicated pregnancies to transplant rejection cannot be ignored. Moreover, their roles along with miRNA need to be probed further. Also the sources of endogenous ligands need to be discovered. Apart from receptors, the other molecules of signalling pathway too need attention to understand the process much better. The need of the time is to push the TLR research into next level where better animal models (knockout) are ready to rule out artefacts. Lastly, to design drugs, vaccines and fine tune them for lesser or ideally no side effects. Therefore, in the light of emerging information about the complexity of TLRs in immune system regulation, it can be concluded that TLRs are in fact a necessary evil. Sometimes, from their usual behaviour as a good cop by being a part of an innate immune system, a first line of defence, may turn rouge due to several compelling reasons and play bad cop. Hence, activation of TLRs is a double edged sword in therapeutics, it has the potential to mount immunity against various autoimmune, inflammatory and cancerous diseases etc. but can also promote their development and dampen immune response against them.

14. References

Akbari, O., Freeman, G.J., Meyer, E.H., Greenfield, E.A., Chang, T.T., Sharpe, A.H., Berry, G., DeKruyff, R.H. & Umetsu, D.T. (2002). Antigen-specific regulatory T cells develop via the ICOS-ICOS-ligand pathway and inhibit allergen-induced airway hyperreactivity. *Nat. Med.*, Vol. 8, pp. 1024–1032.

Akiyama, H. et al. (2000) Inflammation and Alzheimer's disease. *Neurobiol Aging*, Vol.21, pp. 383-421.

Anders, H.J. (2005). A toll for lupus. *Lupus*. Vol. 14, pp. 417–422.

Arancibia, S.A., Beltran, C.J., Aguirre, I.M., Silva, P., Peralta, A.L., Malinarich, F. & Hermoso, M.A. (2007). Toll-like receptors are key participants in innate immune responses. *Biol Res*. Vol.40, pp. 97-112.

Arbour, N.C. (2000). TLR4 mutations are associated with endotoxin hyporesponsiveness in humans. *Nat Genet*, Vol.25, pp. 187–191.

Archer, K.A. & Roy, C.R. (2006) MyD88-dependent responses involving toll-like receptor 2 are important for protection and clearance of *Legionella pneumophila* in a mouse model of Legionnaires' disease. *Infect Immun*, Vol.74, pp. 3325–33.

Arroyo, S.D., Soria, A.J., Gaviglio, A.E., Rodriguez-Galan, C.M., Iribarren,P. (2011) Toll-like receptors are key players in neurodegeneration. *Inter. Immunopharmacology*, Vol.11, pp. 1415–1421.

Asea, A., Kraeft, S.K., Kurt-Jones, E.A., Stevenson, M.A., Chen, L.B. & Finberg RW et al. (2000). Hsp70 stimulates cytokine production through a CD-14-dependent pathway, demonstrating its dual role as a chaperone and cytokine. *Nat Med*, Vol.6, pp. 435–442.

Bafica, A., Scanga, C.A., Feng, C.G., Leifer, C., Cheever, A. & Sher, A. (2005). TLR9 regulates Th1 responses and cooperates with TLR2 in mediating optimal resistance to Mycobacterium tuberculosis. *J Exp Med*, Vol.202, pp. 1715–24.

Baker, B.S., Ovigne, J.M., Powles, A.V., Corcoran, S. & Fry L. (2003) Normal keratinocytes express Toll-like receptors (TLRs) 1, 2 and 5: modulation of TLR expression in chronic plaque psoriasis. *Br J Dermatol*, Vol.148, pp. 670–9.

Banchereau, J. & Steiman, R.M. (1998). Dendritic cells and the control of immunity. *Nature*, Vol.392, pp. 245-52.

Bauer, S., Hangel, D. & Yu, P. (2007). Immunobiology of toll-like receptors in allergic disease. *Immunobiology*, Vol.212, pp. 521-533.

Bell, J. K., Botos, I., Hall, P.R., Askins, J., Shiloach, J., Segal, D.M.,et al (2003).Leucine-rich repeats and pathogen recognition in Toll-like receptors. *Trends Immunol*. Vol.24, pp. 528–533.

Beutler, B. & Rietschel, E. T. (2003). Innate immune sensing and its roots: the story of endotoxin. *Nature Rev. Immunol.*, Vol.3, pp. 169–176.

Beutler, B., Rehli, M. (2002). Evolution of the TIR, tolls and TLRs: functional inferences from computational biology. *Curr. Top Microbial. Immunol.* Vol.270, pp. 1-21.

Bin, L. H., Xu, L. G. & Shu, H. B. (2003).TIRP, a novel Toll/interleukin-1 receptor (TIR) domain-containing adapter protein involved in TIR signaling. *J. Biol. Chem.*, Vol.278, pp. 24526–24532.

Bradley, J. R. & Pober, J. S. (2001).Tumor necrosis factor receptor associated factors (TRAFs). *Oncogene*, Vol.20, pp. 6482–6491.

Bsibsi, M.(2002) Broad expression of Toll-like receptors in the human central nervous system. *J Neuropathol Exp Neurol*, Vol.61, pp. 1013–1021.

Bulut ,Y., Faure, E., Thomas, L., Equils, O. & Arditi M. (2001). Cooperation of Toll-like receptor 2 and 6 for cellular activation by soluble tuberculosis factor and Borrelia burgdorferi outer surface protein A lipoprotein: role of Toll-interacting protein and IL-1 receptor signaling molecules in Toll-like receptor 2 signaling. *J Immunol*, Vol.167, pp. 987–94.

Burns, K., Martinon F., Esslinger C., Pahl H., Schneider P., Bodmer J.L., Marco F.D., French L. & Tschopp J. (1998). MyD88, an adapter protein involved in interleukin-1 signaling. *J. Biol. Chem.*, Vol.273, pp. 12203–12209.

Cario, E. & Podolsky, D.K. (2000). Differential alteration in intestinal epithelial cell expression of toll-like receptor 3 (TLR3) and TLR4 in inflammatory bowel disease. *Infect Immun*, Vol.68, pp. 7010–7.

Carpentier PA, et al. (2005) Differential activation of astrocytes by innate and adaptive immune stimuli. *Glia*, Vol.49, pp. 360-374.

Chen, K., Huang, J., Gong, W., Iribarren P., Dunlop, N.M. & Wang, J.M. (2007). Toll like receptors in inflammation, infection and cancer. *International Immunopharmacology*, Vol.7, pp. 1271-1285.

Chen, X. & Oppenheim, J.J. (2009). Regulatory T cells, Th17 cells, and TLRs: Crucial role in Inflammation, Autoimmunity, and Cancer. *Pathways*, 888.503.3187, Issue 10.

Christensen, S.R. & Shlomchik, M.J. (2007). Regulation of lupus-related autoantibody production and clinical disease by Toll-like receptors. *Seminars in Immunology.* Vol.19, pp. 11–23.

Christensen, S.R., Kashgarian, M., Alexopoulou, L., Flavell, R.A., Akira, S. & Shlomchik, M.J. (2005) Toll-like receptor 9 controls anti-DNA autoantibody production in murine lupus. *Journal of Experimental Medicine.* Vol.202, pp. 321–331.

Curry, J.L., Qin, J.Z., Bonish, B., Carrick, R., Bacon, P. & Panella, J. et al. (2003) Innate immune-related receptors in normal and psoriatic skin. *Arch Pathol Lab Med* ,Vol.127, pp. 178–86.

Drennan, M.B., Nicolle, D., Quesniaux, V.J., Jacobs, M., Allie, N. & Mpagi, J. et al.(2004). Toll-like receptor 2-deficient mice succumb to Mycobacterium tuberculosis infection. *Am J Pathol*. Vol.164, pp. 49–57.

Elizabeth, J., Hennessy, Andrew, E., Parker, Luke A.J.O., Neill. (2010) Targeting Toll-like receptors: emerging therapeutics, *Nature Rev. Drug Discovery*, Vol. 9, pp. 293-307.

Gehring, U., Bischof, W. & Fahlbusch, B., et al. (2002). House dust endotoxin and allergic sensitization in children. *Am J Respir Crit Care Med.*, Vol.166, pp. 939-944.

Gingras, S., Parganas, E., Pauw, A.D., Ihle, J.N. & Murray, P.J. (2004). Re- examination of the role of suppressor of cytokine signaling 1 (SOCS1) in the regulation of toll-like receptor signaling. *J Biol Chem*, Vol.279, pp. 54702-7.

Goldstein, D.R. (2006) Toll like receptors and acute allograft rejection, *Transplant Immuno.* Vol. 17, pp. 211–215.

Harmey, J.H., Bucana, C.D., Lu, W., Byrne, A.M., McDonnell, S. & Lynch, C. et al. (2002). Lipopolysaccharide-induced metastatic growth is associated with increased angiogenesis, vascular permeability and tumor cell invasion. *Int J Cancer* . Vol.101, pp. 415–422.

Hashimoto, C.; Hudson, K. L. & Anderson, K. V. (1988). The *Toll* gene of *Drosophila*, required for dorsal–ventral embryonic polarity, appears to encode a transmembrane protein. *Cell*, Vol.52, pp. 269–279.

Hemmi, H., Kaisho, T., Takeuchi, O., Sato, S., Sanjo, H., Hoshino, K., Horiuchi, T., Tomizawa, H., Takeda, K., Akira, S. (2002). Small anti-viral compounds activate immune cells via the TLR7 MyD88-dependent signaling pathway. *Nat. Immunol.* Vol.3, pp. 196–200.

Hoebe, K., Du, X., Georgel, P., Janssen, E.M., Tabeta, K., Kim, S.O., Goode, J., Lin, P., Mann, N., Mudd, S., Crozat, K., Sovath, S., Han, J. & Beutler, B. (2003). Identification of

Lps2 as a key transducer of MyD88-independent TIR signalling. *Nature,* Vol.424, pp. 743–748.

Horner, A.A., Van Uden, J.H., Zubeldia, J.M., Broide, D. & Raz, E. (2001). DNA-based immunotherapeutics for the treatment of allergic disease. *Immunol. Rev.* Vol.179, pp. 102–118.

Horng, T., Barton, G. M. & Medzhitov, R. (2001). TIRAP: an adapter molecule in the Toll signaling pathway. *Nature Immunol.,* Vol.2, pp. 835–841.

Hsu, Y. C. Rich., Chan, H. F. Carlos, Spicer, D. J., Rousseau, C. M., Giannias, B., Rousseau, S., Ferri, E. L., (2011) *Cancer Res,* Vol. 71(5), pp. 1989-98.

Huang, Q.Q., Sobkoviak, R., Jocheck-Clark, A.R., Shi, B., Mandelin, A.M. & Tak, P.P.et al. (2009). Heat shock protein 96 is elevated in rheumatoid arthritis and activates macrophages primarily via TLR2 signaling. *J Immunol.* Vol.182, pp. 4965-73.

Ishihara, S., Rumi, M.A., Kadowaki, Y., Ortega-Cava, C.F., Yuki, T. & Yoshino N, et al. (2004). Essential role of MD-2 in TLR4-dependent signaling during Helicobacter pylori-associated gastritis. *J Immunol* ,Vol.173, pp. 1406–16.

Iwahashi, M., Yamamura, M., Aita ,T., Okamoto, A., Ueno, A. & Ogawa, N., et al. (2004). Expression of Toll-like receptor 2 on CD16+ blood monocytes and synovial tissue macrophages in rheumatoid arthritis.*Arthritis Rheum.* Vol.50, pp. 1457–67.

Jack, C.S., Arbour, N., Manusow, J., Montgrain, V., Blain, M., McCrea, E., Shapiro, A., Antel JP. (2005) TLR signaling tailors innate immune responses in human microglia and astrocytes. *JImmunol,* Vol.175, pp. 4320-4330.

Jack, C.S. et al. (2007) Th1 polarization of CD4+ T cells by Toll-like receptor 3-activated human microglia.*J Neuropathol Exp Neurol,* Vol.66, pp. 848-859.

Janeway, C. A. & Medzhitov, R. (2002). Innate immune recognition. *Annu. Rev. Immunol.,* Vol.20, pp. 197–216.

Janssens, S. & Beyaert, R. (2003). Functional diversity and regulation of different interleukin-1 receptor-associated kinase (IRAK) family members. *Mol. Cell,* Vol.11, pp. 293–302.

Johnston, D., Zaidi, B., Bystryn, J.C. (2007). TLR7 imidazoquinoline ligand 3M-019 is a potent adjuvant for pure protein prototype vaccines. *Cancer Immunol Immunother,* Vol.58, Issue 8, pp.1133-41.

Kaisho, T., Akira, S., (2002) Toll-like receptors as adjuvants receptors, *Biochimica et Biophysica Acta,* Vol.1589, pp. 1-13.

Kanwar, J.R., Zhou, S.F., Gurudevan, S., Barrow, C.J., Kanwar, R.K. (2011). Toll Like Receptors Play a Role in General Immunity, Eye Infection and Inflammation: TLRs for Nanodelivery. *J Clin Cell Immunol,* Vol.2, Issue 4.

Kasturi, S.P., Skountzou, I., Albrecht, R.A., Koutsonanos, D., Hua, T., Nakaya, H.I. et. al.(2011). Programming the magnitude and persistence of antibody responses with innate immunity. *Nature,* Vol.470, pp.543-547.

Kol, A., Lichtman , A.H., Finberg, R.W., Libby, P. & Kurt-Jones EA. (2000). Cutting edge:heat shock protein (HSP) 60 activates the innate immune response:CD14 is an essential receptor for HSP60 activation of mononuclear cells. *J Immunol,* Vol.164, pp. 13–17.

Krutzik, S.R., Ochoa, M.T., Sieling, P.A., Uematsu, S., Ng, Y.W. & Legaspi A, et al.(2003) Activation and regulation of Toll-like receptors 2 and 1 in human leprosy. *Nat Med,* Vol.9, pp. 525–32.

Le Goffic, R., Balloy, V., Lagranderie, M., Alexopoulou, L., Escriou, N. & Flavell, R. et al. (2006) Detrimental contribution of the Toll-like receptor (TLR)3 to influenza Avirus-induced acute pneumonia. PLoS *Pathog* Vol.2, pp. e53.

Lebouder, E., Rey-Nores, J.E., Rushmere, N.K., Grigorov, M., Lawn, S.D., Affolter, M., Griffin ge, Ferrara, P., Schiffrin, E.J., Morgan, B.P. & Labeta , M.O. (2003) Soluble forms of Toll-like receptor (TLR)2 capable of modulating TLR2 signaling are present in human plasma and breast milk. *J Immunol*, Vol.171, pp. 6680- 9.

Lemaitre, B.; Nicolas, E., Michaut, L., Reichhart, J.M. & Hoffmann, J. A. (1996).The dorsoventral regulatory gene cassette *spatzle/Toll/cactus* controls the potent antifungal response in *Drosophila* adults. *Cell,* Vol.86, pp. 973–983.

Meylan, E., Burns, K., Hofmann, K., Blancheteau, V., Martinon, F., Kelliher, M., et al. (2004).RIP1 is an essential mediator of Toll-like receptor 3-induced NF-κB activation. *Nature Immunol.*, Vol.5, pp. 503–507.

Muzio, M.; Ni, J.; Feng, P. & Dixit, V. M. (1997). IRAK (Pelle) family member IRAK-2 and MyD88 as proximal mediators of IL-1 signaling. *Science,* Vol.278, pp. 1612–1615.

Neill, L.O., (2008) Toll-like receptors in cancer, *Nature Oncogene*, Vol. 27, pp. 158–160s.

Okun, E., Griffioen, J.K., Lathia, D.J., Tang, S., Mattson, P.M., Arumugam, V.T. (2009). Toll like receptors in Neurodegenration, *Brain Res. Rev.* Vol. 59, pp. 278–292.

O'Neill, L. A., Sheedy, F. J., & Claire E. McCoy, C. E. (2011). MicroRNAs: the fine-tuners of Toll-like receptor signalling.*Nature Rev. Immunol.* Vol.11, pp. 163-175.

Parker, L.C., Prince, L.R. & Sabroe, I. (2006). Translational mini-review series on toll like receptors: networks regulated by toll like receptors mediate innate and adaptive immunity. *Clinical and Experimental Immunology.* Vol.147, pp. 199-207.

Pasare, C., Medzhitov, R. (2003). Toll pathway-dependent blockade of CD4+ CD25+ T cell-mediated suppression by dendritic cells. *Science*, Vol.299, pp.1033-1036.

Pessac, B. (2001) Microglia origin and development. *Bull Acad Natl Med*, Vol.185, pp. 346-33.

Poltorak, A., He, X., Smirnova, I., Liu M., Huffel C.V., Du X., Birdwell D., Alejos E., Silva M, Galanos C., Freudenberg M., Castagnoli P.R., Layton B. & Beutler B. (1998). Defective LPS signaling in C3H/HeJ and C57BL/10ScCr mice: mutations in *Tlr4* gene. *Science,* Vol.282, pp. 2085–2088.

Rodriguez, N., Wantia, N., Fend, F., Durr, S., Wagner, H. & Miethke T. (2006) Differential involvement of TLR2 and TLR4 in host survival during pulmonary infection with Chlamydia pneumoniae. *Eur J Immunol*, Vol.236, pp. 1145-55.

Savarese, E., Steinberg, C. & Pawar, R.D., et al. (2008). Requirement of Toll-like receptor 7 for pristane-induced production of autoantibodies and development of murine lupus nephritis. *Arthritis and Rheumatism.* Vol.58, pp. 1107-1115.

Schmausser, B., Andrulis, M., Endrich, S., Muller-Hermelink, H.K. & Eck M. (2005). Toll-like receptors TLR4, TLR5 and TLR9 on gastric carcinoma cells: an implication for interaction with Helicobacter pylori. *Int J Med Microbiol*, Vol.295, pp. 179–85.

Sharma, S., R. tenOever , B., Grandvaux, N., Zhou, G.P., Lin, R. & Hiscott , J. (2003). Triggering the interferon antiviral response through an IKK-related pathway. *Science,*Vol. 300, pp. 1148-1151.

Shibuya, H., Yamaguchi, K., Shirakabe, K., Tonegawa, A., Gotoh, Y., Ueno, N., Irie, K., Nishida, E. & Matsumoto, K.(1996).TAB1: an activator of the TAK1 MAPKKK in TGF-β signal transduction. *Science,* Vol.272, pp. 1179–1182.

Singh, J.C., Cruickshank, S.M., Newton, D.J., Wakenshaw, L., Graham, A. & Lan, J., et al. (2005). Toll-like receptor-mediated responses of primary intestinal epithelial cells during the development of colitis. *Am J Physiol Gastrointest Liver Physiol*, Vol.288, pp. G514–24.

Singh-Jasuja, H., Scherer, H.U., Hilf, N., Arnold-Schild, D., Rammensee, H.G. & Toes, R.E. et al. (2000). The heat shock protein gp96 induces maturation of dendritic cells and down-regulation of its receptor. *Eur J Immunol*; Vol.30, pp. 22 11–221.

Slack, J. L., Schooley, K., Timothy, P. B., Jennifer, L. M., Eva, E. Q., John E. S. & Steven K. D. (2000). Identification of two major sites in the type I interleukin-1 receptor cytoplasmic region responsible for coupling to pro-inflammatory signaling pathways. *J. Biol. Chem.*, Vol. 275, pp. 4670–4678.

Sutmuller, R.P., den Brok, M.H., Kramer, M., Bennink, E.J., Toonen, L.W., Kullberg, B.J., Joosten, L.A., Akira, S., Netea, M.G. & Adema, G.J. (2006). Toll-like receptor 2 controls expansion and function of regulatory T cells. *J. Clin. Invest.* Vol.116, pp. 485–494.

Takaesu, G., Kishida, S., Hiyama, A., Yamaguchi, K., Shibuya, H., Irie, K., Tsuji, J.N. & Matsumot, K. (2000). TAB2, a novel adaptor protein, mediates activation of TAK1 MAPKKK by linking TAK1 to TRAF6 in the IL-1 signal transduction pathway. *Mol. Cell*, Vol. 5, pp. 649–658.

Takeda, K. & Akira, S. (2005). Toll like receptors in innate immunity. *The Japanese Society for Immunology*. Vol.17, pp. 1-14.

Tanaka T, et al. (2008). NF-kappaB independent signaling pathway is responsible for LPS-induced GDNF gene expression in primary rat glial cultures. *Neurosci Lett*; vol.431, pp. 262-267.

Tang SC, et al. (2007). Pivotal role for neuronal Toll-like receptors in ischemic brain injury and functional deficits. *Proc Natl Acad Sci U S A*, Vol. 104, pp. 13798-13803.

Taniguchi, T. & Takaoka, A. (2002).The interferon-α/β system in antiviral responses: a multimodal machinery of gene regulation by the IRF family of transcription factors. *Curr. Opin. Immunol.*, Vol.14, pp. 111–116.

Tjarnlund, A., Guirado, E., Julian, E., Cardona, P.J. & Fernandez C. (2006). Determinant role for Toll-like receptor signalling in acute mycobacterial infection in the respiratory tract. *Microbes Infect*, Vol.8, pp. 1790–800.

Vikki, M., Abrahams, Paulomi B.A., Kim, Y.M., Shawn, L., Chavez, S., Chaiworapongsa, T., Romero, R., Mor G. (2006) *The J. Immunology*, Vol.173, pp. 4286 – 4296.

Walter ,S., et al. (2007) Role of the toll-like receptor 4 in neuroinflammation sin Alzheimer's disease. *Cell Physiol Biochem*, Vol.20, pp. 947-956.

Wang, C., Deng, L., Hong, M., Akkaraju, G.R., Inoue, J. & Chen Z.J. (Jul 2001). TAK1 is a ubiquitin-dependent kinase of MKK and IKK. *Nature*, Vol.412, pp. 346-51.

Wang, J.H., Manning, B.J., Wu, Q.D., Blankson, S., Bouchier-Hayes, D. & Redmond, H.P. (2003). Endotoxin/lipopolysaccharide activates NF-kappaB and enhances tumor cell adhesion and invasion through a beta 1 integrin-dependent mechanism. *J Immunol.* Vol.170, pp. 795–804.

Wang, S., Schmaderer, C., Kiss, E., Schmidt, C., Bonrouhi, M., Porubsky, S., Gretz, N., chaefer, L., Carsten, J., Kirschning, Zoran V., Popovic, Gröne, H.J. (2010) Recipient Toll-like receptors contribute to chronic graft dysfunction by both MyD88- and TRIF-dependent signaling, *Disease Models & Mechanisms*, Vol. 3, pp. 92-103.

Wang, Y., Chen, T., Han, C., He, D., Liu, H., An, H., Cai, Z. et. al. (2007) Lysosome-associated small Rab GTPase Rab7b negatively regulates TLR4 signaling in macrophages by promoting lysosomal degradation of TLR4. *Blood*, Vol. 110, pp. 962-971.

Wesche, H.; Henzel, W. J.; Shillinglaw, W.; Li, S. & Cao, Z. (1997). MyD88: an adapter that recruits IRAK to the IL-1 receptor complex. *Immunity*, Vol.7, pp. 837–847.

Whitmore, M.M., Iparraguirre, A., Kubelka, L., Weninger, W., Hai, T. & Williams, B.R.G. (2007). Negative Regulation of TLR-Signaling Pathways by Activating Transcription Factor-3. *J Immunol* , Vol.179, pp.3622-3630.

Wright, S.D., Ramos, R.A., Tobias, P.S., Ulevitch, R.J. & Mathison, J.C. (1990). CD14, a receptor for complexes of lipopolysaccharide (LPS) and LPS binding protein. *Science*, Vol.249, pp. 1431–1433.

Xu, Y., Tao, X., Shen, B., Horng, T., Medzhitov, R., Manley, J.L. & Tong, L. (2000). Structural basis for signal transduction by the Toll/interleukin-1 receptor domains. *Nature*, Vol.408, pp. 111–115.

Yamaguchi, K. , Shirakabe, K., Shibuya, H., Irie, K., Oishi, I., Ueno, N., Taniguchi, T., Nishida, E. & Matsumoto K. (1995). Identification of a member of the MAPKKK family as a potential mediator of TGF-β signal transduction. *Science*, Vol. 270, pp. 2008-2011.

Yamamoto, M., Sato, S., Hemmi, H., Hoshino, K., Kaisho, T., Sanjo, H., Takeuchi, O., Sugiyama, M., Okabe, M., Takeda, K. & Akira, S. (2003). Role of adaptor TRIF in the MyD88-independent Toll-like receptor signaling pathway. *Science*, Vol.301, pp. 640–643.

Yauch, L.E., Mansour, M.K., Shoham, S., Rottman, J.B. & Levitz ,S.M. (2004).Involvement of CD14, toll-like receptors 2 and 4, and MyD88 in the host response to the fungal pathogen Cryptococcus neoformans in vivo. *Infect Immun* , Vol.72, pp. 5373–82.

Ye, H., Arron, J.R., Lamothe, B., Cirilli, M., Kobayashi, T., Shevde, N.K., Segal, D., Dzivenu, O.K., Vologodskaia, M.,Yim, M., Du, K., Singh, S., Pike, J.W., Darnay, B.G., Choi ,Y. & Wu, H. (2002). Distinct molecular mechanism for initiating TRAF6 signalling. *Nature,*Vol. 418, pp. 443–447.

Yoneyama, M., Suhara, W., Fukuhara, Y., Fukuda, M., Nishida, E. & Fujita, T. (1998). Direct triggering of the type I interferon system by virus infection: activation of a transcription factor complex containing IRF-3 and CBP/p300. *EMBO J.*, Vol.17, pp. 1087–1095.

5

Molecular Aspects of Neutrophils as Pivotal Circulating Cellular Innate Immune Systems to Protect Mammary Gland from Pathogens

Jalil Mehrzad[1,2]
[1]Sections Immunology and Biotechnology, Department of Pathobiology,
Faculty of Veterinary Medicine,
[2]Institute of Biotechnology, Ferdowsi University of Mashhad, Mashhad,
Iran

1. Introduction

As a pivotally cellular and molecular arms of circulating innate immune system, polymorphonuclear cells (PMNs) are the most vital primary mobile phagocytes in the body of mammals; their appropriate function is very essential to enhance animals' and humans' health performance. As the first type of innate immune cells arriving at the site of infection, neutrophils play a key role in initiating an innate, inflammatory, and specific immune responses; their importance for protection of organs in the body from pathogens has long been a crucial concern (Burvenich et al., 1994; Paape et al., 1996; Reeves et al., 2002; Burvenich et al., 2003; Mehrzad et al., 2004; 2005a; Letiember, et al., 2005; Liu et al., 2005; Borregaard et al., 2007; Stevens, et al., 2011a; 2011b; Bruhn et al., 2011). The proof of vital roles of neutrophils is that the neutropenic animals/humans are always highly susceptible to many pathogens. Clearly, the complex phenomenon of PMN chemotaxis, diapedesis, phagocytosis, and eventually microbicidal activity each contributes to the ability of PMN to provide an effective first line defense for the body and organs like udder (Burvenich et al., 2003; Mehrzad et al., 2000; 2001a; 2001b; 2002a; 2002b; 2004; 2005a; 2007; 2008a; 2008b; 2009; Mayadas & Cullere, 2005; Borregaard et al., 2008). In this concept many powerful afferent (sensing) and efferent (effector) arms of the neutrophils inside and outside of the cytoplasm are involved; the most common arms are enzymes, granules, free radicals or reactive oxygen species (ROS) and reactive nitrogen species (RNS) and in phagolysosome, into which microbicidal agents are released, neutrophil extracellular traps (NETs), neutrophils' membrane receptors like pattern recognition receptors (PRRs), opsonin receptors etc. that sense, bind and efficiently kill invading microbes, destroy virulence factors, or prevent them from spreading.

Oscillation and/or impairment of neutrophils' functions, originating from the bone marrow, is a peculiar feature during the physiological and environmental stresses; this impairment might be cumulative upon diapedesis/extravasation of neutrophils (Mehrzad et al., 2001a; 2002a; 2005a, 2004; 2007; 2008a; 2008b; Van Oostveldt et al., 2002a; 2002b; Burvenich et al., 2003). Generalised PMN impairment can be multifactorial, e.g. due to metabolic (Suriyasathaporn et al., 1999) and hormonal (Gray et al., 1982; Alexandrova, 2009; Lai &

Gallo, 2009) changes. The inevitable occurring of general and local immunocompromised conditions in biologically pivotal organ, mammals' udder, (Burvenich et al., 1994; Hoeben et al., 2000a; Burvenich et al., 2003; Mehrzad et al., 2001a; 2004; 2005a; 2008a; 2009) leads to udder infection and/or inflammation and breast disorders, affecting adult mammals, especially high yielding dairy cows, thereby causing neonatal infections, critical public health damage and economic losses to bovine, meat, dairy and food industries and overall human food chains.

Most researchers see the immunocompromised condition in animals and human as a result of neutrophils' dysfunction; this neutrophils' dysfunctional status can be cumulative upon neutrophils' influx into the udder (Mehrzad et al., 2001a; 2004; 2005a; 2008a; 2009). Despite all progresses and advances in the efferent and afferent branches of molecular aspects of neutrophils, the molecular basis of neutrophils interactions with other immune and non-immune cells in the udder is incompletely understood.

This chapter presents the cellular and acellular branches of neutrophils-pathogens interactions and factors affecting the effectiveness of particularly neutrophils' efferent arms of innate molecules in bovine. I chose bovine as a model to update our knowledge and to incorporate new observations that broaden our understanding of 1) overall neutrophils' involvement in innate immunity 2) how neutrophils engulf and kill invading pathogens and 3) how some key mechanisms of neutrophil's oscillatory events occur in bovine model. I discuss various aspects of bovine neutrophils that are absolutely relevant to their pivotal roles in an efficient innate immune response against pathogens. Aspects such as cellular and molecular innate immunity and host-pathogen interactions, biology, biochemistry and biophysics of bovine neutrophils as well as immunotoxicology, especially environmental immunotoxins (Mehrzad et al., 2011) and some nutritional immunology (Ibeagha et al., 2009), applying basic techniques like luminometry and flow cytometry will be schematically addressed to gain more insight into the static and dynamics branches of circulating and post-diapedetic neutrophils' functions. Although it is hardly possible in this chapter to address the breadth of information available on efferent arms of neutrophils in healthy and diseased animals and humans, our readers are therefore referred to many more recent detailed references of the many aspects of neutrophils in healthy and diseased hosts and their impacts on udders' health and performance as well.

2. Fine structure of neutrophils

As the primary and pivotal cells providing innate host defence against pathogens, neutrophils are characterized by their multi-lobed or sometimes picnotic dark-bluish stained nuclei (see figure 1) with the plenty of membrane receptors. The fine structure of bovine PMN has been exclusively demonstrated in classic studies (Paape et al., 2002; Mehrzad et al., 2001a; 2005b). The cell is delineated by a plasma membrane that has a number of functionally important receptors. These include L-selectin and β_2-integrin adhesion molecules associated with the binding of PMN to endothelial cells that are important for migration into sites of infection (Stevens et al., 2011a; 2011b; Pezeshki et al., 2011). Membrane receptors for the Fc component of the IgG_2 and IgM classes of immunoglobulins and C3b are necessary for mediating effective phagocytosis of invading microbes (Paape et al., 1996). Dying or apoptotic PMN express receptors that mark them for quick disposal by macrophages.

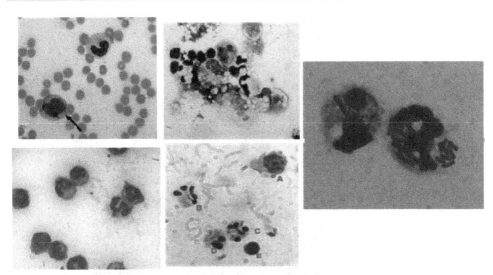

Fig. 1. Upper: Whole blood smear (left), immature neutrophil (arrow); milk neutrohils after
first step of centrifugation (right), which is almost indistinguishable, with the techniques
established in routine laboratories they can easily be distinguishable. A typical
phagocytosed microbes by milk neutrophils (far right); these engulfed microbes must be
destroyed effectively to limit infection. Lower: Isolated bovine blood neutrohils from
healthy animal (left), which is pure, and postdiapedetic udder (right) neutrohils (B, C and D)
macrophage (A) and lymphocyte (E).

The most prominent characteristic of the PMN is the multilobulated nucleus (see figures 1 and
2). The multilobulated nucleus is important because it allows the PMN to line up its nuclear
lobes in a thin line, permitting rapid migration between endothelial cells. Macrophages on the
other hand have a large horseshoe shaped nucleus that makes migration between endothelial
cells more difficult. Thus, the PMN is the first newly migrated phagocytic cell to arrive at an
infection site. Their surface microvilli are also pivotal for their functionality (see figures 2 and
3). Within the cytoplasm there are isles of glycogen that make up 20% of the cell on a dry
weight basis and numerous bactericidal granules that are used by the cell for bactericidal
activity. Generally, human neutrophils have two predominantly distinct granule populations;
azurophilic (primary) granules which are large and appear as electron dense granules on
electron microscopy, and specific (secondary) granules which are small and appear as light
staining granules on electron microscopy. Azurophilic granules are more abundant in
immature lineage of neutrophils than specific granules (Borregaard et al., 2007). Similarly,
bovine PMN contains azurophilic and specific granules (figure 2). They also contain a third
novel granule that is larger, denser and more numerous than the other two granules. These
granules contain lactoferrin, which is also found in secondary granules, but they do not
contain constituents common to azurophilic granules. Instead, they contain a group of highly
cationic proteins and are the exclusive store of powerful oxygen-independent bactericidal
compounds (Gennaro et al., 1983). The most important antibacterial mechanism derived from
azurophilic granules is the MPO-H_2O_2-halide system (Heyneman et al., 1990; Heyneman &
Burvenich, 1992; Mehrzad et al., 2001a; 2002a; 2009). MPO in the presence of hydrogen
peroxide (H_2O_2) and halide ions kills bacteria. The functionality of these ROS producing

granules might be altered during physiological and pathological conditions of animals, and should therefore be further investigated.

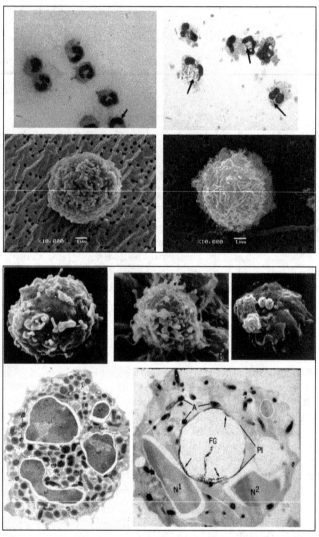

Fig. 2. Upper panel: upper: Isolated neutrophils from blood (left), in which the presence of immature neutrophil (arrow) is distinguishable and post-diapedetic neutrophils in lactating udder (right), in which phagocytosed bacteria (arrows) are visible. Lower: Scanning electron micrograph of PMN isolated from blood (left) and milk (right). Protruding pseudopods needed for phagocytosis in PMN, which is distinguishable in blood and post-diapedetic neutrophils. The blood PMN has higher convulsed cell membrane that forms protruding pseudopods. This might be due to phagocytosis of milk fat globules and casein miscelles. Samples were taken from cows suffering from *E. coli* mastitis. Lower panel: (A) Scanning

electron micrograph of a neutrohil isolated from post-diapedesis in udder. As a result of the cell ingesting its membrane material during phagocytosis of milk fat globules and casein miscelles, the neutrophils lost the protruding pseudopods required for phagocytosis (×20,000). (B) Scanning electron micrograph of a neutrohil isolated from blood. It has a highly convoluted cell membrane that forms protruding pseudopods (×15,000). Far right: Scanning electron micrograph of a PMN isolated from milk with three Staphylococcus aureus (arrows) are present on the surface of the neutrophil; the bacterium at lower left is partially engulfed by a pseudopod (×20,000). Lower left, transmission electron micrograph of bovine neutrophils isolated from blood. The neutrohil, which is limited by the plasma membrane, contains portions of a multilobed nucleus (N1 to N4), glycogen granules (G), specific granules (S), azurophilic granules (A), and large electron dense granules (D). Azurophilic granules are stained more intensely than the specific and large electron dense granules because the neutrophils were incubated with diaminobenzidine and hydrogen peroxide. As a result, an electron-dense product, indicative of peroxidatic activity, has formed in azurophilic granules (×22,000). Lower right, transmission electron micrograph of bovine neutrophils isolated from lactating udder. Deposition of an electron-dense product performed on neutrophils, which was not stained, electron dense product corresponds to areas that are high in peroxidatic activity. These areas represent the azurophilic granules and periphery (arrows) of phagolysosomes containing a milk fat globule. Nuclear lobes (N1, N2), azurophilic granules (A), phagolysosome (PI), fat globule (FG) (×25,000). Partially adapted from (Paape M., Mehrzad j., et al., 2002).

3. Movement of neutrophils from bone marrow to the mammary glands

The issue of life span, mechanomics and biophysics of this dynamically mobile cell, neutrophil, is very pivotal issue in biomedical research. The neutrophilic PMN leukocytes of the blood circulation are specialized terminally differenciated with a short life-span. All blood and immune cells originate from a self-renewing small population of pluripotent stem cells (CFU-S) that can replicate themselves, or can become committed to a particular development pathway. Neutrophils are the major class of leukocytes in peripheral blood of human and domestic animals. The circulation of a healthy human adult contains 4,500-10,000 leucocytes/μl with approximately 60% or more being neutrophils (Nathan, 2006). A healthy adult human produces ~10^{11} neutrophils each day each of which survives about 6-8 hours in the circulation. Almost similar pattern on leukocyte and neutrophils quantities existed in bovine leukocyte and neutrophils (see e.g., Mehrzad et al., 2001a; 200ab; 2001c; 2002a; 2004; 2005a and plenty more). These vital circulating innate immune cells, neutrophils, are formed through the multi-step process of granulopoiesis, from the colony-forming unit of granulocytes (CFU-G) through myeloblasts, promyelocytes, myelocytes, metamyelocytes, and band cells. Precursor cells undergo substantial morphologic, biochemical and functional changes during granulocytic maturation. These changes are associated with significant changes in cell size and nuclear shape, and with the development of stage-specific proteins essential for phagocytosis and microbial killing (Smit et al., 1996; Van Merris et al., 2001a; 2001b; 2002; Burvenich et al., 2003; Mehrzad et al., 2001a; 2001c).

The efficiency of PMN against invading pathogens was previously shown to be highly dependent on the rate of diapedesis into the infection site (Heyneman et al., 1990; Heyneman & Burvenich, 1992; Mehrzad et al., 2001b; 2004; 2005a; 2005b) and on the ability of these PMN to generate ROS (Heyneman & Burvenich, 1992) and Mehrzad et al., 2001a;

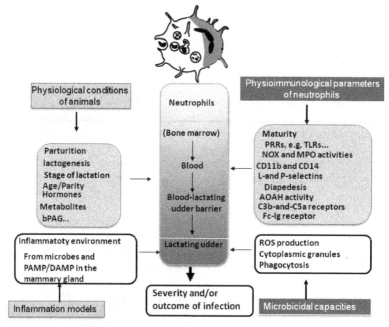

Neutrophil transmigration through blood-milk barrier

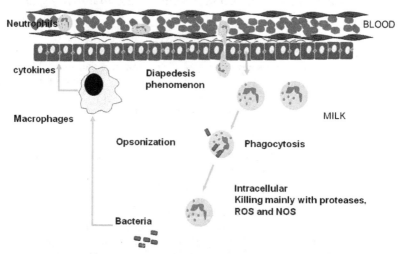

Fig. 3. Upper panel: A schematic representation of the major contributing factors such as some physiological conditions (lactation, parity or age and status of inflammation) to microbicidal capacity of neutrophils in the blood and mammary gland, and the strong link of these conditions to some key immunophysiological parameters of innate host defence in bovine model. This interrelated link happens not only in the blood, but also in the bone marrow, affecting on the most pivotal efferent branches of neutrophil functions in the organs and body, thereby contributing to the outcome or severity of infection. Because

neutrophils are the first cells recruited to the site of infection, their capacity and functionality make this pivotal cell of the circulating innate immune system as one of the cornerstones of the induction and shaping of adaptive immunity in body and organs. Microbicidal activity of neutrophils occurs mainly intracellularly during phagocytosis, with the contribution of many soluble and insoluble proteins, enzymes and ROS produced both inside and outside of the neutrophils. Neutrophils are activated by a wide array of compounds, such as inflammatory mediators, cytokines and ligands for many receptors like pattern recognition receptors (PRRs) (e.g. via Toll-like receptors or TLRs). The activation elicits classic neutrophil functions such as chemotaxis, adherence, ingestion and eventually killing of phagocytosed microbes. Some mediators, cytokines, hormones and metabolites suppress neutrophils' functions throughout the body. Like blood PMN, post-diapedetic PMN functional impairment occurs immediately around parturition; this is coincided with oscillatory events in the cellular and molecular parts of post-diapedetic PMN like viability and killing capacity in the udder. These impairments are more pronounced immediately after parturition and beginning of lactogenesis, which is far more pronounced in older animals. This diagram is based on the author's own studies on bovine PMN functions (see some references appeared in the reference section). The scheme observed in animal model of innate immune system is a fundamental consideration in human, and many molecular aspects of this diagram remains to be further studied in the area of innate immunology in animals and human. Lower panel: Simple scheme of the complex blood-milk barrier showing enterance of invading microbes, which is almost always ascendingly, via teat canal, in the udder cisterna. When microbes enter the gland the triger of innate immune cells in the gland, mainly macrophages and neutrophils, producing veriety of cytokines, chemokins and plenty more immunogenic molecules, creating cell-cell signaling, activating epithelial and endothelial cells, thereby resulting in a masive recruitment of neutrophils in the mammary gland. When real professional phagocytes, neutrophils, reach the site of infection they capture and ingest microbes by phagocytosis and eventually destroy the pathogenic microbes with their microbicidal arsenal, mainly ROS and proteases and RNS (reactive nitrogen species). This final step of first line defence mechanism is the main focus of the future resaerch in the area of molecular immunobiology.

2001c; 2005a; 2005b; 2009). Although the immature neutrophils expressed already the membrane adhesion molecule CD (cluster of differentiation) 11b, they were not capable of rapidly migrating to the infected organs to efficiently ingest and kill the invading pathogens. The impairment of ROS production was attributed to the absence of membrane-bound NADPH-oxidase activity, as myeloperoxidase was already present in the rare azurophilic granules at the promyelocytic stage (Van Merris et al., 2002). Thus, when maturation is impaired due to an increased proliferation rate, a higher number of immature neutrophils will appear in the blood circulation. These findings support the hypothesis postulated by (Heyneman & Burvenich, 1992; Mehrzad et al, 2001a; 2005a; 2005b; 2009) namely that the presence of myelocytes, metamyelocytes and band cells (shift to the left) observed during acute inflammation and sepsis may compromise the animals' resistance by supplying more cells that are morphologically immature and functionally insufficient. Van Werven et al. (1997) and Mehrzad et al. (2001a; 2002a; 2004; 2005a; 2007) demonstrated that the increase of neutrophil functionality was a result of increased enzyme activity per neutrophil, rather than an increase of the number of neutrophils. Therefore, the enhanced enzymatic activity in neutrophils after onset of infection/inflammation was believed to be induced by granulocyte-moncyte colony-stimulating factors (GM-CSF), reflecting an increased proliferation and differentiation of bone marrow granulocytes (Heyneman et al., 1990; Heyneman & Burvenich, 1992; Mehrzad et al., 2001a; 2001b; 2004; 2005a). It has been postulated that myeloid stem cells leave the bone marrow almost by a pipeline mechanism, the older cells being released first (Heyneman & Burvenich, et al., 1992). The molecular mechanisms that control the release of mature PMN from the bone marrow into the circulating pool and then extravasation are very complex and poorly understood (see figures 3 and 4).

Neutrophils circulate in the blood until recruited to sites of infection by chemical signals. This migration begins when neutrophils interact with activated endothelial cells. Inflammatory cytokines like tumor necrosis factor-α (TNF-α), interleukin-1 (IL-1), and interferon-γ (IFN-γ) produced by activated macrophages at sites of infection activate endothelial cells and induce expression of receptors like E-selectin (CD62E) and P-selectin (CD62P) and ligands like Sialyl-Lewis X on glycan-bearing cell adhesion molecule-1 (GlyCAM-1) and P-selectin glycoprotein ligand-1 [PSGL-1]) which interact with neutrophil receptors like L-selectin (CD62L) (Diez-Fraille et al., 2004; Sohn et al., 2007a; 2007b ; Zarbock A & Ley, 2008). Selectin-ligand interactions are of low affinity leading to only "rolling" and slowing of neutrophils on the endothelial cell surface in post capillary venules to enable stronger associations.

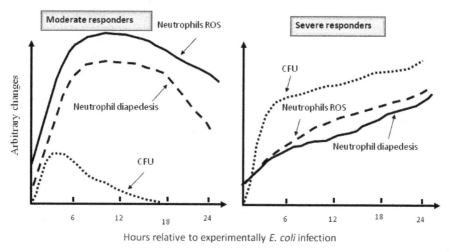

Hours relative to experimentally *E. coli* infection

Fig. 4. This figure shows the overall disparities of neutrophils' diapedesis rate, post-diapedetic neutrophil ROS production capacity and *E. coli* CFU dynamics in modertate and severe responders of animal infection model; it is based on the study of the kinetics of chemiluminescence and intramammary infection/inflammation (Mehrzad et al., 2001b, 2004; 2005a). Moderate responders' neutrophils are functioning much more appropriately than severs'. The fast increase in neutrophils' diapedesis rate and post-diapedetic neutrophil ROS production capacity during acute infection of mammary gland lags exponential growth of *E. coli* in the gland. Compared with severe responders, the fast-strong local response in moderate responders facilitated recovery of acute infection and inflammation. The bacterial growth in the lactating udder is exceeded to the neutrophils' diapedesis and ROS production rates in sever responders. This is very important and basic cellular part of innate immunity of mammary gland. This different response is mainly due to the far stronger pre-infection blood and post-daipedetic neutrophils' functions, especially, ROS production as well as the neutrophils' ROS production during the "early phase" of infection/inflammation. So, the capacity of PMN ROS production (especially intracellular) and quality of pos-diapedetic neutrophils both before and during early infection, is crucial for the severity of the diseases, and leads to a faster elimination of pathogens, becuae the fast-strong local response in moderate responders facilitated recovery of infection/inflammation.

Besides increased expression of selectins, TNF- α and IL-1 also enhance endothelial cell expression of vascular cell adhesion moledule-1 (VCAM-1) and intracellular adhesion molecule-1 (ICAM-1) and ICAM-2, which are ligands for the neutrophil integrins very late antigen-4 (VLA-4) and leukocyte function antigen-1 (LFA-1 or CD11a/18 or $\alpha_L\beta_2$) and macrophage-1 antigen (Mac-1, CD11b/18 or $\alpha_m\beta_2$), respectively. Interactions of neutrophils with these molecules results in firm attachment to the endothelium, followed by their activation, and spreading. Interactions of neutrophil receptors CXCR1 and CXCR2 down a concentration gradient of their ligand chemokine CXCL8 result in transmigration of neutrophils between endothelial cell spaces to the infectious site (Paulsson et al., 2010). Neutrophil LFA-1-endothelial ICAM-1 and CD177-CD31 (platelet endothelial cell adhesion molecule-1 [PECAM-1]) interactions facilitate this migration (Sachs et al., 2007).

A potential role of adhesion molecules like L-selectin in the release of neutrophils from the bone marrow is very critical, because L-selectin is highly expressed on mature PMN in the post-mitotic pool in the bone marrow and in the circulation (Diez-Fraile et al., 2004). The process of granulopoiesis is strictly controlled by regulatory growth factors, comprising cytokines and colony-stimulating factors, which have pleiotropic effects on proliferation, differentiation and functional activation of precursor cells (Burvenich et al., 2003). Using an optimised cell culture assay for the bovine (Smit et al., 1996; Van Merris et al., 2001a; 2001b), it was demonstrated that physiological concentrations of β-hydroxybutyric acid and acetoacetic acid induced remarkable suppression on the proliferation of hematopoietic cells (van Werven et al., 1997; Hoeben et al., 1999). Bovine pregnancy-associated glycoprotein also reduced the proliferative activity of bovine progenitor cells (Hoeben et al., 1999). Therefore, the neutrophil circulating pool is largely depending on the proliferative capacity of the bone marrow. After having exerted their role in immune function, PMN die by senescence (Mehrzad et al., 2001a; Van Merris et al., 2002; Burvenich et al., 2003). Aged PMN undergo spontaneous apoptosis in the absence of pro-inflammatory agents prior to their removal by macrophages (Paape et al., 2002; Burvenich et al., 2003), thus preventing the release of their cytotoxic content. Inflammation and infection hugely increase the rate of PMN production, shortening the maturation time, thereby leading to the release of immature neutrophils in the circulation pool.

Advances in mammary gland immunology of recent decades have provided insights into the mechanisms responsible for the defense of the mammary gland against infection. PMN has a pivotal role in the protection of the gland from infections (Paape et al., 2002; Burvenich et al., 2003; Mehrzad et al., 2001a; 2001b; 2001c; 2002; 2004; 2005a; 2005b; 2009). The life cycle of the bovine PMN is short. Formed in the bone marrow, PMN require 10 to 14 days to mature (Bainton et al., 1971; Burvenich et al., 2003). After maturation, PMN may be stored for a few additional days. Mature PMN leave the hematopoietic compartment of the bone marrow and enters the vascular sinus by travelling in migration channels through endothelial cells. Normally, mature neutrophils circulate in the blood stream briefly (half-life of ~9 hours), then leave the blood stream by diapedesis and enter tissues where they function as strong phagocytes for 1 to 2 days. In healthy animals, production and destruction of PMN is tightly regulated, which keeps their number in blood, milk, and tissue almost constant (Heyneman et al., 1990; Heyneman & Burvenich, 1992; Paape et al., 2002; Burvenich et al., 2003; Mehrzad et al., 2002a) and this is an essential element of their role in the first line of immune defense. Continuous influx of PMN is orchestrated by the local accumulation of chemotactic factors, which may be of endogenous or exogenous origin. Examples of the former include complement derived factors (e.g., C5a), lipid-derived mediators (e.g., leukotriene B4, platelet-activating factor or PAF) and tissue-derived chemokines (in particular IL-8). The dynamic of PMN diapedesis through blood/milk barrier helps to explain the observed PMN activity fluctuations in milk (Smits et al., 1999; Mayadas & Cullere 2005; Pezeshki et al., 2011).

Transendothelial/epithelial concentrations of neutrophils is very critical to effectively kill invading microbes (Li et al., 2002; Mehrzad et al., 2005a; 2005b). The issue of blood and post-diapedetic PMN functions and concentrations in different physiological and pathological conditions remains the focus of most concern. Although the presence of strong chemotactic factors in non-inflamed udder is the subject of debate, their presence in inflammatory environment of udder and milk is indisputable (Manlongat et al., 1998; Rainard, 2002; Stevens et al., 2011a; 2011b; Pezeshki et al., 2011). Most inflammatory chemoattractants are only induced and released during acute infection. However, a restricted number of chemoattractants can be constitutively present in normal plasma at high concentrations, e.g. Regakine-1 (Struyf et al., 2001). During mastitis, inflammatory chemoattractants simply guide PMN toward infection foci. Potent bovine PMN chemoattractants include C5a, an active cleavage product of the C5 in the complement system, various lipopolysaccharides (LPS), IL-1, IL-2 and IL-8 (Gray et al., 1982). These chemoattractants bind to specific receptors on the PMN plasma membrane.

When the completely equipped neutrophils reach the site of infection/inflammation, they with macrophages capture and ingest microbes by phagocytosis and destroy them with their microbicidal arsenal. Neutrophils engage microorganisms through extracellular membrane receptors like PRRs, e.g., TLRs, C-type lectins (mannose receptor), scavenger receptors like CD36, Nod-like receptors (NLRs), and N-formyl Met-Leu-Phe (f- MLP) receptors (Nathan., 2006; Diez-Fraille et al., 2004; Bellocchio et al., 2004; Sohn et al., 2007a; 2007b ; Zarbock A & Ley, 2008; Rainard, 2002; Stevens et al., 2011a; 2011b). Neutrophils also bind to pathogens coated with various opsonins like IgG, complement components (e.g. iC3b), and lectins. Activated neutrophils express the high affinity Fc-receptor, FcγR1, which binds to IgG-Fc of antibody-coated microbes, and β_2 integrins on the neutrophil surface can capture pathogens coated with the iC3b. Bound pathogens are then surrounded by neutrophil membrane projections and engulfed in the cellular cytoplasm inside a phagosome. The phagosome fuses with a lysosome to produce a phagolysosome where the captured pathogens are destroyed.

One of the critically hottest topics in the molecular aspects of inflammation, infection and sepsis in relation to neutrophils in animals and human would be the cross-talk between C5a and neutrophils' surface receptors, e.g., C5a-C5aR, C5aR-TLR4 interactions. Normally, C5aR is up-regulated in inflammatory environment (Bruhn et al., 2011; Stevens et al., 2011a; 2011b). There is considerable evidence for the participation of C5aR in the harmful consequences of experimental infection, sepsis and cancer in human and animals. Therefore, interception of either C5a or C5aR dramatically improves the exaggerated inflammatory reactions which can be good direction to treat and remodel tissue injuries and damages. This evidence would open a new door to the molecular aspects of controlling and treating of inflammation, infection and sepsis. For example, *in vivo* blockade of C5aR resulted in greatly improved survival of animals after sepsis. Similar phenamena could be observed and would be applied for other key molecules like IL-1-IL-1R interactions as well as TLRs antagonists/agonists in the inflammatory environment.

Extravasation of activated PMN occurs after their adhesion to the endothelial surface. This is accomplished by the expression of specific membrane adhesion molecules. The essential role of the CD11/CD18 family of adhesion molecules in bovine PMN-surface adhesion is well-documented (Diez-Fraille et al., 2004). These molecules bind to ICAM-1, ICAM-2 and endothelial leukocyte adhesion molecules (ELAM-1) on the endothelial surface. After binding to these molecules, PMN leave the circulation and are ready to function at the infection site. Down-regulated CD11/CD18 in circulating PMN can cause a harder and slower PMN recruitment into the mammary gland (Burvenich et al., 2003; Diez-Fraille et al., 2004). Inflammatory environment of the udder induces adherence of circulating PMN to the endothelium by up-regulation of CD11b/CD18 (Diez-Fraille et al., 2004), of which activity is crucial to bovine PMN diapedesis across the blood/milk barrier (Smits et al., 2000); in such an environment, blood PMN number, and effective adhesion, migration, opsonization, phagocytosis and killing are of crucial importance to the outcome of the infection and the severity of the disease (Gray et al., 1982; Burvenich et al., 1999; 2003; Mehrzad et al., 2001a; 2001b; 2005a; 2005b; 2009). The impact of fast PMN diapedesis during udder infection/inflammation on PMN quality and their ROS production capability could cause dissimilarities between post-diapedetic PMN from inflamed and non-inflamed quarters (Mehrzad et al., 2001b; 2005a; 2005b; 2009) (see later figures of this chapter). The underlying cellular and molecular mechanisms of this disparity would be pivotal for further investigation in the area of animals and human mammary gland immunobiology and neoplasia.

The source of host and/or pathogen-derived cytokines in udder secretions and their impact on udder PMN function has been a subject of investigation. There is evidence of cytokines secretion by mammary macrophages and epithelial cells during both physiological and pathological conditions of the gland (Boudjellab et al., 1998; Mehrzad et al., 2001b; 2004; 2005a; 2005b; Rainard, 2002; Stevens et al., 2011a; 2011b; Pezeshki et al., 2011). These cytokines influence PMN function. For example, the IL-8 is involved in the recruitment of PMN and T lymphocytes into the gland (Barber et al., 1999). Proinflammatory cytokines, like TNF- α, IL-1β, and LPS suppress the gene expression of cytochrome P-450 1A1 (*cyp1a1*), by activating the transcription nuclear factor κB (NF-κB) (Notebaert et al., 2005). PMN also play a crucial role in the recruitment of other leukocytes such as CD4[+] T lymphocyte and CD8[+] T lymphocyte to the inflammation sites (Mehrzad et al., 2008a; 2008b). From bone marrow to the blood stream and the extravasation, the on time PMN influx to the site of inflammation is important in limiting injury and promoting recovery of severe inflammation (Carey et al., 1997; Mehrzad et al., 2001b; 2004; 2005a; 2005b).

4. Location of microbicidal weaponry in circulating and post-diapedetic neutrophils

Armed with an array of highly microbicidal weapons, such as enzymes that hydrolyze and destroy proteins, lipids and sugars of pathogens, the weaponry is mainly stored in, at least, three different kinds of granules in the cytoplasm as well as outside the cytoplasm. Additionally, neutrophils have powerful systems for generation of large amounts of free radicals or ROS. Microbial pathogens are taken up into an intracellular compartment, called phagolysosome, into which microbicidal agents are released. There are also many new forms of innate effector molecules like neutrophil extracellular traps (NETs), PRRs, opsonin receptors and plenty more that sense, bind and efficiently kill invading microbes, destroy virulence factors, or prevent them from spreading.

Following adherence of opsonized bacteria to surface receptors on the PMN, phagocytosis, respiratory burst and degranulation are triggered. The process of opsonization, though not essential for phagocytosis, certainly promotes the uptake of bacteria by PMN. The phagocytosis process is energy-dependent and requires the presence of a functional cytoskeleton. The cytoskeleton machinery, when sequentially activated following receptor stimulation, is thought to envelope the microorganism in a "zipper mechanism" (Griffin et al., 1975). Immunological recognition is mainly accomplished by specific antibodies (IgG_2 and IgM) which recognize the bacterium through Fab-regions and bind to PMN via Fc-receptors on the PMN plasma membrane (Paape et al., 1996). There is a synergy between the Fcγ and C3b receptors activity and neutrophils' ROS production (Newman & Johnston, 1979).

Neutrophils produce several proteolytic enzymes that degrade and destroy microbes in the phagolysosome. Two important proteases produced by neutrophils are the serine protease, elastase, and cathepsin G (Reeves et al., 2002; Mehrzad et al., 2005b). More importantly, neutrophils also destroy ingested microorganisms with ROS produced by the "phagocyte oxidase system (phox)," or "NADPH oxidase or NOX," which reduces molecular oxygen into ROS in the phagolysosome (Mehrzad et al., 2001a; 2001c; 2005a; Reeves et al., 2002). NOX pumps electrons from the oxidation of NADPH to NADP in the neutrophil cytosol, across the phagolysosome membrane via flavocytochrome b558 (the core component of phox) and onto molecular oxygen (O_2) in the phagolysosome reducing it to superoxide anion (O_2^-), and cascade reaction of respiratory burst starts. NOX activity and K^+ flux are important for provision of acidic pH in the phagolysosome for effective killing of engulfed microbes (Reeves et al., 2002). Normally, during intracellular killing pH of the phagolysosome (initially neutral) rapidly drops to ~4 within <10 min; this change in pH is very important for killing of engulfed microbes, because many enzymes and peptides necessary for microbicidal are activated at acidic pH.

After a complicated cascade of release of biological substances and activation of the endothelium, neutrophils migrate into the mammary gland and finally also appear in the fluid of the lactiferous sinus (Burvenich et al., 1994; 2003). Although several antimicrobial systems exist in the mammary gland (Burvenich et al., 1994; Paape et al., 1996; 2002), but, it is the massive influx of neutrophils that will resolve the infection through efficiently killing of the invading bacteria (Mehrzad et al., 2001b; 2005a; 2005b; Burvenich et al., 2003; Paape et al., 2002). Diapedesis will also affect binding of immunoglobulins to the PMN surface. An increased expression of Fc receptors and phagocytosis happens after *in vitro* migration of bovine PMN through membranes (Berning et al., 1993; and Worku et al., 1994). After *in vivo* migration of PMN into mammary quarters of nulliparous heifers, binding of IgG_1 and IgG_2 increased while binding of IgM decreased. Binding of IgA remained unchanged. The greatest change occurred with the binding of IgM. Seventy-six percent of the blood PMN bound IgM, whereas only 2% of the post-diapedetic PMN bound IgM. Interestingly, phagocytic activity of PMN increased after *in vitro* chemotaxis but not after *in vivo* chemotaxis of neutrophils. Activation of complement also promotes chemotaxis, extravasation, phagocytosis and killing capacities. The C3b and iC3b, generated on the surface of bacteria following antibody union, are recognized respectively by CR1 and CR3 receptors located on the PMN cell membrane. The type of bacteria also affects bovine PMN bactericidal capacity. For example, slime-producing *Staphylococcus aureus* hampers the killing capacity of PMN (Barrio et al., 2000; Mehrzad et al., 2009). The specific interactions between extracellular matrix proteins of *Staphylococcus aureus* and ICAM-1 inhibits further PMN recruitment, boosting anti-inflammatory reactions (Chavakis et al., 2002). This might be counterproductive for the killing activity of PMN. During migration of PMN into milk in response to infection increased binding of C3b was observed (DiCarlo et al., 1996). Thus, PMN are fully armed to confront invading bacteria, resulting in a more rapid ingestion and elimination of the pathogens. Once complement and immunoglobulins bind to receptors on the PMN surface, PMN become activated and generate ROS, such as O_2^-, H_2O_2 and halogen reactive species. This process associated with the respiratory burst is called the "oxygen-dependent" or "oxidative" killing, and that associated with neutrophil granules is also called "oxygen-dependent", but "non-oxidative" killing. Killing classified on the basis of these criteria has been explicitly addressed (e.g., Root & Cohen, 1981; Babior, 1984; Spitznagel & Shafer, 1985; Babior, 1994; Reeves et al., 2002; Mehrzad et al., 2001c; 2009; 2011). The pivotal role of ROS in all further events for killing of engulfed microbes by neutrophils is therefore indisputable.

ROS formed by neutrophils are critical microbicidal agents against infection as evidenced by individuals afflicted with Chronic Granulomatous Disease (CGD). Patients with CGD have mutations in key elements of NOX and are profoundly susceptible to bacterial and fungal infections (Heyworth et al., 2003), though this kind of mutation has not been observed in bovine. In addition, a number of proteolytic enzymes including elastase, cathepsin G, myeloperoxidase, gelatinase, and others contained in the azurophilic and specific granules fuse with the phagolysosome and also contribute to the intracellular killing of microbes and degradation of its contents.

Intracellular killing of phagocytosed microorganisms is accomplished by following adherence to the PMN surface, usually, but not necessarily, via specific receptors (Horwitz et al., 1982). Three different mechanisms are involved for intracellular bacterial destruction: 1) an oxygen-dependent mechanism (production of ROS), 2) a nitrogen dependent mechanism (RNS especially nitrogen oxide (NO) derived from L-arginine) and 3) an oxygen-and nitrogen-independent microbicidal mechanism e.g., lyzozyme, lactoferrin, proteases, pH changes and even neutrophil extracellular traps (NETs). Because of their essentiality for killing, here my prime focus is the oxygen-dependent microbicidal mechanisms and how these mechanisms are generated in neutrophils to efficiently destroy pathogens. Though not predominantly, pathogens are trapped and killed extracellularly, e.g., NETs, as well. Impaired neutrophil NETs formation would be considered as a novel innate immune deficiency of animals and human; the NETs are lattices of DNA, histones, granule enzymes, and antimicrobial proteins that are released by the PMNs in parallel with extrusion of nuclear material. It has been found that defect in NETs formation in neutrophils is substantially rescued by the ROS generation, confirming the broadly essential roles of ROS in NETs-related killing of pathogen. Similarly, NETs-related killing of pathogens and NETs formation occurs via pathways involving both ROS and RNS (Allport et al., 2002). Thus, ROS generation is always the most pivotal and prerequisite for all further events for efficient killing of invading microbes.

Baldridge and Gerard (1933) first reported that an increase in oxygen consumption by neutrophils takes place when phagocytosis is triggered. ROS generated by reduction-oxidation (redox) reactions, have been recognized as one of the major contributors to the killing of pathogens. This phenomenon is accompanied by an increase in oxygen consumption and the hexose monophosphate shunt (HMPS) activity by PMN and has been termed the "respiratory" burst. The oxygen molecule is central for PMN respiratory burst activity (Allen et al., 1972; Babior, 1984; 1994; Reeves et al., 2002); its importance in microbicidal activity of PMN was highlighted by the inefficient PMN bactericidal activity in anaerobic conditions (Mandell, 1974). One example: for each molecule of O_2 consumed 4 O_2^- ions are generated; roughly 0.5 fmol of O_2 is consumed for each bacterium engulfed, resulting in an intravacuolar O_2^- release of about 4 mol.l^{-1} (Reeves et al., 2002). Though still remains inconclusive, the application of ozone gass (O_3) would be further examined in domestic animals for treatment of infections such as mastitis, metritis, arthritis, cancer and increase many cell signaling pathways for tissue remodeling and repair; because it boosts milk PMN ROS production capacity (Ogata & Nagahata, 2000), cleaning pathogen/damage-associated molecular patterns PAMPs/DAMPs from inflamed site (Lai & Gallo., 2009; Alexandrova, 2009).

As shown in figure 5, the first step in the cascade of respiratory burst is the formation of O_2^-, requiring NOX, of which substrate (NADPH) is generated by HMPS to act as an electron donor (Rossi and Zatti, 1964; Babior, 1984; Rossi, 1986).

$$2 O_2 + NADPH \rightarrow 2O_2^- + NADP^+ + H^+$$

Different stimuli (e.g., complement components, immunoglobulin, formyl-methionyl-leucyl-phenylalanine (fMLP), phorbol myristate acetate (PMA) and bacterial peptides) act via different specific receptors and thus have various signal transduction mechanisms to activate the NOX. Extensive research into activation by PMA has followed the identification of protein kinase-c (PK-C) as its cytosolic receptor (Nishizuka, 1984). PMA is a strong NADPH-oxidase and PK-C agonist (Tauber, 1987, Karlsson et al., 2000). Particulate stimuli may also act indirectly via PK-C (Cooke & Hallett, 1985) or via other intermediates such as arachidonic acid and its metabolites and phospholipase-A2 (Tauber, 1987). The next step is the formation of H_2O_2 by dismutation of O_2^-, which is mediated by superoxide dismutase (SOD):

$$2 O_2^- + 2H^+ \rightarrow H_2O_2 + O_2$$

The O_2^- and H_2O_2, generated by NADPH-oxidase and SOD, are the precursors of variety of subsequent powerful ROS. Included among these ROS are a variety of oxidized halogens, including hypohalite ions or HOX (Thomas & Fishman, 1986; Weiss et al., 1986) and a variety of chloramines (Thomas et al., 1982) used by PMN as microbicidal agents. These are

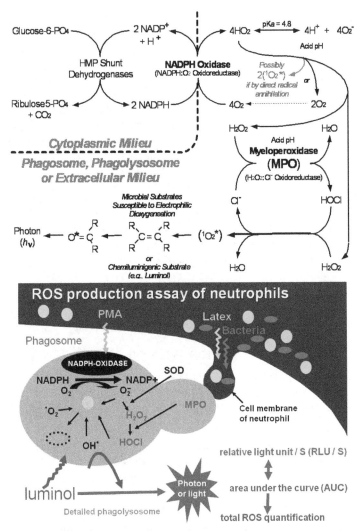

Fig. 5. Upper panel: Diagram depicting the major enzymatic systems responsible for microbicidal metabolism and oxygenation activities and the relationship of these activities to photon emission. In the scheme the activities of the cytoplasmic milieu are separated from those of the phagosome-phagolysosome-extracellular milieu. The superscripted number that precedes each molecular symbol (e.i., [1]for singlet, [2]for doublet, and [3]for triplet multiplicity) depicts the equation: $|2s| + 1$ = multiplicity (n). The diagram adapted from (Allen et al., 2000). Lower panel: Brief scheme of ROS production process by neutrophils during phagocytosis of bacteria. As shown the cell membrane of the neutrophils and bacteria (red). This is non-specefic phagocytosis of bacteria. The bacteria are engulfed by the neutrophils and form phagosome and fussion of phagosome to lysosome and then detialed phagolysosome is highlighted on the scheme. Activation of NADPH-oxidase (NOX) is the triger of neutrophil ROS production, the most fundametally powerful efferent arms of the

innate immune system .When bacteria are attached to the cell membrane ROS production starts and this continues when the pathogen are engulfed. Before engulfment most ROS are produced extracellularly, but afterwards it is produced intracellularly, both of which are pivotal for continuation of innate immune response against pathogens. This is a fundamental concept in the area of ROS-mediated phagocytosis and killing of microbes, in which NOX and MPO are central in this pathway; this is an interestingly big subjetc in innate immunophysiology. These ROS can be measured by chemiluminescence (CL) and this is the main technique that was highlighted in this chapter of the book. To conduct an assay on one of the pivotal efferent arms of neutrophils microbicidal capacity (light or photon produced by ROS), the pure neutrophils are activated artificially with phagocytosis-dependent (latex beads, bacteria etc.) or non-phagocytosis-dependent (PMA...) methods. Researchers routinly use photon enhancer like luminol, isoluminol, lucigenin and plenty more. The metabolites of, e.g., luminol (aminophtalate) is very unstable and can easily and immediately be oxidized by hydrogen peroxide-MPO-halide system and gain to the relaxation state and emit light. This light, which is unequivocal representative of PMN ROS production load, can be easily and precisely quatified by CL assay. The two units, which luminometer gives, are the ROS production in function of time.

generated by the H_2O_2-mediated oxidation of halide ions under catalysis by MPO or eosinophil peroxidase (EPO) and the subsequent oxidation of amines:

$$H_2O_2 + X^- \rightarrow HOX + OH^- \quad (X = Cl^-, Br^-, I^-)$$

$$HOX + R\text{-}NH\text{-}R' \rightarrow R\text{-}NX\text{-}R' + H_2O$$

Though not as crucial as PMN in infection and inflammation, the activity of compound I of EPO to react with H_2O_2 is similar to that of MPO but with substrates like Cl^-, however, it is far higher, yielding more HOX (Arnhold et al., 2001; Mehrzad et al., 2001a, 2005a; 2009; 20011).

Another group of ROS that are produced from O_2^- are the hydroxyl radicals (OH°) generated in a transition metals (Fe or Cu) catalyzed reaction between O_2^- and a hydroxyperoxide (a well-known Haber-Weiss reaction, if R = H):

$$O_2^- + ROOH \rightarrow RO + OH^- + H_2O_2 \qquad (R = H, \text{-}C, C(=O))$$

or in a reaction between previously generated oxidizing radical and another compound:

$$OH° + RH \rightarrow R° + H_2O$$

Eventually, singlet oxygen ($^1O_2$) has been found to be produced by neutrophils, and eosinophils (see e.g., Root & Cohen, 1981; Allen et al., 2000), possibly through a reaction between hypohalyte and H_2O_2:

$$HOX + H_2O_2 \rightarrow {}^1O_2 + X^- + H_2O$$

It is evident that the production of large quantities of ROS with a cascade of reactions will provide an environment that is destructive for any microorganims exposed to it, but it is also harmful to the nearby tissues. That is to say that ROS represent a "double-aged sword". Alternatively, ROS also enhance the activity of natural killer cell, T cell and dendritic cells

(DCs), neutralization of PAMPs and proinflammatory cytokines (Suthanthiran et al., 1984; Cemerski et al., 2002; Reth, 2002; Mehrzad et al., 2008a; 2008b; Lai & Gallo, 2009; Alexandrova, 2009), indicating that PMN ROS may not only damage cells and tissues but may also accelerate recovery of inflammation. The above reactions are tightly regulated so that the PMN releases its ROS under appropriate circumstances, depending on the physiological and pathological conditions of animals. What is not yet clear is whether there is a transient PMN ROS production change during physiopathological conditions, and if so, whether this change is or is not beneficial for animals and humans.

Neutrophils are capable of producing a range of ROS following activation of the membrane bound NOX. It is also generally agreed that ROS boost oxygen-independent microbicidal activity, like proteases (Reeves et al., 2002; Mehrzad et al., 2004; 2005a; 2009; 20011). Antimicrobial peptides especially proteases in the udder which is mainly released by neutrophils (Mehrzad et al., 2005b), will potentially promote angiogenesis, activation of macrophages, neutralization of PAMPs and pro-inflammatory cytokines, initiation of T-cell recruitment (Mehrzad et al., 2008a; 2008b) and immature (i)DCs and block of TLRs on iDCs (Lai & Gallo, 2009). Root and Cohen (1981) have suggested several possible direct sites of action for ROS, related to their microbicidal activity; these include: 1) unsaturated carbon bounds that may lead to toxic lipid peroxidation, 2) sulphydryl groups that lead to the destruction of sulphydryl containing enzymes, 3) amino group and possible peptide bound breakage and 4) nucleic acids. *In vitro* studies with O_2^- generating systems in neutrophils such as xanthine oxidase (Rosen & Klebanoff, 1976) suggests that O_2^- are far more toxic to bacteria if they operate in MPO H_2O_2-halide system (Reeves et al., 2002; Mehrzad et al., 2001a; 2001b; 2005a; 2009; 2011), which leads to the production of powerful chlorinated oxidising agents such as ClO^- which have a microbicidal effect by halogenating microbial proteins (see figure 5). Although the microbicidal mechanisms of neutrophils is very hugely broad and complex, but there are plenty mechanisms by which microbes evade and overcome the host's phagocytosis and killing mechanisms to succeed infections in the udder, like avoiding contact with phagocytes and inaccessible to phagocytes, inhibition of inflammatory responses and phagocyte chemotaxis and engulfment, even survival inside of phagocytes.

5. Techniques for neutrophils' ROS quantification versus their quality in the mammary gland

ROS production capacity of neutrophils is the most powerful efferent arms of the innate immune systems in blood stream and interstitial fluid for provision of further cascade of effective innate and adaptive immune responses. Several techniques of PMN ROS quantification are frequently applied. For example, the cytochrome c reduction test, flow cytometry method (Salgar et al., 1991), the scopoletine test (Root & Cohen, 1981) and chemiluminescence (CL) assay (Allen et al., 1972; Hoeben et al., 2000a; Mehrzad et al., 2000; 2001b; 2001c; 2002; 2004; 2005a; 2009; 20011). Also plenty laboratory kits available for precise neutrophils' functional tests both for genomics, proteomics and mechanomics related to the ROS production. The most widely used technique to quantify neutrophils' ROS production is CL (Mehrzad et al., 2000; 2001a; 2001b; 2002a; 2002b; 2004; 2005; 2009). As phagocytosis-induced and/or non-induced CL reflects intracellular and extracellular oxidation-reduction reactions (Mehrzad et al., 2001a; 2005a; 2009), changes might offer some evidence about the animals'/humans' susceptibility to infections.

Whereas many differential leukocyte count methods for blood leukocytes are available, study on the qualitative role of milk leukocytes in healthy and diseased animals and human is rare. The milk leukocytes differentiation also appears difficult. In addition, little attention has been paid to the standardization of particularly sample preparation procedures. To unequivocally evaluate PMN functional assays (from genomics to proteomics, mechanomics and metabolomics) appropriate isolation, differentiation and quantification of neutrophils in original or purified samples are essential. This is more special for neutrophils in non-inflammatory environment of milk/udder; not merely because a variety of cells e.g., PMN, macrophages, lymphocytes and epithelial cells, are existed but because their shapes, size and population could differ, compared to the blood. Milk sample processing varies from the use of centrifuged whole milk samples to dilution with a hypotonic buffer (Mehrzad et al., 2000; 2001a; 2001b; 2001c; 2002a; 2004; 2005a; 2009). Without microscopic confirmation, flow cytometric identification of milk cells based on forward and side scatter is inconclusive because phagocytosis of milk components may alter both size and intracellular granularity. Cellular debris may also interfere with the scatter pattern of normal milk cells. Even for blood leukocytes, their shapes and population changed significantly during mastitis. All of these changes could interfere with the assessment of PMN function. Therefore, developing an isolation, differentiation and enumeration of leukocytes in blood and milk in the laboratory to better assess PMN function is always critical. Nowadays, the problem of breast cancer in human is rising substantially, and particularly deep focus on the cellular and molecular aspects of interstitial fluid of mammary gland is urgently needed.

A functional udder immune system depends on the existence of high quality neutrophils in the interstitial fluid of mammary gland and/or milk, protecting the gland against invading pathogens (Burvenich et al., 1994; 2003; Mehrzad et al 2001a; 2001b; 2001c; 2002; 2005a; 2005b; 2009; 2011). Investigation on PMN viability can provide suitable information about PMN quality and tissue damage. This is more special for milk PMN, which migrate to the apparently unsuitable environment. PMN life span might be affected by many physiological and pathological factors in the gland. Many cellular and acellular signaling pathways are available in blood and mammary tissue for the modulation or inhibition of PMN survival. Till now, little attention has been paid on the neutrophils viability in the interstitial fluid of mammary gland/milk. Accordingly, the contribution of neutrophil enzymes (e.g., activity of NOX, MPO etc.) to the viability is critical (Mayer et al., 1989; Jankowski et al., 2002). This supports the assumption of the existence of a good correlation between PMN viability and CL. To obtain a better insight into the effects of (patho)physiology of mammary gland on non-specific defense mechanisms of the udder, assessment of viability of blood and milk PMN can be pivotal. Milk PMN viability assessment could also be an index for the detection of inflammation of the mammary gland.

To overcome any problem and to simplify PMN functional assay, researchers, who wants to work on this area in animals/human breast physioimmunology, should properly isolate targeted cells from blood and mammary gland for quantitative and qualitative assays (see figures 1-2 and 6); there are plenty references in these topics, and some appeared in the reference list. CL simplifies PMN ROS production measurement, and is a relatively recent technique. Application of CL technique to study PMN function helps to gain more insight into first line of immune defense mechanisms and the pathophysiology of physiological and environmental stresses-related infections and/or inflammations. For CL quantification, we need viable PMN, a PMN activator (e.g. PMA, fMLP, particles, etc.) and a CL substrate (e.g.,

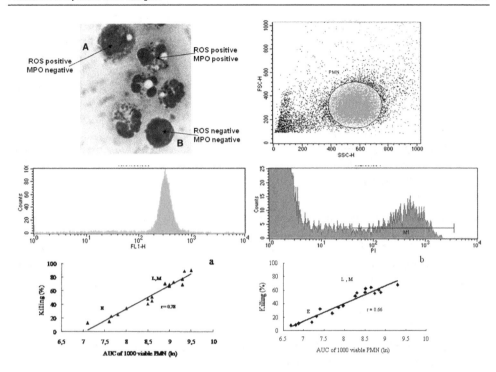

Fig. 6. Upper left: Light microscopic image of PMN (middle), a macrophage (A) and a lymphocyte (B) isolated from non-inflamed lactating udder stained with benzidine dihydrochloride plus H_2O_2 and counterstained with hematoxilin-eosin (× 1000). Because MPO is central to intracellular ROS-associated microbicidal and luminol dependent CL, the contribution of other cells especially macrophages on CL and MPO activity assays should also be considered. Bovine milk macrophages has no MPO activity in our assay, and in case of having mixed cells in the samples their contribution to the CL assay is little. Conversely, bovine post-diapedetic neutrophils has huge MPO activity, and they are main source of CL assay of milk cells. Flow cytometric analysis of isolated bovine milk neutrophils gated in the FS-SS dot plot (upper right). Green fluorescence of PMN labeled with a monoclonal antibody specific against bovine granulocytes and with a secondary FITC-labeled antibody (middle left). Red fluorescence of propidium iodide-incubated PMN selectively gated in the FS-SS dot plot; gate M1 is applied to determine the percentage of dead PMN (for the quantification of viability/quality of post-diapedetic neutrophils) (middle right). Lower panel shows correlation between PMA induced luminol-dependent CL (LDCL) of blood neutrophils (a) and post-diapedetic neutrophils in lactating udder (b) and their effectiveness towards killing of *S. aureus*. E: early lactogenesis period; L, M: late and mid lactogenesis periods, respectively. Partially adapted from (Mehrzad et al., 2001a; 2001c).

luminol, isoluminol, lucigenin etc). Luminol-dependent CL has been described as an appropriate probe for assessment of blood and milk PMN ROS production (Briheim et al., 1984). The PMN metabolic pathways responsible for O_2-dependent bactericidal activity and CL assays are depicted schematically in figure 5.

A flow cytometric technique has also been used to detect ROS production, necrosis, apoptosis and many immunological assays on bovine blood and interstitial fluid neutrophils (Mehrzad et al., 2001a; 2001b; 2001c; Dosogne et al., 2002; Vangroenweghe et al., 2001; Van Oostveldt et al., 2001; 2002a; 2002b Mehrzad et al., 2002; 2004; 2005a; 2009; 2011) applying propidium iodide (PI) exclusion method, Anexi V and JC-1 solution (5,5',6,6'-tetrachloro-1,1',3,3'-tetraethylbenzimidazolylcarbocyanine iodide) (Merhzad et al., 2001a; 2001b; 2001c; 2011; Van Oostveldt et al., 2002a; 2002b) (figures 6). Although many immunological assays can be done with flow cytometry, the assay of neutrophils' ROS production with flow cytometry has revealed some challenging results, compared to luminometry technique; also, with the flow cytometry it is hardly possible to measure the kinetics and the dynamics of the neutrophil-pathogen interaction 'during' neutrophil-pathogen interaction.

Methodological studies reveal a very well correlation between PMN viability and CL activity and killing capacities. Isolated blood and milk PMN can appropriately be identifiable on FS-SS dot plot (see figures 5, 6). Flow cytometry is an accurate and reproducible technique for the rapid quantification of PMN apoptosis and necrosis in physiological and pathological conditions of animals and human (figure 6). This can effectively facilitate further PMN functional assay, hence boosting insight into the first line defense mechanism of the host.

6. Lipopolysaccharide, TLR4, TNF-α and NO levels in inflammatory environment of the mammary gland

The compound of the bacterial outer membrane, peptidoglycan monomers and lipopolysaccharide (LPS) or endotoxins, are unique to all Gram-negative bacterial cell walls. In the case of Gram negative bacteria, the principal stimulator of the innate immune system is the LPS; this LPS evokes several functional responses in these short-lived, bone marrow myeloid-derived cells, neutrophils, to the site of inflammation or infection.

The PRRs are the main sensors of pathogens and danger signals in innate immunity. Though they are mainly highly expressed by macrophages and DCs of different organs, neutrophils also highly express these sensor molecules inside and outside their surface. Toll like receptors/proteins, homologues of the *Drosophila* protein Toll, are the most studied and best characterized PPRs, which are responsible for sensing PAMPs and also products of inflamed tissues, DAMPs. TLRs activation triggers signaling pathways that lead to activation of transcription factors such as NF-κB and the interferon regulatory factors. This, in turn, leads to induction of immune and inflammatory genes, including such important cytokines as TNF-α and type I interferons. The contribution of PRRs to inflammation induced by microbial infection, tissue damage and cancer are a hot topic in immunology, immunopathology and immunotherapy. Much evidence points to the role for PRRs and especially TLRs in immune and inflammatory diseases and increasingly in cancer detection and therapy (Bellocchio et al., 2004; Simons et al., 2008). For example, cancerous cell lines are one of the best models to study the biological roles of PRRs in cancer and tumor biology. Role of neutrophils on those points remained deeply unnoticed. Study also reports how, e.g., TLR2 expression by endothelia is locally upregulated by the action of activated neutrophils via an unprecedented mechanism involving cell-cell interaction and NOX, emphasizing yet another way in which the primordial innate immune system is remarkably complex.

The interaction of neutrophils in the sites of inflamed/infections with these key elements of the PAMPs, LPS, and bind to PRRs is pivotal to overcome pathogen and limit the severity of infection. The PRRs are present on a variety of defence cells of the body causing them to synthesise and release a variety of cytokines. Synergistically, the LPS interacts with LPS-binding protein and CD14, which in turn promotes the ability of particularily TLR4 on neutrophils and macrophages to respond to the LPS with the release of various pro-inflammatory cytokines and chemokines (Sohn et al., 2007a; 2007b; Rinaldi et al., 2010; Stevens et al., 2011a ; 2011b). These pro-inflammatory molecules bind on target cells via specific receptors and initiate inflammation. TLRs have been detected on the surface of mammalian cells (Beutler, 2002). They are important in the responses of phagocytes to bacterial, viral, and fungal antigens. TLR2 and TLR4 have candidate genes for resistance to several diseases as they recognise broad classes of PAMPs, such as peptidoglycans and LPS (Werling & Jungi, 2003; Bellocchio et al., 2004). Bovine and human neutrophils express substantial amounts of TLR4 and other TLRs, critical for response to PAMPs/DAMPs (Kurt-Jones et al., 2002 ; Hayashi et al., 2003; Werling. & Jungi, 2003; Rinaldi et al., 2010; Stevens et al., 2011a ; 2011b). TLR4 activates the inflammatory gene expression through NF-κB (Hayashi et al., 2003). GM-CSF and and G-CSF dramatically up-regulate TLR2 and CD14 expression (Kurt-Jones et al., 2002). Recent *in vitro* studies have shown that mammary epithelial cells actively participate in the immunoregulation during inflammation via mainly cytokine production (Sohn et al., 2007a; 2007b; Rinaldi et al., 2010; Stevens et al., 2011a; 2011b). A MAC-T cell line was utilised to investigate the expression of many innate immune mRNAs like IL-1 and its subsequent secretion after stimulation with PAMPs showed that these cells secrete IL-1 in response to LPS. IL-1 also appeared to be an important mediator for the release of the IL-8 and many other chemokines (Huynh et al., 1991; Boudjellab et al., 1998; 2000; Pezeshki et al., 2011).

During infection of mammary gland, IL-1, IL-6 and IL-8 (Shuster et al., 1997), platelet-activating factor (PAF), (Pezeshki et al., 2011), prostaglandins (Pezeshki et al., 2011; Shuster et al., 1997), activated complement C5 (C5a; Shuster et al., 1997; Rinaldi et al., 2010) NO (Blum et al., 2000), many ROS (Mehrzad et al., 2001; 2004; 2005a) and proteases (Mehrzad et al., 2005b) are released locally. In milk, an increase in TNF-α, a cytokine of particular interest in the pathogenesis of mastitis, is observed (Blum et al., 2000; Hoeben et al., 2000b; Shuster et al., 1997). The kinetics of cytokines in the inflammatory environment of udder shows that the increase in TNF-α and IL-1, the mother of proinflammatory cytokines, occurs faster during inflammation from endotoxins than from *E. coli* mastitis, though more pronounced in *E. coli* infection (Blum et al., 2000; Hoeben et al., 2000b). Absorption of this cytokine from the udder into the blood circulation is highest during *E. coli* mastitis. The level of these key cytokines in milk correlated well with the pyrexia and the severity of the udder infection (Shuster et al., 1997; Blum et al., 2000; Hoeben et al., 2000b; Pezeshki et al., 2011).

Many of the biological activities of LPS are mediated by TNF-α. LPS and cytokines stimulate the synthesis of NO, which is a vasodilator. Synthesised from L-arginine, this diatomic free radical, NO, is lipid soluble and easily diffuses through the cell membrane. It is short lived and usually reacts and degrades fast. The natural form is a gas that reacts with a variety of innate immune molecules and mediates a large spectrum of immunobiological effects in the body. An inducible NO synthase (E.C. 1.14.13.39, iNOS) is expressed by a variety of cells, especially phagocytes, as a result of triggering with substances of microbial origin such as LPS and TNF-α. In response to invading pathogens and PAMPs like LPS, bovine phagocytes produce NO (Adler et al., 1995; Stich et al., 1998), functioning as a strong anti-PAMP agent. When the NO is produced in excessive amounts, it can also induce cytotoxic and apoptosis in the cells (Moncada et al., 1991; Anggard, 1994)

Several studies on ruminants have shown a relationship between LPS, TNF-α and production of NO. The increase in TNF-α is followed by a delayed increase in NO_x (NO_2 + NO_3) (Blum et al., 2000; Bouchard et al., 1999). The NO_x production lasts longer in the udder. A causal relationship between TNF-α and NO_x production was observed in studies in which *E. coli* LPS was injected intravenously. It seems that severe forms of udder's inflamed environment are accompanied by the highest increase in blood stream's levels of both TNF-α and NO_x; the increase in NO_x and TNF-α during infection is not inhibited by antibiotics (Blum et al., 2000), supporting the notion that the release of NO_x is PAMP dependent rather than *E. coli*. Initially called endothelium derived factor (EDRF), NO causes many other vital physiological phenomena like vasodilation and subside of inflammation. It is released after the fever peak, and is involved in this delayed phase of hyperemia.

7. Neutrophil AOAH as a potent protector of mammary gland from pathogens

The contribution of circulating and postdiapedetic neutrophils' acyloxyacyl hydrolase (AOAH) to the outcome of infection in animals has recently been highlighted (Dosogne et al., 1998; Mehrzad et al., 2007). Apart from existence of many bactericidal mechanisms in the bovine neutrophils (Barrio et al., 2000; Burvenich et al., 2003; Mehrzad et al., 2001a; 2001b; 2001c; 2002; 2004; 2005a; 2005b; 2007; 2008a; 2009), there are many other soluble and insoluble proteins on the neutrophils in the mammary gland that protect the gland from invading pathogens. One of them is AOAH molecules. Endotoxins or LPS are released during bacterial growth and lysis of Gram-negative bacteria have been recognized as important mediators for the treatment and outcome of coliform mastitis (Pyörälä et al., 1994; Dosogne et al., 2002; Mehrzad et al., 2007). The role of the absorption of free LPS into the circulation is controversial (Dosogne et al., 2002; Mehrzad et al., 2004; 2005a; 2007). Conversely, it is accepted that the amount of released LPS into the mammary gland, its subsequent detoxification and TNF-α production significantly contribute to the outcome of coliform infection (Blum et al. 2000; Hoeben et al. 2000b; Mehrzad et al., 2007). Severity of *E. coli* infection seems to be related to the enhanced release of secondary induced inflammatory mediators such as TNF-α (Blum et al., 2000; Mehrzad et al., 2007), as a result of impaired LPS detoxification mechanisms in inflamed organ. It has been suggested (Burvenich et al., 1996; 2003; Paape et al., 1996; 2002) that local CD14 expression alleviates the toxic effects of LPS in the mammary gland. AOAH, an enzyme hugely produced by bovine neutrophils, hydrolyses LPS (McDermott et al., 1991; Mehrzad et al., 2007) and alleviate the inflammation. This neutrophils' arsenal, AOAH, hydrolyses two acyl chains of the lipid A of LPS, leading to substantial decreased toxicity of LPS while retaining much of the immunostimulatory potency of native toxicity of LPS (Munford and Hall, 1986).

Although there are some rare investigation of bovine blood PMN AOAH activity, but little has been done on post-diapedetic neutrophils' AOAH activity either during physiological or pathological conditions. Immediately after parturition, there is a

Molecular Aspects of Neutrophils as Pivotal Circulating Cellular Innate Immune Systems to
Protect Mammary Gland from Pathogens

173

decreased blood PMN AOAH activity (Dosogne et al., 1998) that coincides with the decreased PMN ROS production and number in circulation (Mehrzad et al., 2001b; 2002a; 2004; 2005a). This coincidence could be considered as a risk factor for Gram negative bacterial infections during especially physiological stress (Mehrzad et al., 2001b; 2004; 2005a). Indeed, intravenous LPS administration to rabbits resulted in a rapid (within 90 min) increase of plasma AOAH activity (Erwin and Munford, 1991). The finding that PMN AOAH activity is increased upon LPS stimulation may indicate the existence of a PMN-dependent self-regulatory protection mechanism against endotoxemia and sepsis. It is suggested that a decreased AOAH activity in post-diapedetic PMN can also contribute to the outcome of organ failure and even death, as we observed in bovine (Mehrzad et al., 2007).

Apart from AOAH, bovine neutrophils granules also contain different LPS binding cationic proteins such as lactoferrin, and a huge variety of cationic antimicrobial proteins (Levy et al., 1995; Mehrzad et al., 2005b). These proteins do not degrade the LPS molecule, but binding to LPS results in a decreased LPS bioavailability and hence may attenuate its toxicity during Gram-negative bacterial infections. In a recent study, oral lactoferrin administration attenuated spontaneous TNF-α production by peripheral blood cells in human (Zimecki et al., 1999). Study on this topic would be very interesting for immunobiologists.

Several classes of phagocyte-derived antimicrobial peptides have been purified from mammalian phagocytes, and it is now clear that next to their production of ROS, bovine PMN also inactivate microorganisms by exposing them to these antimicrobial peptides and proteins within the phagolysosomal vacuoles. Bovine PMN granules contain a group of highly cationic proteins. Beta-defensins, a family represented by 13 cationic, tridisulfide-containing peptides with 38-42 residues, have potent antibacterial activities against both S. aureus and E. coli in vitro. Similar molecules have also been isolated from specialized epithelia. These polypeptides are structured through disulfide bonds of cysteine but can also be linear and unstructured; they remarkably contribute to host defense against pathogens. Because many bactericidal peptides like β-defensins etc. are stored in the dense granules of neutrophils, it is likely that they are discharged simultaneously during PMN activation. Although co-packaged in the dense granules, cathelicidins, but not β-defensins, are stored as inactive propeptides. Following PMN stimulation with PMA, the cathelicidins Bac5 and Bac7 are cleaved from their respective propeptides and released extracellularly. In contrast, β-defensins exist as fully processed peptides in bovine PMN.

The 46 kDa soluble CD14 (sCD14), which is shedding of membrane CD14 (mCD14) from phagocyte, is also available in interstitial fluid/milk (Wang et al., 2002; Sohn et al., 2007a; 2007b), and can bind LPS directly and prevent LPS from binding to mCD14, thus preventing over-secretion of TNF-α, thereby silencing the severity of inflammation and clinical symptoms. This potentially plays a role in neutralizing LPS and controlling the clinical symptoms associated with acute infection. In vitro incubation of recombinant bovine (rbo) sCD14 with PMN and LPS prevented LPS induced upregulation of CD18 adhesion receptors (Wang et al., 2002; Sohn et al., 2007a). Intramammary and systemic use of rbosCD14 may provide a means of eliminating the potential damaging effects of LPS during acute infection and sepsis; this approach would also be applicable in human inflammatory and infectious diseases.

Furthermore, iron-binding protein, lactoferrin, is small protein synergizes neutrophils' functions and LPS detoxification. Bovine lactoferrin does far beyond the binding of iron, and has considerable inhibitory effect on bacterial growth (Bishop et al., 1976). Lysozyme or muramidase can cleave the mucopeptide layer of most non-encapsulated Gram-positive bacterial cell walls resulting in cytoplasmic blebbing of the bacterial cell wall, leading to direct bacterial lysis, especially when the osmolarity of the infected microenvironment is sufficiently low. Lysozyme has also the capacity to neutralise and strongly interact with *E. coli* LPS; another non-oxidative antimicrobial agent in PMN, which directly/indirectly enhances LPS degradation, is PMN elastase. Elastase, cathepsin G and other granule-proteases degrade the outer membrane protein A of *E. coli*, which is located on the surface of the bacteria (Belaaouaj et al., 1998). PMN ROS production synergises activity of all above mentioned antimicrobial and anti-PAMP compounds. Overall, apart from the role of bovine PMN granules and enzymes, it is fully accepted that the PMN ROS production plays a major role in protection of udder from Gram negative bacterial infection (Burvenich et al., 2003; Mehrzad et al., 2004; 2005a) and detoxification of LPS.

8. Oscillatory events on neutrophils functions

Neutrophil dysfunction in animals and human has been associated with decreased immunocompetence, resulting in the suppression of host defense mechanisms and increased susceptibility to many infectious and non-infectious diseases. Nowadays, potential increasingly environmental stresses and worldwide-food scarcity issues have resulted in unstoppably intensive feed/food and dairy production. The intensive production system leads to unstoppable oscillatory events on innate immune systems, especially neutrophils in bone marrow, blood and udder of high yielding dairy cows, compromising innate defence system in udder, thereby making animals particularly sensitive to infections. Oscillatory events on neutrophils occurs in all stages of maturation and functions (see figures 7 and 8), not only in mature animals but also in neonate, e.g., in bovine (Mehrzad et al., 2001a; 2001c; 2002a; 2008a 2008b; 2008c). Relative magnitude of circulating and post-diapedetic PMN impairment differed from different physiopathological status of animals and humans. A dramatic reduction in random migration, iodination and ROS production of blood PMN were observed during the first week after parturition (Heyneman et al., 1990; Hoeben et al., 2000a; Mehrzad et al., 2001a; 2001b; 2001c). It was recently discovered that the adhesion molecule L-selectin is shed from the surface of bovine PMN at parturition (Diez-Frail et al., 2004). Surface expression of L-selectin remains low for several days following parturition and could contribute to the reported defect in bovine PMN chemotaxis during the period immediately following parturition (Berning et al., 1993; Diez-Frail et al., 2004). Regulation of bovine PMN adhesion molecules during mammary gland infection and possible use of immunomodulators has recently been studied (Diez-Frail et al., 2004).

Cumulative deficiencies in opsonin levels (IgG₁ and conglutinin) were observed in peak of physiological stress in animals, which closely coincided with impaired PMN oxidation-reduction reactions capacity (Detilleux et al., 1994; Burvenich et al., 2003). The proportion of all cases of infections especially mastitis, metritis, arthritis and laminitis that develop during period at which the animals encounter with maximal stress status; these period is coincided with maximal oscillatory events in circulating and post-diapedetic neutrophils (Burvenich et al., 1994; 2003; Mehrzad et al., 2001a; 2001c; 2002a; 2008b; 2008c).

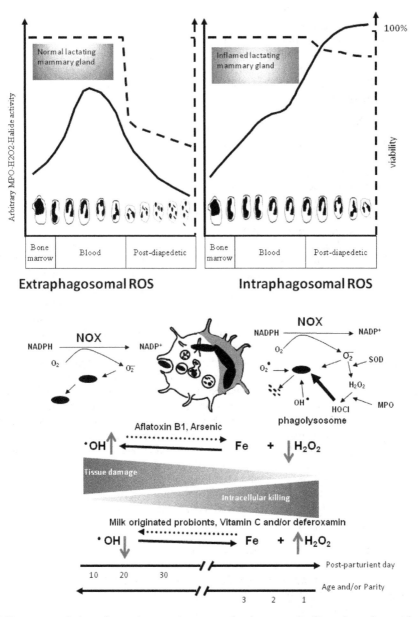

Fig. 7. Upper panel: An schematic overview on author's recent findings (together with literatures) about changes in neutrophils' MPO-H_2O_2-Halide system (solid lines), viability (dashed lines) and dynamics of neutrophils structure and maturity in healthy and mastitis dairy cows. Formed in bone marrow, blood neutrophils function and structure changed after normal extravasation. These changes differed in inflammatory environments. The most probable reason for these disparities would be the "rate of diapedesis", which is faster

during inflammation; pinpointing the aspects of molecular mechanisms of this classically mechanomical phenomenon of neutrophils in different physiological and pathological conditions in animals and humans is very interesting topics for further fundamental research in the area of innate immune system. Lower panel: Diagram illustrating the oscillatory events on neutrophils and some potential nutritional and environmental interventions (Ibeagha et al., 2009; Mehrzad et al., 2008c; 2011) in animals and human to modulate their neutrophils' ultimate functions. These provocative hypotheses address the points that during severe infection/inflammation of the udder extracellular production of ROS by neutrophils may be impaired and could lead to tissue damage in mammary gland. Normally, ROS for bactericidal activity is produced intracellularly for effective destruction of microbes with a minimal tissue damage. The hypothesis is based on the study of the kinetics of chemiluminescence: 1) there is a difference between extracellular and intracellular ROS production of both blood and post-diapedetic neutrophils during different stages of lactogenesis, and 2) in blood and milk, extracellular ROS production by neutrophils is more pronounced in old animals. This may lead to an impaired bactericidal capacity of resident udder neutrophils and boost tissue damage in aged animals (Mehrzad et al., 2001a; 2001b; 2002; 2004; 2005a; 2005b) and partially adapted from (Burvenich et al., 2003). Further, many environmental toxins cause oscillations on neutrophils' ultimate functions (Mehrzad et al., 2011); conversely potential nutritional intervention could reverse the oscillatory events in neutrophils (Ibeagha et al., 2009; Mehrzad et al., 2008c); what happens on the impacts of nanotubes, nanovectors, nanoneedles, nanoparticles and nanoadjuvants on this casecade of events can be very interesting to work. Promising photoredox and antioxidant properties of vitamin C, probionts and deferoxamin with huge quenching capacity mainly on OH$^\bullet$ with much less pronounced on H_2O_2 and $O_2^{\bullet-}$ (Mehrzad et al., unpublished data), and dietary supplementation with probiotics and peptides originated from bovine milk augments neutrophils' functions (Gill et al., 2000; 2001a; 2001b; Mehrzad et al., 2002b). Reverse results have been observed with aflatoxin B1 (Mehrzad et al., 2011), Arsenic, Lead (Mehrzad et al., unpublished data) and plenty more with marked oscillatory effects on neutrophils' ultimate functions. Both in animals and humans due to many environmental and physiological stresses influencing on the overall immune system of the body, switching the oxidant-antioxidant systems on the body from antioxidant status to prooxidant ones and excessive extracellular ROS will accumulate in the body. To remove excessive and unwanted ROS, especially OH$^\bullet$ in the body some antioxidants like vitamins C, E, A..., deferoxamin and probionts can be promisingly helpful and here immunobiologists are strongly encouraged to focus on those novel topics of nutritional and environmental immunology in animals and humans.

One of the most critically physiological associated stress periods would be periparturient period and early lactogenesis. Both in milk and blood PMN function is substantially decreased around parturition (Van Oostveldt et al., 2001; Mehrzad et al., 2001a; 2001c, 2002; 2009; Burvenich et al., 2003). Up till now the underlying mechanisms involved in periparturient immunosuppression remain unknown. However, metabolites (e.g. β-hydroxybutyrate) (Suriyasathaporn et al., 1999) and hormones (e.g. growth hormone, cortisol, pregnancy associated glycoprotein) (Gray et al., 1982; Burvenich et al.,1994; Suriyasathaporn et al., 1999) have been reported as attributable factors.

There are many reports demonstrating that at least some of hormones and metabolites contribute to the oscillatory events in PMN function, targeting both the afferent and efferent arms of PMN functions (Gray et al., 1982; Burvenich et al., 1994; Suriyasathaporn et al., 1999; Hoeben et al., 1999; 2000a). As these studies suggest, the link between periparturient immunosuppression and hormonal and metabolic changes is nevertheless apparent; most of which directly/indirectly affect PMN functions. Hormonal and metabolic changes such as glucocorticoids, ketone bodies and pregnancy associated glycoproteins play a causative role in oscillatory events on key efferent arms of PMN function, ROS production/microbicidal capacity (Dosogne et al., 1998; Hoeben et al. 2000a). These hormones and metabolites also inhibit the proliferation of bone marrow cells *in vitro* (Hoeben et al. 1999; Van Merris, et al., 2001a; 2001b 2002).

Our understanding of the precise ways in which the complex cascade of ROS production occurs in blood or milk PMN during physiological and pathological conditions is still in its infancy. This is especially true for the mechanism of in vivo effect of PMN functions by hormones and metabolites, especially the metabolomics aspects of neutrophils' dysfunction. Based on current understanding of impact of hormones on PMN function, the membrane, cytosolic and nuclear effects of hormones (e.g. growth hormone, sex hormones, cortisol, pregnancy associated glycoprotein) and metabolites (β-hydroxybutyrate, non-esterified fatty acid) on blood and post-diapedetic PMN functions are to be more fundamentally investigated.

Recombinant bovine somatotropin (bST) has been shown to boost cows' milk production and compositional performance following experimentally induced *E. coli* and *Streptococcus uberis* infection (Hoeben et al., 1999). Recombinant bST also prevented severe local and general clinical symptoms in cows suffering from *E. coli* mastitis, especially in severe responders. Prolactin, bST, and insulin-like growth factor-I (IGF-I) are thought to be involved in several immune functions (Elvinger et al., 1991; Hooghe et al., 1993; Kooijman et al., 1996). The function of bST on PMN can either be directly or indirectly mediated through IGF-I. Plasma and milk concentrations of IGF-I increase after bST administration (Zhao et al., 1992). Their concentration differs throughout lactation in milk (Campbell et al., 1991). An increased number of circulating leukocytes, band neutrophils, and an enhanced PMN functions in cows treated with bST after stress related to parturition. Also PMN ROS generation, chemotaxis, random migration, phagocytosis towards IgG-opsonised microorganisms is boosted by IGF-I and bST (Fu et al., 1991; Wiedermann et al., 1993; Warwick-Davies et al., 1995; Mehrzad et al., unpublished). The expression of complement receptors on neutrophils can be upregulated by bST and IGF-I. Increased chemotaxis and random migration (Wiedermann et al., 1993), increased numbers of circulating neutrophils (Clark et al., 1993), and increased proliferation of granulocyte and monocyte precursors (Merchav et al., 1993); *in vivo* bST administration leads to elevation in blood IGF-I lovel. Though *in vivo* might be different from *in vitro*, many recent studies revealed an increased PMN ROS production capacity after *in vivo* administration of bST in healthy animal model; similar results were observed *in vitro* (Mehrzad et al., 2002b). Thus, there is ample evidence that bST and IGF-I can boost neutrophils' functions. Concentration of some biomolecules like β-lactoglobulin in udder secreta is minimal during maximal stress condition of lactaogenssi (Caffin et al., 1984); this means that the β-lactoglobulin can be a potential immunomodulator in the mammary gland and good topic to further focus and apply in human breast and milk physioimmunobiology (Wong et al., 1998; Mehrzad et al., 2000). Hence the insight into PMN activators and/or inhibitors in milk during physiological and pathological conditions is crucial concern for udder's first line defense mechanism and neonatal passive immunity in animals and humans.

As explained before, blood and post-diapedetic neutrophils have the potential to produce substantial amounts of ROS to kill engulfed bacteria (Hoeben et al., 2000a; Mehrzad et al., 2001a; 2001c; 2002a; 2004; 2005a; 2005b; 2009). ROS production can be measured in resting (non-stimulated) neutrophils and after stimulation with e.g., PMA, zymosan, bacteria and latex beads.

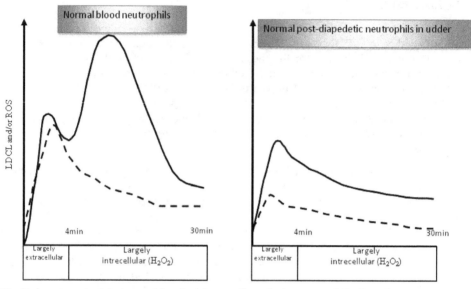

Fig. 8. A comparison between blood and post-diapedetic neutrophils chemiluminescence (CL) profiles of PMA-activated luminol-enhanced neutrophils during different physiological status of animals. The intra-and-extra-cellular ROS production of neutrophils and the concept of biphasic versus monophasic CL pattern of neutgrophils are overviewed. The first peak is the result of mainly initial extracellular reactions and the second peak is mainly a result of subsequent intracellular reactions of the MPO-H$_2$O$_2$ system. The Y-axes are the cumulative RLU / s in function of time, and the X-axes are the entire measurement period of CL. Based on the author's previous studies, curves are arbitrarily depicted to show how neutrophils microbicidal capacity changes after diapedesis through blood-milk barrier and during different physiological status. Oscillatory phenomenon observed in the postdiapedetic neutrophils specially the monophasic pattern with minimal ROS production peak. Throughout lactogenesis period of the lactating mammary gland, the kinetics of post-diapedetic PMN CL never exhibited double phase patterns. Further, blood PMN CL kinetics immediately after parturition gave neither double phase nor high intensity as in later phase of lactogenesis period. The plateau and shape of the blood and- post-diapedetic neutrophils' CL curves shows a biphasic pattern of the blood neutrophils CL during minimal stress condition (like later period of lactogenesis). The intensity of ROS production is lower in post-diapedetic neutrophils than in blood neutrophils, the plateau and shape of the milk- and blood CL curves were similar during maximal physiological and environmental

stresses. Thus, the oscillatory phenomenon of milk PMN ROS production/microbicidal capacity during parturition and lactation seems to be directly related to that of the blood PMN. This animal model of ineffectiveness of the oxygen-dependent intracellular killing mechanisms of neutrophils during inevitable physiological and environmental stresses is very interesting topic of efferent arms of neutrophils for further research in animals and human.

Production of ROS is effective in killing engulfed microbes (Burvenich et al., 1994; 2003; Reeves et al., 2002; Mehrzad et al;, 2001a; 2001c; 2002a; 2004; 2005a; 2005b; 2009). Also the most widely used technique to estimate oscillatory events in bovine and human PMN ROS production is the elegantly simple CL assay (Hoeben et al., 2000a; Mehrzad et al., 2001a; 2001b; 2001c; 2002a; 2004; 2005a; 2009; 2011).

Little comparison has been made between CL of circulating and post-diapedetic neutrophils. To interpret and assess the responsiveness of PMN to stimulating agents such as PMA, it is necessary to distinguish between stimulated and non-stimulated PMN. This offers information about the activity of protein kinase C and NADPH-oxidase, as PMA is a protein kinase C and NADPH-oxidase agonist (Karlsson et al., 2000; Mehrzad et al., 2001a; 2001b; 2001c; 2002; 2004; 2005a; 2009) in the lactating mammary gland. Ingestion of milk fat globules and casein micelles affects milk PMN quality (Mehrzad et al., 2001a; 2001b; 2004; Paape et al., 2002; Burvenich et al., 2003) and subsequent degranulation. No such a problem in blood stream is existed. Smits et al, (1999) have shown that *in vitro* transepithelial/endothelial diapedesis of PMN across mammary gland reduces ROS production of PMN. It has also been shown that the function of post-diapedetic neutrophils in udder differs from their blood counterparts (Smits et al., 2000; Mehrzad et al., 2001a; 2001b; 2001c; 2002a; 2009). Some physiological influencing factors such as lactogenesis (Mehrzad et al., 2001a; 2001c) and ageing (Mehrzad et al., 2002a; 2008b; 2009) are involved in overall PMN impairment. Some other contributing factors would be β-lactoglobulin (Mehrzad et al., 2000b), of which concentration in milk is minimal during maximal stress condition like early lactogenesis (Caffin et al., 1984). The PMN function impairment generally coincides with cow's susceptibility for environmental infection (van Werven et al., 1997; Burvenich et al., 1994; Burvenich et al., 2003; Mehrzad et al., 2004; 2005a). Dynamically, the topic is very important especially for human medicine and further research on this topic of mammary gland innate defence system is deeply needed.

Apart from the involvement of environmental and nutritional factors in hosts' PMN functions and resistance to infection, plenty of many other factors contribute to PMN oscillatory events and the outcome of infection/inflammation in humans and animals; one of the key and interestingly dynamic attributing factors would be the effect of genetics on the quantity and quality of circulating and and post-daipedetic neutrophils (Dietz et al., 1997; Riollet et al., 2000; Wall et al., 2005; Radwan et al., 2007; Rupp et al., 2007; Bannerman et al., 2008). Undoubtedly, all of above mentioned factors could become an important alternative for prophylactic measures of infectious and inflammatory diseases in animals and humans.

Another future increasingly challenging issue in the area of innate immunotoxicity is the environmental and artificial nanoparticles (Karathanasis et al., 2009; Sadikot & Rubinstein, 2009; Gonçalves et al., 2010; Paulsson et al., 2010; and plenty more), which can be both friend and foe for the innate immune system and cancer development. This can be more special for the oscillatory events on both afferent and efferent arms of blood and post-diapedetic neutrophils. Exposures to airborne nanosized particles have been frequently experienced by animals/humans throughout their evolutionary stages, affecting on, e.g., portals of body's entry (respiratory and gastrointestinal tracts and skin). To highlight potential mechanisms of nanotubes, nanovectors, nanoneedles, nanoparticles and nanoadjuvants and cancer nanomedicine, researchers should always focus on immune systems especially the issue of genomics, proteomics and mechanomics aspects of free radicals production of the phagocytes. Application of those potentially promising idea and hypotheses in relation to the neutrophils' oscillatory events versus neutrophils the medicines, eg, topical wound protectant and antiseptics for the treatment of human/animals blister wounds contaminated with microbes or to kill abnormal cells in the body would be very challengingly promising. The challenge is to integrate effectively all information from cellular to molecular events anthropogenically happening for animals/humans' health and performance may contribute to further oscillatory in neutrophils.

9. Conclusions and future perspectives

The issues on animals and humans' diseases are many; among them is neutrophil function that has been the researchers' past, current and future concern. It is clear that appropriate function of neutrophils in the body of animals and humans is very vital to enhance their health and performance. The concepts of neutrophil recruitment at the site of microbial invasion and the interesting phenomenon of nonspecifically engulfing and killing of microbes by neutrophils is still a complex cascade of many cellular and molecular events; molecularly, afferent (sensing) and efferent (effector and/or highly intracellular-and-extracellular microbicidal compounds) weapons of neutrophils are vital in protection of the hosts. Inevitable occurring of general and local immunocompromised conditions especially on the effector weaponry of neutrophils leads to countless infectious and non-infectious diseases. Most researchers see the immunocompromised condition of the organs like udder as a result of neutrophils' dysfunction in bone marrow, bloodstream and interstitial fluid. This chapter would make the complex oscillatory events happening in neutrophils a little bit more comprehensible.

Despite intense progress in molecular biology, medicine, nutrition, genetics and nanomedicine, animals and humans are still susceptible -more than before- to environmental bacteria; this susceptibility is maximal during stress, of which neutrophils dysfunction can be one of the most central attributable factors. Immunomodulation is still far from assured. The long-term and fundamental solution for the oscillatory event on neutrophils is to strengthen their functions by means of attainable physio-immunological approaches. This requires a comprehensive study on molecular and cellular aspects of physio-immunological alterations throughout gestation, lactation and diseases.

One of the focuses of the chapter was a comparative overview of blood and post-diapedetic neutrophils' functions. To uncover further evidence on neutrophils' oscillatory events during stress conditions the shape of blood and post-diapedetic PMN CL proven one more reason for high susceptibility of animals/humans to infections. On this topic, many more questions remain open for future research. Future research is also necessary to pinpoint the physiopathological influencing factors on post-diapedetic neutrophils' necrosis and apoptosis. The hypotheses of contribution of antioxidants like vitamins C, E, A, GHS and dynamic of phagolysosomal pH on post-diapedetic neutrophils' quality and first line defense during stress condition could be tested in the future research.

It is conclusive that blood PMN had stronger weaponry than that of post diapedetic PMN, when encountered with pathogens. It is also concluded that the relative magnitude of blood and post-diapedetic neutrohpils' oscillation/impairment differ from different physiopathological status of animals. For example, post-diapedetic PMN quality impairment is more pronounced in older animals/humans. This impairment coincided with the impairment of PMN microbicidal capacity in bloodstream; PMN ineffectiveness against invading pathogens not merely resulted from the quantity of PMN, but, more importantly, from the quality of PMN, which was identified via PMN CL kinetics and PMN viability. In healthy animals the lowest post-diapedetic PMN quality is found during stress conditions, which is more pronounced in older ones, proving one more reason for high susceptibility of aged animals and humans to infections during environmental and physiological stresses. The explanations in this chapter aimed to increase the insight into the first line defense mechanism of organs like mammary gland/breast, could further deepen our understanding at the complex physiopathology of mammary gland infections, cancers and other stress-related infectious and non-infectious diseases. It is conceivable, however, more novel findings and views on these topics remain for future research.

With the existed knowledge, it is clear that stressed animals and humans are relatively immunosuppressed. This could boost their susceptibility to environmental bacterial infections. Nowadays, the overstressed animals/humans are more susceptible to environmental pathogens than before. The main concern now is how to control and enhance these non-specific aspects of immune system. Clearly, the most appropriate treatment for infectious and non-infectious diseases is preventive treatment. The chapter clearly demonstrates that the severity of mammary gland infections is highly related to pre-infection neutrophils' functions, quick recruitment of neutrophils in the gland and their quality after diapedesis. All of these neutrophils' functions impaired during stress conditions. Therefore, preventive measures on animals around stress should be thoroughly performed. The preventive measures should be aimed at lowering stressful conditions and ensuring a high standard of nutrition and hygiene. Both in animals and humans zero stress status must be implemented for the future; this is hardly achievable. The long-term, environmentally friendly ways and fundamental solution for stress-related infectious diseases in animals/humans is "to strengthen their first line defense" by means of attainable physio-immunological approaches. This requires more insight into the first line defense mechanism, which is absolutely crucial. Perhaps one exciting and environmentally acceptable approach for infection/inflammation control would be application of "probionts". Protection of the organ from pathogens with less/non-pathogen bacteria, then further research on host-bacteria interactions would be promising.

As addressed, the protruding psuedopodes in blood differs from those of post-diapedetic neutrophils; it would be worth studying the impact of stress, age and infections on surface morphology of blood and post-diapedetic neutrophils. To further mimic the first line defense mechanism similar study should be conducted on "bone marrow-blood-barrier". Positive role of transient PMN impairments during parturition and early lactation in animals and humans should not be ignored as a good event, because this might be responsible for less damage on biomolecules, cells and tissue during periparturient period, potentially providing better passive immunity to neonates from invading pathogens. Study should also be focused on molecular mechanisms of higher blood and milk neutrophil's functions (both efferent and afferent arms) in younger animals and humans.

10. Acknowledgment

The author gratefully acknowledges the bureau (area) for Research & Technology of Ferdowsi University of Mashhad for granting the basic research studies in connection with neutrophil functions in animals and human. The author also gratefully thanks Prof. Dr. Christian Burvenich for his encouraging support.

11. References

Adler H., Frech B., Thony M., Peterhans E. & Jungi T.W. (1995). Inducible nitric oxide synthase in cattle. Differential cytokine regulation of nitric oxide synthase in bovine and murine macrophages, J. Immunol. 154: 4710-4718.

Alexandrova M. L. (2009). What happens with ageing: decline or remodeling of opsonin-independent phagocyte oxidative activity? Luminescence, 24: 340-347.

Allen R.C., Stjernholm R.L. & Steele R.H. (1972). Evidence for the generation of an electronic excitation state(s) in human polymorphonuclear leukocytes and its participation in bactericidal activity. Biochem. Biophys. Res. Commun. 47: 679-684.

Allen R.C., Dale D.C. & Taylor F.B. Jr. (2000). Blood phagocyte luminescence: gauging systemic immune activation. Method in Enzymol. 305: 591-629.

Allport J.R., Lim Y.C., Shipley J.M., Senior R.M., Shapiro S.D., Matsuyoshi N., Vestweber D. & Luscinskas F.W. (2002). Neutrophils from MMP-9- or neutrophil elastase-deficient mice show no defect in transendothelial migration under flow in vitro. J. Leukoc. Biol. 71: 821-828.

Anggard E. (1994). Nitric oxide: mediator, murderer, and medicine. The Lancet. 343 : 1199-1206.

Arnhold J., Furtmüller P.G., Regelsberger G. & Obinger C. (2001). Redox properties of the couple compound I/native enzyme of myeloperoxidase and eosinophil peroxidase. Eur. J. Biochem. 268: 5142-5148.

Babior B. (1984). The respiratory burst of phagocytes. J. Clin. Invest. 73: 599-601.

Babior B.M. (1994). Activation of the respiratory burst oxidase. Environmental Health Ptospectives. (suppl 10) 102: 53-56.

Baldridge C.W. & Gerard R.W. (1933). The extra respiration of phagocytosis. Am. J. Physiol. 103: 235-236.

Bannerman D.D., Springer H.R., Paape M.J., Kauf A.C. & Goff J.P. (2008). Evaluation of breed-dependent differences in the innate immune responses of Holstein and Jersey cows to Staphylococcus aureus intramammary infection. J. Dairy Res., 75:291-301.

Barber M.R., Pantschenko A.G., Hinckley L.S. & Yang T.J. (1999). Inducible and constitutive in vitro neutrophil chemokine expression by mammary epithelial and myoepithelial cells. Clin. Diagn. Lab. Immunol., 6: 791-798.

Barrio B., Vangroenweghe F., Dosogne H. & Burvenich C. (2000). Decreased neutrophil bactericidal activity during phagocytosis of slime-producing Staphylococcus aureus strain. Vet. Res., 31: 603-609.

Belaaouaj A., McCarthy R., Baumann M., Gao Z., Ley T.J., Abraham S.N. & Shapiro S.D. (1998). Mice lacking neutrophil elastase reveal impaired host defence against gram negative bacterial sepsis. Nature Med., 4: 615-619.

Bellocchio S, Moretti S, Perruccio K, Fallarino F, Bozza S, Montagnoli C, Mosci P, Lipford GB, Pitzurra L, & Romani L. (2004). TLRs govern neutrophil activity in aspergillosis. J Immunol. 173:7406-7415.

Berning L.M., Paape M.J. & Peters R.R. (1993). Functional variation in endogenous and exogenous immunoglobulin binding to bovine neutrophils relative to parturition. Am. J. Vet. Res., 54: 1145-1153

Beutler B., (2002). TLR4 as the mammalian endotoxin sensor, Curr.Top.Microbiol.Immunol. 270 108-120.

Bishop J., Schanbacher F., Ferguson L. & Smith K. (1976). In vitro growth inhibition of mastitis-causing coliform bacteria by bovine apo-lactoferrin and reversal of inhibition by citrate and high concentrations of apo-lactoferrin. Infect. Immun., 14 : 911-918.

Blum J.W., Dosogne H., Hoeben D., Vangroenweghe F., Hammon H.M., Bruckmaier R.M. & Burvenich C. (2000). Tumor necrosis factor-α and nitrite/nitrate responses during acute mastitis induced by Escherichia coli infection and endotoxin in dairy cows. Dom. Anim. Endocrinol., 19: 223-235.

Borregaard N., Sørensen O.E. & Theilgaard-Monch K. (2008). Neutrophil granules: a library of innate immunity proteins. TRENDS in Immunology, 28: 340-345.

Bouchard L., Blais S., Desrosiers C., Zhao X. & Lacasse P. (1999). Nitric oxide production during endotoxin-induced mastitis in the cow, J.Dairy Sci. 82: 2574-2581.

Boudjellab N., Chan-Tang H.S., Li X. & Zhao X. (1998). Bovine mammary epithelial cells secrete interleukin-8 in response to lipopolysaccharide stimulation. Am. J. Vet. Res., 59: 1563-156.

Boudjellab N., Chan-Tang H.S. & Zhao X. (2000). Bovine interleukin-1 expression by cultured mammary epithelial cells (MAC-T) and its involvement in the release of MAC-T derived interleukin-8, Comp. Biochem. Physiol. A. Mol. Integr. Physiol. 127: 191-199.

Bruhn O., Grötzinger J., Cascorbi I., & Jung S. (2011). Antimicrobial peptides and proteins of the horse - insights into a well-armed organism. Veterinary Research 2011, 42:98-120.

Burvenich C., Paape M.J., Hill A.W., Guidry A.J., Miller R.H., Heyneman R., Kremer W.D.J. & Brand A. (1994). Role of the neutrophil leukocyte in the local and systemic reactions during experimentally induced E. coli mastitis in cows immediately after calving. Vet. Q., 16: 45-50.

Burvenich C., Paape M.J., Hoeben D., Dosogne H., Massart-Leën A.M. & Blum J. (1999). Modulation of the inflammatory reaction and neutrophil defence of the bovine lactating mammary gland by growth hormone. Domest. Anim. Endocr., 17: 149-159.

Burvenich C., Van Merris V., Mehrzad J., Diez-Fraile A. & Duchateau L. (2003). Severity of E. coli mastitis is mainly determined by cow factors. Vet. Res., 34, 521-562.

Caffin J.P., Poutrel B. & Rainard P. (1984). Physiological and pathological factors influencing bovine α-lactalbumin and β-lactoglobulin concentrations in milk. J. Diary Sci., 68: 1086-1094.

Campbell P.G., Skaar T.C., Vega J.R. & Baumruker C.R. (1991). Secretion of insulin-like growth factor-I (IGF-I) and IGF-binding proteins from bovine mammary tissue in vitro. J. Endocr., 128: 219-228.

Carey L.A., Perkowski S.Z., Lipsky C.L., Cirelli R.A., Spath J.A. Jr. & Gee M.H. (1997). Neutrophil recruitment as a factor limiting injury or promoting recovery from acute lung injury. Am. J. physiol., 272: (Heart Circ. Physiol. 41) H179-H289.

Cemerski S., Cantagrel A., van Meerwijk J.P.M. & Romagnoli P. (2002). Reactive oxygen species differently affect T cell receptor signaling pathways. J. Biol. Chem. 277: 19585-19593.

Chavakis T., Hussain M., Kanse S.M., Peters G., Bretzel R.G., Flock J.I., Herrmann M. & Preissner K.T. (2002). Staphylococcus aureus extracellular adherence protein serves as anti-inflammatory factor by inhibiting the recruitment of host leukocytes. Nature Medicine. 8: 687-693.

Clark R., Strasser J., McCabe S., Robbins K. & Jardieu P. (1993). Insulin-like growth factor-1 stimulmation of lymphopoiesis. J. Clin. Invest., 92: 540-548.

Cooke E. & Hallett M.B. (1985). The role of C-kinase in the physiological activation of the neutrophil oxidase. Biochem. J. 232: 323-327.

Detilleux J.C., Koehler K.J., Freeman A.E.F., Kehrli M.E. & Kelley D.H. (1994). Immunological parameters of periparturient Holstein cattle: genetic variation. J. Dairy Sci., 77: 2640- 2645.

DiCarlo A.L., Paape M.J. & Miller R.H. (1996). Reactivity of purified complement component 3b with bovine neutrophils and modulation of complement receptor 1. Am. J. Vet. Res. 57: 151-156.

Dietz A.B., Cohen N.D., Timms L. & Kehrli M.E. Jr (1997). Bovine Lymphocyte Antigen Class II Alleles as Risk Factors for High Somatic Cell Counts in Milk of Lactating Dairy. J Dairy Sci., 80:406–412.

Diez-Fraille A., Mehrzad J., Meyer E., Duchateau L. & Burvenich C. (2004). Comparison of L-selectin and Mac-1 expression on blood and milk neutrophils during experimental Escherichia coli-induced mastitis in cows. Am. J. Vet. Res., 65:1164-1171.

Dosogne H., Capuco A.V., Paape M.J., Roets E., Burvenich C. & Fenwick B. (1998). Reduction of acyloxyacyl hydrolase activity in circulating neutrophils from cows after parturition. J. Dairy Sci., 81: 672-677.

Dosogne H., Meyer E., Sturk G., Van Loon J., Massart-Leën A.M. & Burvenich C. (2002). Effect of enrofloxacin treatment on plasma endotoxin during bovine Escherichiacoli mastitis. Inflammation Res., 51: 201-205.

Elvinger F., Hansen P.J., Head H.H. & Natzke R.P. (1991). Actions of bovine somatotropin on polymorphonuclear leukocytes and lymphocytes in cattle. J. Dairy Sci., 74: 2145-2152.

Erwin A.L. & Munford R.S. (1991). Plasma lipopolysaccharide-deacylating activity (acyloxyacyl hydrolase) increases after lipopolysaccharide administration to rabbits. Lab. Invest., 65: 138-144.

Fu Y. K., Arkins S., Wang B.S. & Kelley K.W. (1991). A novel role of growth hormone and insulin-like growth factor-I. Priming neutrophils for superoxide anion secretion. J. Immunol., 146: 1602-1608.

Gennaro R.B., Dewald B., Horisberger U., Gubler H.U. & Baggiolini M.A. (1983). A novel type of cytoplasmic granule in bovine neutrophils. J. Cell Biol., 96: 1651-1661.

Molecular Aspects of Neutrophils as Pivotal Circulating Cellular Innate Immune Systems to
Protect Mammary Gland from Pathogens

185

Gill H.S., Doull F. & Rutherfurd K.J. (2000). Immunoregulatory peptides in bovine milk. Br. J. Nutr. 84 Suppl 1: S111-S117.

Gill H.S. &, Rutherfurd K.J. (2001a). Immune enhancement conferred by oral delivery of Lactobacillus rhamnosus HN001 in different milk-based substrates. J. Dairy Res. 68:611-616.

Gill H.S., Cross M.L., Rutherfurd K.J. & Gopal P.K. (2001b). Dietary probiotic supplementation to enhance cellular immunity in the elderly. Br. J. Biomed Sci. 58:94-96.

Gonçalves D.M, Chiasson S. & Girard D. (2010). Activation of human neutrophils by titanium dioxide (TiO2) nanoparticles. Toxicology in Vitro 24 (2010) 1002–1008.

Gray G.D., Knight K.A., Nelson R.D. & Herron M.J. (1982). Chemotactic requirements of bovine leukocytes. Am. J. Vet. Res., 43: 757-759.

Griffin F.M. Jr., Griffin J.A.., Leider J.E. & Silverstein S.C. (1975). Studies on the mechanism of phagocytosis. I. Requirements for circumferential attachment of particle-bound ligands to specific receptors on the macrophage plasma membrane. J. Exp. Med. 142: 1263-1282.

Hayashi F., Means T.K., & Luste A. D. (2003). Toll-like receptors stimulate human neutrophil function. Blood, 102: 2660-2669

Heyneman R., Burvenich C. & Vercauteren R. (1990). Interaction between the respiratory burst activity of neutrophil leukocytes and experimentally induced E. coli mastitis in cows. J. Dairy Sci., 73: 985-994.

Heyneman R. & Burvenich C. (1992). Kinetics and characteristics of bovine neutrophil alkaline phosphatase during acute Escherichia coli mastitis. J. Dairy Sci., 75: 1826-34.

Heyworth P.G., Cross A.R. & Curnutte J.T. (2003). Chronic granulomatous disease. Curr. Opin. Immunol. 15: 578-584.

Hoeben D., Burvenich C., Eppard P.J. & Hard D.L. (1999). Effect of recombinant bovine somatotropin on milk production and composition in bovine Streptococcus uberis mastitis. J. Dairy Sci., 82: 1671-1683.

Hoeben D., Monfardini E., Opsomer G., Dosogne H., De Kruif A., Beckers J.F. & Burvenich C. (2000a). Chemiluminescence of bovine polymorphonuclear leukocytes during the periparturient period and relation with metabolic parameters and bovine pregnancy-associated glycoprotein. J. Dairy Res., 67: 249-259.

Hoeben D., Burvenich C., Trevisi E., Bertoni G., Hamann J. & Blum J.W. (2000b). Role of endotoxin and TNF-α in the pathogenesis of experimentally induced mastitis in periparturient cows. J. Dairy Res., 67: 503-514.

Horwitz M.A. (1982). Phagocytosis of microorganisms. Rev. Infect. Dis. 4: 104-123.

Huynh H.T., Robitaille G. & Turner J.D. (1991). Establishment of bovine epithelial cells (MAC-T): an in vitro model for bovine lactation, Exp. Cell. Res. 197: 191-199.

Ibeagha A.E., Ibeagha-Awemu E.M., Mehrzad J., Baurhoo B., Kgwatalala P. & Zhao X. (2009). The effect of selenium sources and supplementation on neutrophil functions in dairy cows. Animal, 3: 1037-1043.

Jankowski A., Scott C.C. & Grinstein S. (2002). Determinants of phagosomal pH in neutrophils. J. Biol. Chem. 277: 6059-6066.

Karathanasis E., Geigerman C.M., Parkos C.A., Chan L., Bellamkonda R.V. & Jaye D.L. (2009). Selective Targeting of Nanocarriers to Neutrophils and Monocytes Annals of Biomedical Engineering, 37: 1984–1992

Karlsson A., Nixon J.B. & Mcphail L.C. (2000). Phorbol myristate acetate induces neutrophils NADPH-oxidase activity by two separate signal transduction pathways: dependent or independent of phosphatidylinositol 3-kinase. J. Leukocyte Biol. 67: 396-404.

Kurt-Jones E.A., Mandell L., Whitney C., Padgett A., Gosselin K., Newburger P.E., Finberg R.W., (2002). Role of toll-like receptor 2 (TLR2) in neutrophil activation: GM-CSF enhances TLR2 expression and TLR2-mediated interleukin 8 responses in neutrophils, Blood. 100: 1860-1868.

Lai Y., & Gallo R.L. (2009). AMPed up immunity: how antimicrobial peptides have multiple roles in immune defense. Trends in Immunology, 30: 131-141

Li Y., Karlin A., Loike J.D. & Silverstein S.C. (2002). A critical concentration of neutrophils is required fro effective bacterial killing in suspension. PNAS. 99: 8289-8294.

Liu Y, Walter S, Stagi M, Cherny D, Letiembre M, Schulz-Schaeffer W, Heine H, Penke B, Neumann H, & Fassbender K (2005). LPS receptor (CD14): a receptor for phagocytosis of Alzheimer's amyloid peptide. Brain. 128:1778-89.

Mandell G.L. (1974). Bactericidal activity of aerobic and anaerobic polymorphonuclear neutrophils. Infect. Immun. 9: 337-341.

Mayadas T. N. & Cullere X. (2005). Neutrophil β2 integrins: moderators of life or death decisions. Trends in Immunology. 26: 388-395.

Mayer S.J., Keen P.M., Craven N. & Bourn F.J. (1989). Regulation of phagolysosome pH in bovine and human neutrophils: the role of NADPH oxidase activity and an Na+/H+ antiporter. J. Leukocyte Biol. 45: 239-248.

Mehrzad J., Dosogne H., Meyer E., Hoeben D. & Burvenich C. (2000). Effect of α-lactalbumin and β-lactoglobulin on the supperoxide production of bovine milk neutrophils. Biotechnol. Argronomy Soc. Environ., 4: 22 (abstract).

Mehrzad J., Dosogne H., Meyer E., Heyneman R. & Burvenich C. (2001a). Respiratory burst activity of blood and milk neutrophils in dairy cows during different stages of lactation. J. Dairy Res., 68:399-415.

Mehrzad J., Dosogne H., Meyer E. & Burvenich C. (2001b). Local and systemic effects of endotoxin mastitis on the chemiluminescence of milk and blood neutrophils in dairy cows. Vet Res., 32:131-144.

Mehrzad J., Dosogne H., Vangroenweghe F. & Burvenich C. (2001c). A comparative study of bovine blood and milk neutrophil functions with luminol-dependent chemiluminescence. Luminescence., 16:343-356.

Mehrzad J., Duchateau L., Pyörälä S. & Burvenich C. (2002a). Blood and milk neutrophil chemiluminescence and viability in primiparous and pluriparous dairy cows during late Pregnancy, around parturition and early lactation. J. Dairy Sci., 85:3268-3276.

Mehrzad J., Dosogne H., Vangroenweghe F. & Burvenich C. (2002b). Effect of bovine somatotropin (bST) on bactericidal activity of bovine neutrophil. Biotechnol. Argronomy Soc. Environ. 6: 15 (abstract).

Mehrzad J., Duchateau L. & Burvenich C. (2004). Viability of milk neutrophils and severity of bovine coliform mastitis. J Dairy Sci., 87:4150-4162.

Mehrzad J., Duchateau L. & Burvenich C. (2005a). High milk neutrophil chemiluminescence
limits the severity of bovine coliform mastitis. Vet. Res., 36:101-116.

Mehrzad J., Desrosiers C., Lauzon K., Robitaille G., Zhao X. & Lacasse P. (2005b). Proteases
involved in mammary tissue damage during endotoxin-induced mastitis in dairy
cows. J Dairy Sci., 88:211-222.

Mehrzad J., Dosogne H., De Spiegeleer B., Duchateau L. & Burvenich C. (2007). Bovine
blood neutrophil acyloxyacyl hydrolase (AOAH) activity during endotoxin and
coliform mastitis. Vet. Res., 38:655-668.

Mehrzad J., Janssen D., Duchateau L. & Burvenich C. (2008a). Increase in Escherichia coli
inoculum dose accelerates CD8+ T-cell trafficking in the primiparous bovine
mammary gland. J. Dairy Sci., 91:193-201.

Mehrzad J. & Zhao X. (2008b). T lymphocyte proliferative capacity and CD4+/CD8+ ratio in
primiparous and pluriparous lactating cows. J. Dairy Res., 75:457-465.

Mehrzad J., Mohri M. & Burvenich C. (2008c). Excessive extracellular chemiluminescence
and necrosis of neutrophils in bovine neonates and potentially supportive role of
vitamin C. In: Bioluminescence and Chemiluminescence, Light Emission: Biology and
scientific applications. Shen X., Yang, XL, Zhang XR, Cui ZJ, Kricka LJ and Stanley
PE, (Ed.), (233-336), Published by World Scientific Publishing Co. Pte. Ltd, ISBN
978-912-8395-72, Shanghai, China

Mehrzad J., Duchateau L. & Burvenich C. (2009). Phagocytic and bactericidal activity of
blood and milk-resident neutrophils against Staphylococcus aureus in primiparous
and multiparous cows during early lactation. Vet. Microbiol., 134:106-112.

Mehrzad J., Klein G., J Kamphues., Wolf P., Grabowski N. & Schuberth H.J. (2011). In vitro
effects of very low levels of aflatoxin B1 on free radicals production and
bactericidal activity of bovine blood neutrophils. Vet. Immunol. Immunopathol.
141: 16–25.

Merchav S., Lake M. & Skottner A. (1993). Comparative studies of the granulopoietic
enhancing effects of biosynthetic human insulin-like growth factors I and II. J. Cell
Physiol., 157: 178-183.

Moncada S., Palmer R.M.J. & Higgs E.A. (1991). Nitric oxide: physiology, pathophysiology,
and pharmacology, Pharmacol.Rev. 43: (1991) 109-142.

Nathan C. (2006). Neutrophils and immunity: challenges and opportunities. Nat. Rev.
Immunol. 6: 173-182.

Newman S.L. & Johnston R.B. (1979). Role of binding through C3b and IgG in
polymorphonuclear neutrophil function: studies with trypsin-generated C3b. J.
Immunol. 123: 1839-1846.

Nishizuka Y. (1984). The role of protein kinase C in cell surface signal transduction and
tumour promotion. Nature (London) 308: 693-698.

Ogata A. & Nagahata H. (2000). Intramammary application of ozone therapy to acute
clinical mastitis in dairy cows. J. Vet. Med. Sci. 62: 681-686.

Paape M.J., Lillius E.M.P., Wiitanen A. & Kontio M.P. (1996). Intramammary defence against
infections induced by Escherichia coli in cows. Am. J. Vet. Res., 57: 477-482.

Paape M.J., Mehrzad J., Zhao X., Detileux J. & Burvenich C. (2002). Defense of the bovine
mammary gland by polymorphonuclear neutrophil leukocytes. J. Mammary Gland
Biol. Neoplasia., 7: 109-121.

Paulsson J.M., Jacobson S.H. & Lundahl J. (2010). Neutrophil activation during transmigration in vivo and in vitro A translational study using the skin chamber model. J. Immunol. Methods. 361:82-88.

Pezeshki A., Stordeur P., Wallemacq H., Schynts F., Stevens M., Boutet P., Peelman L.J., De Spiegeleer B., Duchateau L., Bureau F. and Burvenich C. (2011). Variation of inflammatory dynamics and mediators in primiparous cows after intramammary challenge with Escherichia coli. Vet. Res. 42:15-25.

Pyörälä S., Kaartinen L., Käck H. & Rainio V. (1994). Efficacy of Two Therapy Regimes for Treatment of Experimentally Induced Escherichia coli Mastitis in the Bovine. J. Dairy Sci., 77: 453-461.

Rainard P. (2002). Bovine milk fat globules do not inhibit C5a chemotactic activity. Vet Res. 33(4):413-419.

Reth M. (2002). Hydrogen peroxide as second messenger in lymphocyte activation. Nature Immunol. 3: 1129-1134.

Rinaldi M., Li R.W., Bannerman D.D., Daniels K.M., Evock-Clover C., Silva M.V., Paape M.J., Van Ryssen B., Burvenich C. & Capuco A.V. (2010). A sentinel function for teat tissues in dairy cows: dominant innate immune response elements define early response to E. coli mastitis. Funct. Integr. Genomics. 10:21-38.

Root R.K. & Cohen M.S. (1981). The microbicidal mechanisms of human neutrophils and eosinophils. Rev. Infect. Dis. 3: 565-598.

Rosen H. & Klebanoff S.J. (1976). Chemiluminescence and superoxide production by myeloperoxidase deficient leukocytes. J. Clin. Invest. 58: 50-60.

Rossi F. and Zatti M. (1964). Changes in the metabolic pattern of polymorphonuclear leukocytes during phagocytosis. Br. J. Exp. Pathol. 45: 548-559.

Rossi F. (1986). The O_2^- forming NADPH oxidase of the phagocytes: nature, mechanisms of activation and function. Biochem. Biophys. Acta. 853: 65-89.

Sachs U.J., Andrei-Selmer C.L., Maniar A., Weiss T., Paddock C., Orlova V.V., Choi E.Y., Newman P.J., Preissner K.T., Chavakis T. & Santoso S. (2007). The neutrophil-specific antigen CD177 is a counter-receptor for platelet endothelial cell adhesion molecule-1 (CD31). J. Biol. Chem. 282: 23603-13612.

Sadikot R. T. & Rubinstein I. (2009). Long-Acting, Multi-Targeted Nanomedicine: Addressing Unmet Medical Need in Acute Lung Injury. Journal of Biomedical Nanotechnology. 5: 614-619.

Shuster D.E., Kehrli M.E.J., Rainard P. & Paape M. (1997). Complement fragment C5a and inflammatory cytokines in neutrophil recruitment during intramammary infection with Escherichia coli. Infect. Immun. 65: 3286-3292.

Simons, M. P., O'Donnell, M. A. & Griffith, T. S. (2008). Role of neutrophils in BCG immunotherapy for bladder cancer. Urol. Oncol. 26, 341–345

Smits E., Burvenich C., Guidry A.J., & Massart-Leen A. (2000). Adhesion receptor CD11b/CD18 contributes to neutrophil diapedesis across the bovine blood-milk barrier. Vet. Immunol. Immunopathol., 73: 255-265.

Smits E., Burvenich C., Guidry A.J., Heyneman R. & Massart-Leen A. (1999). Diapedesis across mammary epithelium reduces phagocytotic and oxidative burst of bovine neatrophils. Vet. Immunol. Immunopathol., 68: 169-176.

Spitznagel J.K. & Shafer W.M. (1985). Neutrophil killing of bacteria by oxygen-independent mechanisms: A historical summary. Rev. Infect. Dis. 7: 398-403.

Stevens MG, Peelman LJ, De Spiegeleer B, Pezeshki A, Van De Walle GR, Duchateau L &
    Burvenich C. (2011a). Differential gene expression of the toll-like receptor-4 cascade
    and neutrophil function in early- and mid-lactating dairy cows. J. Dairy Sci.
    94:1277-1288.
Stevens MG, Van Poucke M, Peelman LJ, Rainard P, De Spiegeleer B, Rogiers C, Van de
    Walle GR, Duchateau L, & Burvenich C. (2011b). Anaphylatoxin C5a-induced toll-
    like receptor 4 signaling in bovine neutrophils. J. Dairy Sci. 94:152-164.
Stich R., Shoda L., Dreewes M., Adler B., Jungi T. & Brown W. (1998). Stimulation of nitric
    oxide production in macrophages by Babesia bovis, Infect. Immun. 66: 4130-4136.
Suriyasathaporn W., Daemen A.J.J.M., Noordhuizen-Stassen E.N., Nielen M., Dieleman S.J.,
    & Schukken,YH (1999). ß-hydroxybutyrate levels in peripheral blood and ketone
    bodies supplemented in culture media affect the in vitro chemotaxis of bovine
    leukocytes. Vet. Immunol. Immunopathol., 68: 177-186.
Suthanthiran M., Solomon S.D., Williams P.S., Rabin A.L., Novogrodsky A. & Stenzel K.H.
    (1984). Hydroxyl radical scavengers inhibit human natural killer cell activity.
    Nature (Lond.). 307: 276-278.
Tauber A.I. (1987). proten kinase C and the activation of the human neutrophil NADPH-
    oxidase. Blood. 69: 484-488.
Thomas E.L., Jefferson M.M. & Grishman M. (1982). Myeloperoxidase-catalyzed
    incorporation of amino acids into proteins: role of hypochlorous acid, and
    chloramines. Biochemistry. 21: 6299-6308.
Thomas E.L. & Fishman M. (1986). Oxidation of choloride, and thiocyanate by isolated
    leukocytes. J. Biol. Chem. 261: 9694-9702.
Van Merris V., Lenjou M., Hoeben D., Nijs G., Van Bockstaele D. & Burvenich C. (2001a).
    Culture of bovine bone marrow cells in vitro. Vet. Q., 23: 170-175.
Van Merris V., Meyer E., Dosogne H. & Burvenich C. (2001b). Separation of bovine bone
    marrow into maturation related myeloid cell fractions. Vet. Immunol.
    Immunopathol., 83: 11-17.
Van Merris V., Meyer E. & Burvenich C. (2002). Functional maturation during bovine
    granulopoiesis. J. Dairy Sci., 85: 2859-68.
Van Oostveldt K., Vangroenweghe F., Dosogne H. & Burvenich C. (2001). Apoptosis and
    necrosis of blood and milk polymorphonuclear leukocytes in early and
    midlactating healthy cows. Vet. Res., 32: 617-22.
Van Oostveldt K., Paape M.J. & Burvenich C. (2002a). Apoptosis of bovine neutrophils
    following diapedesis through a monolayer of endothelial and mammary epithelial
    cells. J. Dairy Sci., 85: 39-147.
Van Oostveldt K., Tomita G.M., Paape M.J. & Burvenich C. (2002b). Apoptosis of
    neutrophils during Eschericha coli and endotoxin mastitis. Am. J. Vet. Res., 63: 448-
    453.
Van Werven T., Noordhuizen-Stassen E.N., Daemen A.J.J.M., Schukken Y.H., Brand A. &
    Burvenich C. (1997). Preinfection in vitro chemotaxis, phagocytosis, oxidative burst,
    and expression of CD11/CD18 receptors and their predictive capacity on the
    outcome of mastitis induced in dairy cows with Escherichia coli. J. Dairy Sci., 80:
    67-74.

Vangroenweghe F., Dosogne H., Mehrzad J. & Burvenich C. (2001). Effect of milk sampling techniques on milk composition, bacterial contamination, viability and functions of resident cells in milk. Vet. Res., 32: 565-579.

Wall R.J., Powell A.M., Paape M.J., Kerr D.E., Bannerman D.D., Pursel V.G., Wells K.D., Talbot N. & Hawk H.W. (2005). Genetically enhanced cows resist intramammary Staphylococcus aureus infection. Nat. Biotechnol., 23:445-451.

Wang Y., Zarlenga D.S., Paape M.J. & Dahl G.E. (2002). Recombinant bovine soluble CD14 sensitizes the mammary gland to lipopolysaccharide. Vet. Immunol. Immunopathol., 86: 115-124.

Warwick-Davies J., Lowrie D.B. & Cole P.J. (1995). Growth hormone is a human macrophage activating factor. Priming of human monocytes for enhanced release of H_2O_2. J. Immunol., 154: 1909-1918.

Weiss S.J., Test S.T., Eckmann C.M., Roos D. & Regiani S. (1986). Brominating oxidants generated by human eosinophils. Science. 234: 200-202.

Werling D. & Jungi T.W. (2003). Toll-like receptors linking innate and adaptive immune response, Vet.Immunol.Immunopathol. 9 : 1-12.

Wiedermann C.J., Reinisch N. & Braunsteiner H. (1993). Stimulation of monocyte chemotaxis by human growth hormone and its deactivation by somatostatin. Blood., 82: 954-960.

Wong K.F., Middleton N., Montgomery M., Dey M. & Carr R.I. (1998). Immunostimulation of murine spleen cells by materials associated with bovine milk protein fraction. J. Dairy Sci., 81: 1825-1832.

Worku M., Paape M.J., Filep R. & Miller R., (1994). Effect of in vitro and in vivo migration of bovine neutrophils on binding and expression of Fc receptors for IgG2 and IgM, Am.J.Vet.Res. 55: 221-226.

Zarbock A & Ley K. (2008). Mechanisms and consequences of neutrophil interaction with the endothelium. Am. J. Pathol.172: 1-7.

Zhao X., McBride B.W., Trouten-Radford L.M. & Burton J.H. (1992). Specific insulin-like growth factor-1 receptors on circulating bovine mononuclear cells. J. Recept. Res., 12: 117-129.

Zimecki M., Spiegel K., Wlaszczyk A., Kubler A. & Kruzel M.L. (1999). Lactoferrin increases the output of neutrophil precursors and attenuates the spontaneous production of TNF-alpha and IL-6 by peripheral blood cells. Arch. Immunol. Ther. Exp. Warsz., 47: 113-118.

6

An Ag-Dependent Approach Based on Adaptive Mechanisms for Investigating the Regulation of the Memory B Cell Reservoir

Alexandre de Castro

Laboratory of Computational Mathematics, National Center of Technological Research on Informatics for Agriculture (Embrapa Agriculture Informatics), Brazilian Agricultural Research Corporation (Embrapa), Campinas, Brazil

1. Introduction

Twenty years ago, Farmer, Packard, and Perelson presented an elegant dynamical model [1] to study Idiotype Network theory [2-19], in which they showed that every molecular and cellular binding site (cell receptor) can be modeled by binary *bit-strings* of length ℓ. In such a model, an antibody molecule can always recognize an antigen when there is complementarity between their *bit-strings*. The coincidence of antigens and lymphocyte receptors (lock-and-key model) is determined by considering the number of complementary bits [8,20]. For instance, if a B lymphocyte is represented by a binary string 00010101 ($\ell = 8$) and an antigen is represented by the 11101010 binary string, the immune response is activated (Fig. 1). The match between bit-strings does not need to be perfect, however; some bit positions are allowed in which two strings differ. These differences between strings (mismatches) reflect the degree of affinity between the entities of the immune system in mammals and determine the quality of the response.

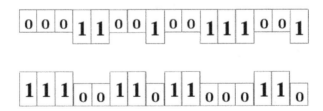

Fig. 1. Pictorial representation of the binding site (cell antigen) by means of a bit-string frame [6].

In another work, Lagreca *et al.* (2001) [21] also proposed a dynamic model that was based on the recognition of shapes or patterns using bit-strings, but used the iterative solution of a coupled map system that enabled the treatment of high dimensions. In the model created by

Lagreca *et al.* (2001), the B cell and the antibody populations are treated as a clone pools because their receptors are represented by the same bit-strings. Because a bit-string can be considered as the binary representation of an integer, the model indexes each clone to an entire σ, and the temporal evolution of the populations is described by the $N(\sigma, t)$ concentration. The model also considers a source term that simulates the role played by the bone marrow, where new bit-strings are presented. The death or depletion of clones occurs in two ways: 1) by means of natural death (apoptosis), described by the parameter d; and 2) by means of a general suppression mechanism, described by a Verhulst-like factor [22]. This factor is widely used in simulations of biological systems, because it limits the maximum population that can survive in a particular environment [22]. The Lagreca *et al.* model (2001) considers this maximum B cell population (N_{max}) to be the same for every clone, and the populations are normalized by the $y(\sigma,t) = N(\sigma,t) / N_{max}$ function.

Thus, considering a discrete temporal evolution, the following coupled map set proposed by Lagreca *et al.* [21] allows part of an adaptive immunological system to be simulated:

$$y(\sigma,t+1) = (1 - y(\sigma,t)).$$

$$\cdot \left\{ m + (1-d)y(\sigma,t) + b\frac{y(\sigma,t)}{y_{tot}(t)} \left[(1-a_h)(y(\overline{\sigma},t) + y_F(\overline{\sigma},t)) + a_h \sum_{i=1}^{B} (y(\overline{\sigma_i},t) + y_F(\overline{\sigma_i},t)) \right] \right\}, \quad (1)$$

where $(1-y(\sigma,t))$ is the Verhulst-like factor; $y_F(\sigma,t)$ describes the antigen population, characterized by a σ bit-string which, in this case, represents distinct antigenic determinants; $\overline{\sigma}$ represents the perfect complementary shape of σ; and $\overline{\sigma_i}$ are the nearest neighbors of $\overline{\sigma}$ in a B-dimensional hypercube. The term m represents the population of cells produced by bone marrow; the $(1-d)$ term represents the percentage of the lymphocyte population that survives a natural cell death (apoptosis); and the other terms describe the clonal proliferation $y(\sigma,t)$ that occurs because of interaction with complementary B cells and/or antigens.

The b parameter is a clonal proliferation constant (typically related to the mean number of new cells produced by the pre-existing cells), and $y_{Tot}(t)$ is the total population, given by equation 2:

$$y_{tot}(t) = \sum_{\sigma} \left[y(\sigma,t) + y_F(\sigma,t) \right] \quad (2)$$

The parameter a_h is the connectivity factor between a specific *bit-string* and the specular image of its neighbors. When $a_h = 0.0$, only a perfect coincidence of complementary shapes is valid. When $a_h = 0.5$, a bit-string can recognize equally both its own specular image and the nearest neighbors of its specular image. The temporal evolution of the antigen pool is defined by equation 3.

$$y_F(\sigma,t+1) = y_F(\sigma,t) - k\frac{y_F(\sigma,t)}{y_{tot}(t)} \left\{ (1-a_h)y(\overline{\sigma},t) + a_h \sum_{i=1}^{B} y(\overline{\sigma_i},t) \right\}, \quad (3)$$

where k is an antigen removal parameter that represents the interactions with the clonal populations.

In fact, it is well-known that the soluble antibody population is one of the essential mechanisms of immunological response regulation [23-25]. However, despite the pioneering work of Lagreca et al. (2001) in developing a coupled map for studying the behavior of the mammalian immune system, their model did not consider these populations [1-6], which makes the model incomplete with respect to the regulation of the immune response by adaptive mechanisms. This omission opens up the possibility of extending their work by taking the soluble antibody populations into account. We have performed that work and present our immunological modeling and simulation findings in this paper.

2. Materials and methods

In this section, we briefly describe the Verhulst approach and provide details of an extension to the Lagreca et al. (2001) model, which includes an antibody variable to address the regulation of the structural mechanisms that are mediated by the immunoglobulin population. This variable was not considered in the simplified model proposed by Lagreca et al. [21].

2.1 The Verhulst approach

Since the early nineteenth century, studies on population dynamics have been developed to identify possible nonlinear behaviors. One of the first efforts aimed at predicting biological population behavior was made by Pierre François Verhulst (1804-1849), a Belgian mathematician. He proposed a nonlinear model in which the death rate was proportional to the square of the number of individuals in the population. The model can be expressed by differential equations [26-30], as follows:

$$\frac{dN}{dt} = AN - BN^2$$

where N is the number of individuals, and A and B are constants related to the growth rate and the population growth limitation, respectively.

The Verhulst model was used again in 1976, by Robert May [27], to study insect population dynamics. In his experiments, he replaced the original differential method by what is now known as the *map* methodology, in which each value is obtained by its anterior value:

$$N_1 = AN_0 - B\,N_0^2$$

$$N_2 = AN_1 - BN_1^2$$

$$N_{n+1} = AN_n - BN_n^2$$

At the limit of saturation, $AN_{max} - BN_{max}^2 = 0$, then $N_{max} = 0$ or $N_{max} = A/B$.

Solving $\dfrac{N_{n+1}}{N_{máx}} = A\dfrac{N_n}{N_{máx}} - B\dfrac{N_n^2}{N_{máx}}\dfrac{N_{máx}}{N_{máx}}$ and inserting $x_n = \dfrac{N_n}{N_{máx}}$ results in the following:

$x_{n+1} = Ax_n - Bx_n^2.A/B$. Defining the parameter A (birth rate) $= r$ (control parameter), we obtain:

$$x_{n+1} = rx_n(1 - x_n), \quad x_n \in [0,1] \tag{4}$$

In equation (4), known as a *logistic map*, the values for $x_n \in [0,1]$ and r are dimensionless and represent population fractions as a function of each of the n iterations, respectively, while r is a constant that represents the population growth rate in each new iteration. The term (1– x_n) is known as the Verhulst factor [21,31,32].

The bifurcation diagram of the logistic map is built by the iterative resolution of the logistic equation, starting with an arbitrary x_0 initial value and choosing sequential values for the parameters $r, r \in [r_{min}, r_{max}]$. The bifurcation diagram of the logistic equation is shown in Fig. 2.

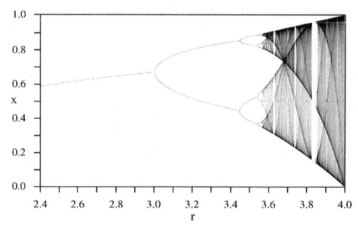

Fig. 2. Classical bifurcation diagram of a logistic map as a function of the parameter r [33].

In Fig. 2, the attractor is a fixed point up to the first bifurcation. For each bifurcation, there occurs a period of duplication before the system reaches the chaotic phase. However, to illustrate the dynamics of this simple model, it is important to show that, for r between 0 and 1, the population death rate is not dependent on the initial population. With r between 1 and 3, the population is prone to an attractor of a fixed point type. For r greater than 3.54, the population wiggles between values of 8, 16, 32, and so on. At approximately r=3.57, the end of the cascade duplication period occurs and chaos begins. From this value, small variations in the initial population produce very different results over time, which is the fundamental characteristic of chaos. For r greater than 4, the populations are outside the [0,1] interval.

It is possible to demonstrate that the Lagreca *et al.* (2001) model for clonal populations reduces to equation 4 when there is no further exposure of the system to the antigens. This reduction occurs because, under this one condition, the additive term (*m*) in equation 1, which represents the bone marrow contribution for the immune repertoire, is very small when compared with the clonal proliferation parameter (*b*) [34,35]. A detailed demonstration of this assertion is presented in subsection 3 of the section on the model parameters.

2.2 Simulation model

As in the Lagreca *et al.* (2001) model [21], our extended Ag-dependent model has molecular receptors of B cells that are represented by bit-strings with 2^B of diversity, where B is the number of bits in the string. The individual components of the immune system represented in the extended model are B cells, antibodies, and antigens located at the vertices of hypercubes of size B. B cells (clones) are characterized by their surface receptors and are modeled by a binary bit-strings. The epitopes [1,8,17-19], which are portions of an antigen that can be connected by the B cell receptor (BCR), are also represented by bit-strings. The antibodies have receptors (paratopes) [1,8,17-19] that are represented by the same bit-string models as the BCR B cell that produced them. Thus, the new dynamic equations that describe the behavior of the adaptive immune system, taking into account the inclusion of antibody populations, are the following:

$$y(\sigma,t+1) = (1-y(\sigma,t))\left\{ m+(1-d)\, y(\sigma,t)+b\frac{y(\sigma,t)}{y_{tot}(t)}\zeta_{a_h}\left(\overline{\sigma},t\right)\right\}, \tag{5}$$

for a clonal population, with complementary shapes included in the term $\zeta_{a_h}(\overline{\sigma},t)$,

$$\zeta_{a_h}(\overline{\sigma},t) = (1-a_h)(y(\overline{\sigma},t)+y_F(\overline{\sigma},t)+y_A(\overline{\sigma},t)) + a_h\sum_{i=1}^{B}(y(\overline{\sigma_i},t)+y_F(\overline{\sigma_i},t)+y_A(\overline{\sigma_i},t)).$$

The clonal populations can range from the value generated by bone marrow (m) up to its maximum value (unity) because the Verhulst factor is a limiting factor [21,31,32].

In the model presented in this paper, the $y_{Tot(t)}$ term represents the sum of the components that belong to an adaptive subset of the immune system, as described in the introduction to this work. Such elements, when added to antibody populations, are expressed as bit-string *concentrations*.

Therefore, the sum of every adaptive component considered by our model is given by equation (6).

$$y_{tot}(t) = \sum_{\sigma}\left[y(\sigma,t)+y_F(\sigma,t)+y_A(\sigma,t)\right] \tag{6}$$

The temporal evolution of the antigens can be defined by equation (7).

$$y_F(\sigma,t+1) = y_F(\sigma,t) - k\frac{y_F(\sigma,t)}{y_{tot}(t)}\left\{(1-a_h)\left[y(\overline{\sigma},t)+y_A(\overline{\sigma},t)\right]+a_h\sum_{i=1}^{B}\left[y(\overline{\sigma_i},t)+y_A(\overline{\sigma_i},t)\right]\right\}, \tag{7}$$

The antibody population is described by a group of 2^B variables, also defined by a B-dimensional hypercube, interacting with the antigen populations of equation (8).

$$y_A(\sigma,t+1)=y_A(\sigma,t)+b_A\frac{y(\sigma,t)}{y_{tot}(t)}\left[(1-a_h)\,y_F(\overline{\sigma},t)+a_h\sum_{i=1}^{B}y_F(\overline{\sigma_i},t)\right]-k\frac{y_A(\sigma,t)}{y_{tot}(t)}\zeta_{a_h}(\overline{\sigma},t)\ ,(8)$$

where b_A is the antibody proliferation parameter; and k is the parameter related to the antibodies and antigens that will be removed.

In our model, equation 8, which considers the adaptive interactions that have been described in the specialized literature, is included. Thus, antibody proliferation is given by the recognition $y_A(\sigma,t)\Leftrightarrow y_F(\overline{\sigma},t)$ [1,8,17-19]. The antibody population is regulated by the intersection of $y_A(\sigma,t)\Leftrightarrow y(\sigma,t)$ [1,8,17-19], $y_A(\sigma,t)\Leftrightarrow y_F(\sigma,t)$ [1,8,17-19], and $y_A(\sigma,t)\Leftrightarrow y_A(\overline{\sigma},t)$ [19,36]. In all cases, the connectivity between the first two neighbors was

considered. The factors $\frac{y_F(\sigma,t)}{y_{TOT}(t)}$ and $\frac{y_A(\sigma,t)}{y_{TOT}(t)}$ also help to regulate the antigen and antibody

populations, while the term $\frac{y(\sigma,t)}{y_{TOT}(t)}$ is the corresponding clonal regulation factor involved

in the formation of immunological memory.

The role performed by the clonal regulation factor, in addition to helping with the B cell response regulation, is fundamental to the regulation of the memorization ability and clonal homeostasis [37-39]. The importance of the effect of the clonal regulation factor over immune system memory evolution is shown in Fig. 3. Three distinct situations are possible:

1. antibody populations are included in the model (which corresponds to the model proposed in this work);
2. antibody populations are not included in the model (which corresponds to the Lagreca et al. [21] model);
3. memory expansion is not limited by the clonal regulation factor (which corresponds to the results obtained by P. G. Etchegoin [40]).

Fig. 3 illustrates the situation in which growth capacity increases indefinitely, which is when the clonal regulation factor is suppressed in the modeling phase. This shows that clonal regulation can be fundamental to the immune system reaching clonal homeostasis.

In the proposed Ag-dependent model, each bit-string is associated with an integer that is situated in an interval , $0\le M\le 2^B-1$, and each represents a clonal population, antigen, or antibody located in the B-dimensional hypercube vertex. The neighbors i of a specific σ or $\overline{\sigma}$ are expressed by the Boolean functions $\sigma_i=(2^i-1xor\sigma)$ or $\overline{\sigma_i}=(2^i-1xor\overline{\sigma})$, respectively. The complementary way of obtaining σ is obtained by $\overline{\sigma}=M-\sigma$ [21].

An example of the way in which the B cell, antibody, or antigen populations are localized in 3-dimensional space is shown in Fig. 4.

For the cubic configuration in Fig. 4, the following algorithm describes how to obtain the first neighbors and the complementary shape of the B cell population identified by the integer $\sigma=4$:

- For a cubic configuration (B=3), there exists a repertoire containing $2^B=8$ integer numbers arranged in the cube vertex. These integer numbers represent the 8 different B cell populations;

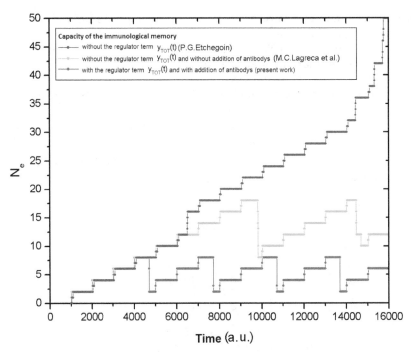

Fig. 3. Capacity of immune system memory in three distinct situations.

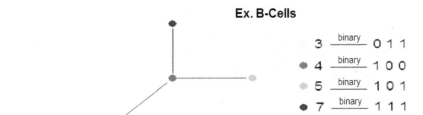

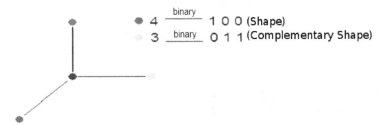

Fig. 4. Spatial arrangement of a B cell population that is identified by 4 integers. Antigens and antibodies also are spatially arranged in the same way, in various cubes.

- Each integer number M must be restrained in the interval $0 \leq M \leq 2^B - 1$; thus, each cube vertex is identified [16];
- With this condition, the smallest value of M is equal to 0 and the largest value is equal to 7. Consequently, the shape space S is equal to $\{0,1,2,3,4,5,6,7\}$;
- To represent the reactions of the lock-and-key type described in the introduction, every cell population in a cubic configuration needs to be represented by 8 bit-strings;

$$\sigma = 4 = \sum_{i=0}^{2} 2^i a_i = 2^0 a_0 + 2^1 a_1 + 2^2 a_2 = 4$$

If, for example, $a_2 = 1$, $a_1 = 0$ and $a_0 = 0$, then in this case 4 in the decimal base corresponds to (1 0 0) in the binary base;

- For the other 7 vertices of the cube:

$$\sigma = 0 = (000),$$

$$\sigma = 1 = (001),$$

$$\sigma = 2 = (010),$$

$$\sigma = 3 = (011),$$

$$\sigma = 4 = (100),$$

$$\vdots$$

$$\sigma = 7 = (111);$$

- For a lock-and-key reaction to occur, there must be another shape $\overline{\sigma}$ that is complementary to $\sigma = 4$, i.e., $\overline{\sigma} = M - \sigma$ [16,21]. Then, $M = 2^B - 1 = 7$ and $\sigma = 4 \rightarrow \overline{\sigma} = M - \sigma = 7 - 4 = 3$, or (0 1 1), in a binary base. This complementary shape is, in principle, an antigen population. However, based on Immune Network Theory, B cells also recognize antibodies and other complementary lymphocytes [1,8,17-19,36];
- Last, search for the first neighbors of the complementary shape $\overline{\sigma} = 3$. If $\sigma_i = (2^i - 1 xor \sigma)$ [16,21], then, for B = 3 (i = 1,2,3), we get the following:

$$\sigma_1 = (2^1 - 1 xor 3) = 2(010),$$

$$\sigma_2 = (2^2 - 1 xor 3) = 0(000),$$

$$\sigma_3 = (2^3 - 1 xor 3) = 4(100).$$

In this example, a B cell population identified by $\sigma = 4$ or (1 0 0) would have recognized an antigen population that is perfectly complementary and is identified by $\overline{\sigma} = 3$ (0 1 1). The antigen populations identified as the first neighbors for $\overline{\sigma} = 3$ are 0, 2, and 4 and can be recognized by the $\sigma = 4$ B cell population, depending on the value of the connectivity parameter a_h, which is included both in our proposed model and in the Lagreca et al. model [21].

Also, for better visualization, we used a 3-dimensional spatial configuration. Similar constructions for this work were made for B-dimensional spaces. Therefore, equations (5) to (8) constitute a set of maps that describes the main interactions of the immune system between the entities that interact through the lock-and-key type of connection, in other words, adaptive immune system entities that self-recognize. Such an equation set is iteratively resolved, considering various initial conditions.

2.3 Simulation dynamics

In this section, we present the dynamics of the simulations that were used to reproduce the proposed experiments *in silico*, and we evaluate the behavior of the proposed model.

To simulate the behavior of the immune system by means of the proposed mathematical model, we developed computational applications in the Fortran programming language (IBM's Mathematical FORmula TRANslation System). The source code was compiled with GFortran (GNU Fortran Compiler) on a Linux Operating System platform. Simulations were performed by a 2 GHz processor, with 4 GB of random-access memory (RAM).

To establish the relationship between antigen mutation and the memory of the lymphocyte population, we performed 3 *in silico* experiments with 30 samples $E_{j,k} = E(j = 1, \beta)(k = 1, \gamma)$.

The same parameters were used in every $E_j = E(j = 1, \beta)$ experiment to represent identical individuals. The antigens were identified by the following expression: $V_i E_{j,k} = V(i = 1, \alpha)E(j = 1, \beta)(k = 1, \gamma)$, where the i, j, and k indexes describe the inoculation order, the experiment, and the sample, respectively. The number α is the number of inoculations in each experiment, β is the number of experiments, and γ is the number of samples in each experiment.

The antigen injection simulations were performed every 1,000 temporal steps (in arbitrary units – a.u.), representing the administration of a new antigen dose in a hypothetical mammal. In the first experiment, we injected 110 different antigen populations in the sample, in the second, 250, and, in the third, 350. To represent the mutation within a population of the same antigen, we used 10 different seeds for the pseudo-random number generator. In the first experiment, a seed was associated with each sample, and the same set of seeds was used to perform the other experiments. In this way, to represent the mutation, we considered that inoculated antigens in the same position belonged to the same species and underwent a mutation for each different sample. The difference between the samples is in the bit-string variation of the inoculated antigens, and the difference between the experiments is in the duration of the time steps. The design of the experiments and the antigen identification used in this work are shown in Fig. 5.

In the schematic diagram shown in Fig. 5, the antigen (i.e., a virus strain) is identified as V1E12, which is the mutation of the antigen V1E11 (belonging to an antigen population of the same species), and the antigen V2E11 is different from the V1E11 antigen (which belongs to various antigen populations).

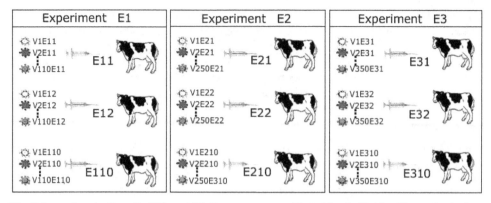

Fig. 5. In each experiment, different lifetimes were considered for individual hypothetical mammals. The lifetime ("lifespan") for E1, E2, and E3 is 110000, 250000, and 350000 respectively.

2.4 Model parameters

The following table shows the ranges for the parameters used in our simulations, based on the literature.

Symbol	Function	Value used in the model	Information obtained from the literature
d	Apoptosis	0.99	De Boer *et al.* [41] (2001): 0.95 Bueno *et al.*[42] (1999): 0.95 Lima *et al.* [43] (2007): $d > 0.95$
m	Source term	$10^{-7} if\ p < 0.1 \quad 0.0 if\ p \geq 0.1$	Lagreca *et al.*[21] (2001): 0.0005 von Laera *et al.* [34] (2005): 0.01 Monvel *et al.*[38] (1993): $m \approx 0.0$
b	Clonal proliferation	2.0	De Boer *et al.* [41] (2001): 2.5-3.0 Utzny *et al.* [44] (2001): 2.0 von Laera *et al.* [34] (2005): 1.2
k	Removal of antibodies and antigens	0.1	von Laera *et al.* [34] (2005): 0.01-0.1

Table 1. Parameters used in the proposed model.

2.4.1 The apoptosis clonal parameter (*d*)

In the extended model presented in this paper, d represents the fraction of cells that is subjected to natural death (apoptosis) or programmed death; thus, $s + d = 1$, where $s = 1 - d$

is the fraction of cells that avoids apoptosis. In the literature, the apoptosis of lymphocytes is typically assumed to occur in percentages not less than 95% [41.43]. For the simulations developed in this study, the natural death parameter was fixed at 0.99 (99%). To give an idea of the effect of varying this parameter, the performances of the model for two different apoptotic events and for the first inoculation antigen were compared (See Fig. 6).

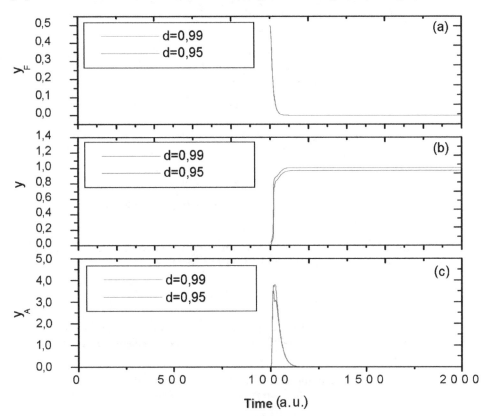

Fig. 6. Evolution of populations of antigens, B lymphocytes, and antibodies with respect to natural death parameter d = 0.99 and d = 0.95. The parameter $b_A = 100$ and initial antigen dosing $Ag_{inicial} = 0.5$. The virgin state of the system is the range of 0 to 1000.

2.4.2 The source term (*m*)

The source term *m* simulates the stochastic behavior of the bone marrow in the production of new lymphocytes [21.38].

In the model described in this work, if the pseudo-random number generator returns a value less than o r equal to $p = 0.1$, the source term takes the value $m = 10^{-7}$, because *m* is experimentally small compared with the levels of lymphocytes produced in the immune response [34,35,38]. If the generator returns values greater than $p = 0.1$, the source term takes the value $m = 0.0$ [21].

2.4.3 The clonal proliferation parameter (b)

Both the pioneering work and the recent work in the literature on theoretical immunology present results on the dynamics of the immune system and the search for attractors of the fixed point type to determine *in machine* clonal homeostasis (equilibrium) in the virgin state (antigen without inoculation) and in the excited state (when an antigen is recognized by some clonal population) [37,38,40].

The condition $y_F = y_A = 0$ is satisfied when the virgin state of the immune system is considered, i.e., without the presentation of antigens, no antibodies are produced. Also, considering that the system only allows high-affinity connections (connections between perfectly complementary shapes), the connectivity factor $a_h = 0$.

In the virgin state, the sum total of the immune populations is restricted to B lymphocytes:

$$y_{Tot}(t) = \sum_\sigma [y(\sigma,t) + y_F(\sigma,t) + y_A(\sigma,t)] = \sum_\sigma y(\sigma,t)$$

Hence, equation 5 reduces to the following:

$$y(\sigma,t+1) = [1 - y(\sigma,)]\{m + (1-d)y(\sigma,t) + b\frac{y(\sigma,t)}{\sum_\sigma y(\sigma,t)} y(\overline{\sigma},t)\}.$$

As in the dynamic simulation used in this work, the virgin state occurs in the interval of 0 to 1000 time steps, and only a pseudo-random number is drawn. Then,

$$\sum_\sigma y(\sigma,t) = y(\sigma,t) = y(\sigma^*,t) = y(t) = y_t \text{ and } y_t = y(\overline{\sigma},t),$$

because, according to Immune Network Theory, for each lymphocyte population, there is another complementary population [17,18,19]. A more detailed explanation can be found in the results section.

Because the bone marrow term in the absence of infection (virgin state of the immune system) is much smaller than the clonal proliferation parameter (m<<b) [34,35], we have the following:

$$y_{t+1} = [(1-d)y_t + by_t](1 - y_t) \text{ or } [1 - d + b]y_t(1 - y_t).$$

Defining $r \equiv 1 - d + b$, the equality results in the following: ($y_{t+1} = ry_t(1 - y_t)$, a logistic map-type equation). Moreover, for the system under study to evolve to a fixed point, the condition $1 < 1 - d + b < 3$ must be satisfied.

Consequently, taking into account an apoptosis parameter equal to $d = 0.99$, the clonal proliferation parameter b must be located within the following range: $1 < 1 + b - 0.99 < 3 \rightarrow 0.99 < b < 2.99$. In the simulations presented in this paper, the clonal proliferation parameter b was set to 2.0.

2.4.4 The antibody and antigen removal parameter (k)

The parameter for the removal of antigens and antibodies k was set to 0.1, to ensure that the populations of antigens and antibodies decay to zero before the antigen is presented.

This procedure, which is adopted for a new antigen, is applied only after the previous antigen has been completely removed [21.45].

2.4.5 Connectivity (a_h)

The connectivity parameter used was 7, so that 99% of the populations are coupled to their perfect complement, and only 1% of the populations are coupled to the first neighbors of their complement. The quality of the immune response is directly related to the degree of affinity among the elements of the adaptive system [8].

2.4.6 Bit-string length (*B*)

Considering the available hypercube immune populations represented by the model, the length of the bit-string B was set at 12. This value corresponds to $2^{12} = 4,096$ different antigens.

2.4.7 Antibody proliferation parameter (b_A)

In the model presented in this work, the initial antigenic dose $(Ag_{initial})$ was set to study the influence of parameter b_A on the immune memory in some simulations.

In other simulations, this parameter was set to study the consequences to the memory of varying the antigen dosage. To clarify, the limit value of $b_A = 0.0$ corresponds to the model previously proposed by Lagreca et al. [21], and the limit value of $Ag_{initial} = y_F = 0.0$ corresponds to the virgin state of the immune system.

3. Results

The clonal populations that were excited after selection by an antigen (or an antigen population) are shown in Fig. 7, as follows: (a) for the first antigen inoculation; and (b) for the second antigen inoculation, with a dosage of 0.1. In this evolution, two populations were excited with the first antigen inoculation at step 1000: the clonal population that recognized the specific antigen (B1 – Burnet idiotypic cells [18.19]) and the clonal population (J1 – Jerne anti-idiotypic cells [18.19]) complementary to B1. At step 2000, the second antigen was inoculated, and four populations survived: the clonal population that was selected by the second antigen (B2), the clonal population (J2) that is complementary to B2, the clonal population that was selected by the first antigen (B1), and the clonal population (J1) that is complementary to B1.

At step 1000, clonal populations B1 and J1 are excited when they are selected by the first antigen, as shown in Fig. 7 (a). However, in step 2000, when populations B2 and J2 are excited, the clonal populations B1 and J1 are already memories of the first antigen. To maintain the homeostasis of the system, there is a decrease in the concentrations of the four remaining populations, as shown in Fig. 7 (b).

3.1 Antigen persistence

The temporal evolution (kinetics) of the Burnet cells is shown in Fig. 8 for each antigen i. Fig. 8 shows that the population selected by the first antigen begins to decrease after the second inoculation.

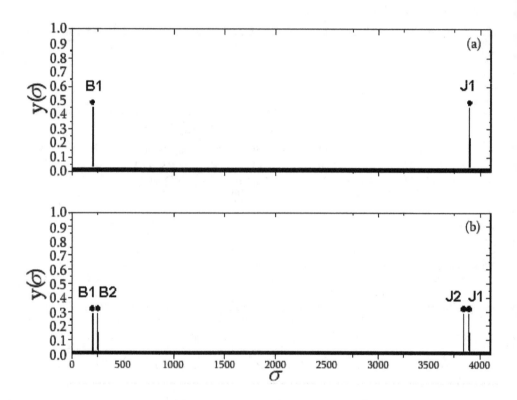

Fig. 7. Surviving clonal populations: (a) for the first antigen inoculated, and (b) for the first and second antigens inoculated.

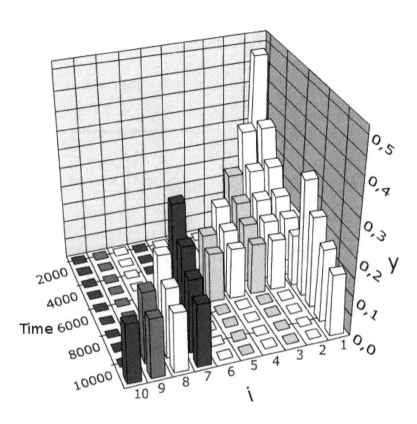

Fig. 8. Evolution of populations in memory, up to 11,000 time steps (concentration of antigens equal to 0.10 a.u.). The first and seventh clonal populations remain excited, while the others disappear – except for the last populations, which were excited near the end of the range.

This behavior occurs because the immune system has a maximum number of cells that it can support; in other words, when new antigens are memorized, others need to be forgotten (immune homeostasis turnover). At time step 7,000, when the seventh inoculation is performed, the first population begins to increase, indicating that it can be stored for a long period. In our Ag-dependent approach, this behavior indicates that an increase in the lifetime (lifespan) of memory can be generated by antigen survival (antigenic dependence).

3.2 Antigen mutation

To study the influence of antigenic mutation on memory (B cell antigen-dependent memory), simulations of inoculations of the 30 samples were also performed, with an antigenic dosage of

$Ag_{initial} = 0.1 a.u.$. The durations of memory populations in each experiment (E1, E2, and E3) are shown in Fig.9.

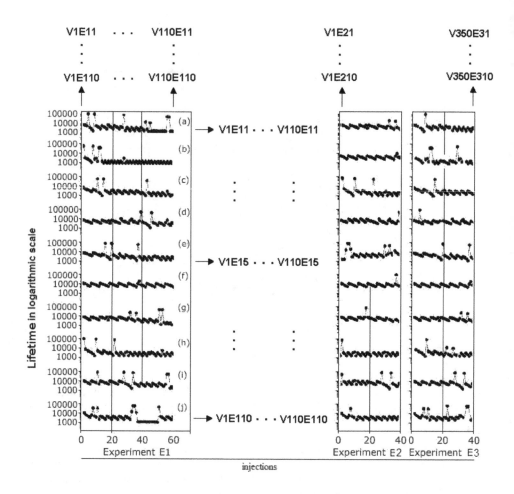

Fig. 9. Lifetime on a logarithmic scale for the clonal populations in each sample and in three experiments. For best viewing results, the graphs were truncated at 60 time steps (experiment E1) and 40 time steps (experiments E2 and E3). The arrows indicate the antigen populations that led to the production of immune memory.

In Fig. 9 (a), for example, all of the lifetimes (lasting memories) are related to antigens of different species (V1E11...V110E11). In contrast, the first lifetime in Fig. 9 (a)-(j) refers to an antigen that has already undergone mutation (V1E11...V1E110). Similar memory developments for experiments E2 and E3 are also shown in Fig. 9. The behavior of the average durability of the memories is shown in Fig. 10 (a) - (c).

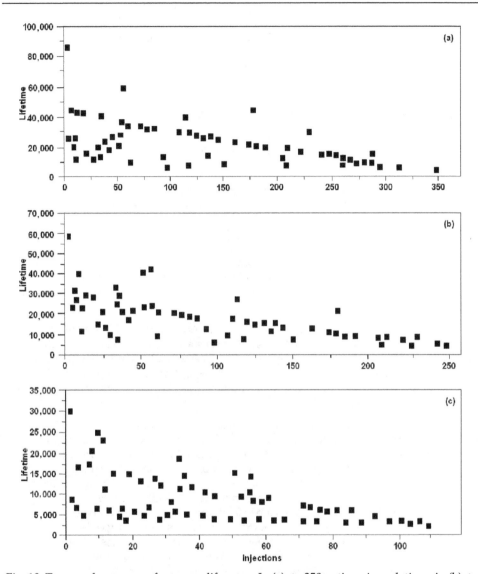

Fig. 10. Temporal averages of memory lifespans. In (a), to 350 antigen inoculations; in (b), to 250 antigen inoculations; and in (c), to 110 antigen inoculations.

The average lifespans are calculated from the memory lifespans generated by each mutated antigen, as follows:

-   For experiment E1 (Fig. 10 (c)), the first average lifetime is obtained by $\dfrac{1}{10}\sum\limits_{k=1}^{10} V_1 E_{1,k}$ and

    the last average lifetime is obtained by $\dfrac{1}{10}\sum\limits_{k=1}^{10} V_{110} E_{1,k}$;

- For experiment E2 (Fig. 10 (b)), the first average lifetime is obtained by $\dfrac{1}{10}\sum_{k=1}^{10} V_1 E_{2,k}$ and the last average lifetime is obtained by $\dfrac{1}{10}\sum_{k=1}^{10} V_{250} E_{2,k}$;

- For experiment E3 (Fig. 10 (a)), the first average lifetime is obtained by $\dfrac{1}{10}\sum_{k=1}^{10} V_1 E_{3,k}$ and the last average lifetime is obtained by $\dfrac{1}{10}\sum_{k=1}^{10} V_{350} E_{3,k}$.

From Figs 9 and 10, the resulting set for this dynamics suggests that different antigens, and mutated antigens, generate different lifespans for immunological memory.

4. Discussion and conclusion

In this paper, an Ag-dependent mathematical model was used to explore how the key elements of the adaptive immune system function. The same model was also used to investigate the factors that are potentially responsible for maximum immunization capacity [40-55].

Inspired by the following statement of Elgueta et al.: "After 20 years, the role for persisting antigens, immune complexes, and FDCs is still not satisfactorily resolved [...] It is completely unknown how the memory B cell compartment is sustained [...] The role of antigens, FDCs, and immune complexes is still open to further investigation" [56], we have paid special attention to the phenomenon of immune memory and its relationship to antigen mutation and antigenic persistence.

Our results suggest that not only antigen type but also antigen mutation can influence the durability of immunizations, indicating that the role of antigen persistence is important for prolonging immune memory. These results were discussed with respect to recent work, and we refer to the adoption of parameter values chosen among data gathered from the literature. The model used in this study took into consideration that the immune system is a network of molecules and cells that can recognize itself [1-6,17]. The cells that recognize antigens select a complementary set of clones (anti-idiotypic antibodies) that can react with the idiotypes of other cells. Thus, the clonal expansion of complementary cells can also occur when these two types of cells interact through lock-and-key connections [8]. In the results presented here, such behavior was observed when an antigen was inoculated into the system and two B cell populations were excited: the population of cells that recognized the antigen and the population of cells that recognized its complementary shape, as shown in Fig. 7.

The results also show that an important factor in the durability of immunological memory is the mutation of antigen populations. In 2009, Tarlinton et al. [49] published a review paper, suggesting that the homeostasis of immune memory can only occur if new memory populations arise over others, i.e., to create dynamic equilibrium among memory cells, some need to disappear for others to arise, because the immune system has a maximum memory capacity [40-55]. Choo et al., in a recent paper published in *The Journal of Immunology* [57], reported the same finding, based on the Ag-independent premise. Choo et al. (2010) have determined, by means of a quantitative analysis, that the homeostatic turnover of Ag-specific CD8 memory T cells is stochastic rather than deterministic.

Then, the results we show in Fig. 8 indicate, in part, an alignment with the work of Choo *et al.*(2010) and with that of Tarlinton et al., because some populations were "forgotten" so that others could be "memorized", thereby complying with the principle of homeostatic turnover. However, Tarlinton *et al.*(2008) [49] and Choo *et al.* (2010) [57] suggest that the mechanism for achieving homeostasis is stochastic, contrary to earlier work of Matzinger (1995)[50] and Nayak *et al.* (2001)[19], who indicated that the durability of memory depends on the antigen type.

The results presented in Figs. 9 and 10 suggest that the homeostatic turnover of a memory B cell depends on the antigen type and also on their mutation(s). Thus, our model aligns best with the earlier work of Nayak *et al.*(2001) and Matzinger *et al.* (1995), and it also aligns to some extent with the work of Tarlinton *et al.*, specifically with respect to storage capacity (homeostatic turnover). However, our results do not line up with a hypothesis of randomness (stochastically) for the kinetics of immune memory, as inferred by Choo *et al.*

The results presented here considered a pool of B cells, but similar conclusions can be drawn from a pool of CD4 T cells. In our simulations, memory lifespan is dependent on the antigen, and the dynamic behavior of memory is strongly deterministic. These results are especially interesting, because they may suggest a deterministic chaotic behavior for the immune memory. In chaotic behavior, there is a mix of stochasticity and determinism, i.e., there exists a well-defined mathematical function for the problem, but small changes in initial conditions can lead to unpredictable results. In conclusion, our results have shown that Choo *et al.*(2010) may have inferred an "apparent" stochastic behavior for homeostatic turnover in their work; however, this behavior may be linked to a deterministic-chaotic dynamic equilibrium. Nevertheless, this finding also indicates that, although the memory behavior is deterministic, just is possible to predict the durability of immunization inferred by a vaccine within a limited interval of antigenic concentration, i.e., outside chaotic region.

5. References

[1] Farmer, J. D., Packard, N. H., Perelson, A. S. *The Immune System, Adaptation, and Machine Learning.* Physica D, Amsterdam, v. 22, pp. 187-204, July 1986.

[2] Roitt, I., Brostoff, J., Male, D. *Immunology.* 4th Ed. New York: Mosby, 1998.

[3] Hofmeyr, S. A. *An Interpretative Introduction to the Immune System Design. In: Principles for the Immune System and Other Distributed Autonomous Systems.* Cohen, I., Segel, L. A. (eds.). Oxford: Oxford University Press, pp. 302-340, 2000.

[4] Klein, J. *Immunology.* Oxford: Blackwell Scientific Publications, 1990.

[5] Lederberg, J. *Ontogeny of the Clonal Selection Theory of Antibody Formation.* Annals of the New York Ac. of Sc., v. 546, pp. 175-182, 1988.

[6] Perelson, A. S., Weisbuch, G. *Immunology for Physicists.* Rev. of Modern Physics, Seattle, v. 69, n. 4, pp. 1219-1267, Oct. 1997.

[7] Celada, F., Seiden, P. *A computer model of cellular interaction in the immune system.* Immunology Today, Amsterdam, pp. 1356-1362, February 1992.

[8] Perelson, A. S., Mirmirani, M., Oster, G. F. *Optimal Strategies in Immunology II. B Memory Cell Production.* J. Math. Biol., Oxford, v. 5, pp. 213-256, October 1978.

[9] Kaufman, M., Urbain, J., Thomas, R. *Towards a logical analysis of the immune response*. J. Theor. Biol., Amsterdam, v. 11, pp. 527-561, January 1985.

[10] Kaufman, M., Weinberg, E. D. *The NK Model of Rugged Fitness Landscapes and Its Application to Maturation of the Immune Response*, J. Theor. Biol., Amsterdam, v. 141, pp. 211-245, December 1989.

[11] Celada, F., Seiden, P. *Affinity maturation and hypermutation in a simulation of the humoral immune response*. Eur. J. Immunol., Weinheim, v. 26, pp. 1350-1358, June 1996.

[12] Menchón, S. A., Ramos, R. A., Condat, C. A. *Modeling subspecies and the tumor-immune system interaction: Steps toward understanding therapy*. Physica A: Statistical Mechanics and its Applications, v. 386, pp. 713-719.

[13] MO, H. *Review of Modeling and Stimulating Human Immune Sysytem. Artificial Intelligence Applications and Innovations*. IFIP International Federation for Information Processing, 2005, v. 187/2005, pp. 845-854.

[14] Rapin, N., Lund, O., Bernaschi, M., Castiglione, F. *Computational Immunology Meets Bioinformatics: The Use of Prediction Tools for Molecular Binding in the Simulation of the Immune System* . PLoS One. v. 5(4), p. e9862, 2010.

[15] Lundegaard, C., Lund, O., Kesmir, C., Brunak, S., Nielsen, M. *Modeling the adaptive immune system: predictions and simulations*. Bioinformatics. v. 23, pp. 3265-3275, 2007.

[16] Boer, R. J., Oprea, M., Rustom. A., Murali-Krishna, K., Ahmed, R., Perelson, A. *Recruitment Times, Proliferation, and Apoptosis Rates during the CD8+ T-Cell Response to Lymphocytic Choriomeningitis Virus*. JOURNAL OF VIROLOGY, v. 75, pp. 10663-10669, 2001.

[17] Jerne, N. K. *Towards a Network Theory of the Immune System*. Ann. Immunol. v. 125C, pp. 373-389, October 1974.

[18] Shibani Mitra-Kaushik, S., Shaila, M. S., Anjali K. Karande, A. K., Nayak, R. *Idiotype and Antigen-Specific T Cell Responses in Mice on Immunization with Antigen, Antibody, and Anti-idiotypic Antibody*. Cellular Immunology v. 209, pp. 109-119, 2001.

[19] Nayak, R., Mitra-Kaushik, S., M. S. Shaila. *Perpetuation of immunological memory: a relay hypothesis*. Immunology v. 102, pp. 387-395, 2001.

[20] Castro, L. N. *Fundamentals of Natural Computing: Basic Concepts, Algorithms, and Applications*. Chapman & Hall/CRC Computer & Information Science Series, 2006.

[21] Lagreca, M. C., Almeida, R. M. C., Santos, R. M. Z. A Dynamical Model for the Immune Repertoire, Physica A, v. 289, pp. 191-207, 2001.

[22] Ausloos, M., Dirickx, M. *The Logistic Map and the Route to Chaos*. 413 p. Springer, 2006.

[23] Heyman, B. *Feedback regulation by IgG antibodies*. Immunology Letters, v. 88, pp. 157-161, 2003.

[24] Hjelm, F., Carlsson, F., Getahun, A., Heyman, B. *Antibody-Mediated Regulation of the Immune Response*. Scandinavian Journal of Immunology, v. 64, 177-184, 2006.

[25] Nimmerjahn, F., Ravetch, J. V. *Antibody-mediated modulation of immune responses*, v. 236, pp. 265-275, 2010.

[26] Ferrari, P. C., Angotti, J. A. P., Tragtenberg, M. H. R. *Introdução ao Caos em Sistemas Dinâmicos*. Mini-curso. Instituto de Física – UFG, 2006.

[27] May, R. M. *Simple Mathematical Models with Very Complicated Dynamics*. Nature, V. 261, p. 459, 1976.

[28] Aubin, D., Dalmedico, A. D. *Writing the History of Dynamical Systems and Chaos: Longue Dureé and Revolution, Disciplines and Cultures.* Historia Mathematica, v. 29, pp. 273-339, 2002.

[29] Erneux, T. *Applied delay differential equations.* In: Surveys and Tutorials in the Applied Mathematical Sciences. Springer, p. 210, 2009.

[30] Moreira, I. C. *Os primórdios do Caos Determinístico.* Ciência Hoje, v. 14, pp. 10-16, 1992.

[31] Dudek, M. R. *Lotka-Volterra PopulationModel of Genetic Evolution.* Communications in Computational Physics, v. 2, pp. 1174-1183, 2007.

[32] Bagnoli, F., Bezzi, M. Eigen's Error Threshold and Mutational Meltdown in a Quasi-species Model, International Journal of Modern Physics C, v. 9, pp. 1-7, 1998.

[33] Gould, H., Tobochnik, J. *An Introduction to Computer Simulation Methods: Applications to Physical Systems.* Addison-Weley Publishing Company. 1996.

[34] von Laer, D., Hasselmannb, S., Hasselmannb, K. *Impact of gene-modified T cells on HIV infection dynamics.* Journal of Theoretical Biology, v. 238, pp. 60-77, 2008.

[35] Walker, R. E., Carter, C. S., Muul, L., Natarajan, V., Herpin, B. R., Leitman, S. F., Klein, H. G., Mullen, C. A., Metcalf, J. A., Baseler, M., Falloon, J., Davey, R. T., Kovacs, J. A., Polis, M. A., Masur, H., Blaese, R. M., Lane, H. C. *Peripheral expansion of pre-existing mature T cells is an important means of CD4þ T-cell regeneration HIV-infected adults.* Nat. Med. v. 4, pp. 852-856, 1998.

[36] Heyman, B. *Regulation of Antibody Responses via Antibodies, Complements, and FC Receptors.* Annu. Rev. Immunol. v. 18, pp. 709-737, 2000.

[37] Rustom Antia, r., Pilyugin, s. s., Ahmed, r. *Models of immune memory: On the role of cross-reactive stimulation, competition, and homeostasis in maintaining immune memory.* Immunology, v. 95, pp. 14926-14931, 1998.

[38] Monvel, J. H. B., Martin, O. M. *Memory capacity in large idiotypic networks.* Bulletin of Mathematical Biology. v. 57, pp. 109-136, 1995.

[39. Vani, J., Elluru, S., Negi, V., Lacroix-Desmazes, S.. Michel D. *Role of natural antibodies in immune homeostasis: IVIg perspective.* Autoimmunity Reviews, *v. 7, pp. 440-444, 2008.*

[40] Etchegoin, P. G. *Vaccination pattern affects immunological response.* Physica A: Statistical Mechanics and its Applications, v. 354, pp. 393-403, 2005.

[41] Boer, R. J., Oprea, M., Rustom. A., Murali-Krishna, K., Ahmed, R., Perelson, A. *Recruitment Times, Proliferation, and Apoptosis Rates during the CD8+ T-Cell Response to Lymphocytic Choriomeningitis Virus.* Journal of Virology, v. 75, pp. 10663-10669, 2001.

[42] Bueno, V., Pacheco-Silva, A. *Tolerância oral: uma nova perspectiva no tratamento de doenças autoimunes.* Revista da Associação Médica Brasileira, v. 45, pp. 79-85, 1999.

[43] Lima, F. A., Carneiro-Sampaio, M. *The role of the thymus in the development of the immune system.* Reviews and Essays, v. 29, pp. 33-42, 2007.

[44] Utzny, C., Burroughs, N. J. *Long-term Stability of Diverse Immunological Memory.* J. Theor. Biol., v. 211, pp. 393-402, 2001.

[45] Yao, W., Hertel, L., Wahl, L. M. *Dynamics of recurrent viral infection.* Proc. R. Soc. B, v. 273, pp. 2193-2199, 2006.

[46] Dimitrijevic, L., Zvancevic-Simonovic, S., Istojanovic, M., Inic-Kanada, A., Ivkovic, I. *The Possible Role of Natural Idiotopes in Immune Memory.* Clinical & Developmental Immunology, v. 11, pp. 281-285, 2004.

[47] Obukhanych, T. V., Nussenzweig, M. C. *T-independent type II immune responses generate memory B cells.* Journal of Experimental Medicine, v. 203, pp. 305-310, 2006.

[48] Lanzavecchia, A., Sallusto, F. *Human B cell memory.* Current Opinion in Immunology, v. 21, pp. 298-304, 2009.

[49] Tarlinton, D., Radbruch, A., Hiepe, F., Thomas Dorner, T. *Plasma cell differentiation and survival.* Current Opinion in Immunology, v. 20, pp. 162-169, 2008.

[50] Matzinger, P. *Immunology: memories are made of this?* Nature, pp. 369-605, 1995.

[51] Hendrikxa, L. H., Berbersa, G. A. M., Veenhovenb, R. H., Sandersc, E.A.M., Buismana, A. M. *IgG responses after booster vaccination with different pertussis vaccines in Dutch children 4 years of age: Effect of vaccine antigen content.* Vaccine, v. 27, pp. 6530-6536, 2009.

[52] Tizard, I. R. *Immunology: An Introduction.* 4th ed. Philadelphia: Saunders College Publishing, 1995.

[53] Abbas, A. K., Lichtman, A. H., Pober, J. S. *Cellular and Molecular Immunology.*

[54] Kamradt, T., Avrion, M. N. *Advances in immunology: Tolerance and Autoimmunity.* N Engl J Med, v. 344, pp. 655-64, 2001.

[55] Peter, D., Roitt, I. M. *Advances in immunology: The Immune System.* New Engl. J. Med., v. 343, pp. 37-49, 2000.

[56] Elgueta, R., Vries, V. C., Noelle, R. J. The immortality of humoral immunity. Immunological Reviews, v. 236, pp. 139-150, 2010.

[57] Choo, D. K., Murali-Krishna, K., Anita, R., Ahmed, R. Homeostatic Turnover of Virus-Specific Memory CD8 T Cells Occurs Stochastically and Is Independent of CD4 T Cell Help. Journal of Immunolody, v.185, pp. 3436-44, 2010. Esta precisa ser a referência número 1.

7

Immunology of Leishmaniasis and Future Prospective of Vaccines

Rakesh Sehgal[1], Kapil Goyal[1], Rupinder Kanwar[2],
Alka Sehgal[3] and Jagat R. Kanwar[2]
[1]Department of Parasitology, Postgraduate Institute
of Medical Education & Research, Chandigarh,
[2]Nanomedicine-Laboratory of Immunology and Molecular Biomedical Research (LIMBR),
Centre for Biotechnology and Interdisciplinary Biosciences (BioDeakin), Institute for
Technology & Research Innovation (ITRI), Deakin University, Geelong, Technology
Precinct (GTP), Waurn Ponds, Geelong, Victoria,
[3] Government Medical College & Hospital, Sector 32, Chandigarh,
[1,3]India
[2]Australia

1. Introduction

Leishmaniasis causes human suffering on a global scale and there are more than 12 million current cases with 2 million additional cases annually. There is a serious threat to get infected cases of 350 million in endemic areas specifically in South East Asia. The epidemiological studies revealed that there are 20 protozoan parasite species of the genus *Leishmania* known to cause leishmaniasis in humans (Table 1)(WHO 2004). Leishmaniasis is prevalent in tropical and subtropical regions and endemic in more than 88 countries where annually 2 million new cases are reported. The geographic distribution of each *Leishmania* species affects the type of disease that occurs in each region of the world. Visceral leishmaniasis (VL; commonly known as kala-azar) is caused by *Leishmania donovani* in South Asia and Africa, while *Leishmania infantum* causes VL in the Mediterranean, the Middle East, Latin America and parts of Asia too (Table 2)(WHO 2010). Other mammals can also be infected with *Leishmania* spp., dogs develop canine visceral leishmaniasis (CaVL) and they serve as an important parasitic reservoir in these regions. Cutaneous leishmaniasis (CL) is caused by *L. major* in Africa, the Middle East and parts of Asia, by *Leishmania tropica* in the Middle East, the Mediterranean and parts of Asia, and by *Leishmania aethiopica* in parts of Africa. Many different species may be involved in the Americas, where CL can be found throughout South America and as far as Mexico in the north (Table 1 and 2). Infection have also been reported in Canada and the US. Australia is free of *Leishmania* spp. but infection among local animals like captive kangaroos, wallabies and other marsupials have been reported recently and there are chances of transmission of this disease to human through infected meat and also due to close proximity with these native animals (Gelanew, Kuhls et al. 2010).

Old world, subgenus Leishmania	
Visceral leishmaniasis	*Leishmania donovani, L. infantum*
Cutaneous leishmaniasis	*L. major, L. tropica, L. aethiopica*
New world, subgenus Leishmania	
Visceral leishmaniasis	*L. infantum*
Cutaneous leishmaniasis	*L. infantum, L. mexicana, L. pifanol, L. amazonensis*
Diffuse cutaneous leishmaniasis	*L. mexicana, L. amazonensis*
New world, subgenus Viannia	
Cutaneous leishmaniasis	*L. braziliensis, L. guyanensis, L. panamensis, L. peruviana*
Mucocutaneous leishmaniasis	*L. braziliensis, L. panamensis*

Table 1. Main species of *Leishmania* that affect humans.

2. Immunology of leishmaniasis

Leihmaniasis is caused by one of several species of *Leishmania*. The clinical spectrum depends upon both the parasite species and the host's immune response. Some *Leishmania* spp. cause cutaneous, mucocutaneous or diffuse cutaneous leishmaniasis whereas others may disseminate to internal organs such as the liver, spleen and bone marrow to cause visceral leishmaniasis. The main species of *Leishmania* that affect humans are given Table 1&2.

Leishmania parasite exists in two different morphological forms i.e. promastigotes (flagellate form) and amastigote (aflagellated form). Promastigotes develops inside the midgut of sandfly and become infective, non-dividing metacyclic promastigotes which are located near stomodeal valve (an invagination of the foregut into midgut). During blood feeding metacylic promastigotes are regurgitated along with immunomodulatory parasite-derived proteophosphoglycans and various salivary components. The metacyclic promastigotes are rapidly phagocytosed by one of several possible cell types that are found in the local environment. The various cell types may include neutrophils, tissue-resident macrophages or dendritic cell (DC) or monocyte derived DCs (moDCs). After establishing an intracellular niche, metacyclic promastigotes are transformed to non motile amastigote form. These amastigotes replicate within the host cells, which rupture to release too many amastigotes, allowing reinfection of phagocytes. The transmission is complete when infected phagocytes are taken up by another sandfly with the blood meal and amastigotes then convert into promastigotes in the sandfly midgut. (Fig 1: Life cycle of *Leishmania* parasite)

Disease	*Leishmania sp.(CFSPH 2009)*	Geographical burden
Cutaneous Leishmaniasis (CL)	*L. mexicana* complex (ZCL)	Argentina, Belize, Bolivia, Brazil. Colombia, Costa Rica, Ecuador, French Guiana, Guatemala, Mexico, Peru, Suriname, USA, and Venezuela
	L. tropica complex (ACL)	Afghanistan, Azerbaijan, India, Iran, Iraq, Israel, Morocco, Pakistan, Syria, Turkey, and Uzbekistan
	L. major complex (ZCL)	Afghanistan, Algeria, Azerbaijan, Burkina Faso, Cameroon, Chad, Egypt, Ethiopia, Gambia, Georgia, Ghana, Guinea Bissau, India, Iran, Iraq, Israel, Jordan, Kazakhstan, Kenya, Kuwait, Libya, Mali, Mauritania, Mongolia, Morocco, Niger, Nigeria, Oman, Pakistan, Saudi Arabia, Senegal, the Sudan, Syria, Tunisia, Turkey, Turkmenistan, Uzbekistan, and Yemen
	L. aethiopica complex (ZCL)	Ethiopia, Kenya, and Uganda
	L. brazilensis complex (ZCL)	Argentina, Belize, Bolivia, Brazil. Colombia, Costa Rica, Ecuador, French Guiana, Guatemala, Honduras, Mexico, Nicaragua, Panama, Paraguay, Peru, and Venezuela
	L. guyanensis complex (ZCL)	Argentina, Belize, Bolivia, Brazil. Colombia, Costa Rica, Ecuador, French Guiana, Guatemala, Guyana, Honduras, Nicaragua, Panama, Peru, Suriname, and Venezuela
Mucosal/mucocutaneous Leishmaniasis (ML)	*L. braziliensis* complex	Argentina, Belize, Bolivia, Brazil. Colombia, Costa Rica, Ecuador, French Guiana, Guatemala, Honduras, Mexico, Nicaragua, Panama, Paraguay, Peru, and Venezuela
	L. guyanensis complex	Colombia, Costa Rica, Ecuador, Guatemala, Honduras, Nicaragua, and Panama
Visceral Leishmaniasis (VL; Kala-azar)	*L. donovani* complex (AVL, ZVL)	Afghanistan, Albania, Algeria, Argentina, Armenia, Azerbaijan, Bangladesh, Bhutan, Bolivia, Bosnia & Herzegovina, Brazil, Bulgaria, Chad, Central African Republic, China, Colombia, Croatia, Cyprus, Djibouti, Egypt, El Salvador, Eritrea, Ethiopia, France, Gambia, Georgia, Greece, Guatemala, Honduras, India, Iran, Iraq, Israel. Italy, Jordan, Kazakhstan, Kenya, Kyrgyzstan, Lebanon, Libya, Macedonia, Malta, Mauritania, Mexico, Monaco, Montenegro, Morocco, Nepal, Nicaragua, Oman, Pakistan, Paraguay, Portugal, Romania, Saudi Arabia, Senegal. Slovenia, Somalia, Spain, Sri Lanka, the Sudan, Syria, and Yemen
Post-Kala-azar Dermal Leishmaniasis (PKDL)	*L. donovani* complex	Bangladesh, China, Nepal, India, Iran, Iraq, Kenya, Pakistan, the Sudan

Table 2. Disease phenotype and geographical burden attributed to various *Leishmania* species (WHO 2010).

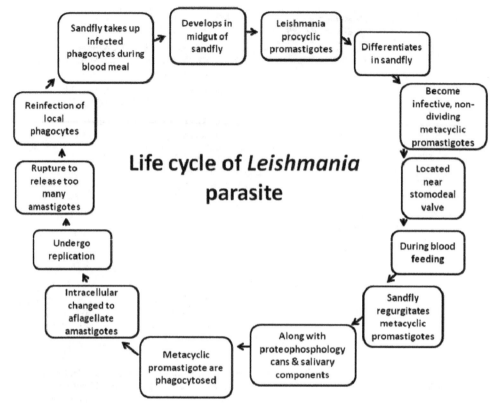

Fig. 1. Life cycle of Leishmania parasite.

3. Host cells for *Leishmania* parasites

Leishmania spp. is an obligate intracellular pathogen which mainly infects macrophages. Recent studies have shown that it can infect multiple cell types. Neutrophils have been regarded as Trojan Horses which help promastigotes to establish intracellular niche in macrophages without triggering their antimicrobial defences. The promastigotes are phagocytosed by neutrophils and they reside in their phagosomes. They become phagocytic meal for the macrophages when undergo apoptosis. Since these apoptotic bodies are phagocytosed through receptor mediated pathways that fail to trigger antimicrobial defences.(Ravichandran and Lorenz 2007) The neutrophils are attracted at local site of sandfly bite due to alarmins(IL-33,IL1β,high mobility group protein B1-HMGB1), which are endogenous molecules that provide signal of tissue damage.(Haraldsen, Balogh et al. 2009) Mononuclear phagocytes which are infected with Leishmania parasites also produce various chemokines which help in recruitment of neutrophils.(Lopez Kostka, Dinges et al. 2009; Xin, Vargas-Inchaustegui et al. 2010)

Leishmania promastigotes have a dense covering of glycocalyx which is attached to the plasma membrane with the help of GPI (glycophosphoinositol). Lipophosphoglycan (LPG) is an important molecule which promotes the infectivity of the parasite in mammalian host.

It is a long phosphoglycan molecule having repeated sugar residues, glycan side chains and a capping oligosaccharide. It shows a great variability in its structure which helps in immune evasion. Another important surface glycoprotein is zinc metalloproteinase(GP-63) which acts as a virulence factor (Gomez, Contreras et al. 2009). *Leishmania donovani* promastigotes stimulate neutrophil extracellular traps (NETs) by a LPG independent pathway (Gabriel, McMaster et al. 2010). These NETs are filamentous DNA which are decorated with antimicrobial peptides.

Though the neutrophils play an important role but mononuclear phagocytes are equally essential for the replication and long term survival of parasites. Dermal DCs uptake the parasite within first few hours of infection by pseudopodium formation (Ng, Hsu et al. 2008). As the number of resident macrophages and dendritic cells is limited in the skin, the parasitic multiplication is accompanied by the recruitment of monocytes (precursor of DCs) (Charmoy, Brunner-Agten et al. 2010). Infected inflammatory moDCs may facilitate parasite to reach the draining lymph node. *Leishmania* parasite can hide itself in skin and lymph node fibroblasts.

In human neutrophils, phagosomes containing promastigotes fuse with myeloperoxidase(mpo) containing primary granules. It is an additional fusion of phagosome with tertiary and specific granules which lead to parasite degradation. These tertiary and specific granules are responsible for acidification and superoxide generation (Fig 2).

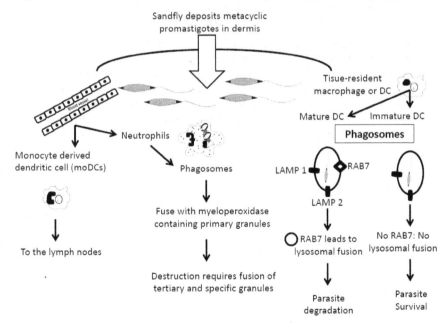

Fig. 2. Different cell types involved in Leishmaniasis and fate of phagosome. Metacyclic promastigotes are deposited in the dermis and taken up by various cells like neutrophils, monocyte derived dendritic cells, macrophages. Small GTPase RAB 7 helps in lysosomal fusion and its degradation. This fusion is inhibited in immature dendritic cells. This could be a mechanism to ensure the transport of live parasites to lymphnodes. Adapted from (Kaye and Scott 2011).

Inside macrophages parasite containing phagosomes mature to form phagolysosome but promastigotes inhibit this process. Lysosomal-associated membrane protein 1 (LAMP 1) and LAMP 2 are found in phagosomes containing *Leishmania* promastigotes in both immature DCs and mature DCs. Maturation of parasite containing phagosomes is arrested at late endosomal stage. Fusion of lysosome occurs with the help of GTPase RAB7 which is observed in mature DCs only. Thus, inhibition of RAB7 recruitment could be a mechanism used by *Leishmania* to transport the live parasites safely to lymph nodes (Lippuner, Paape et al. 2009).

LPG also provides an opportunity for the parasite to survive inside phagosomes by altering acidification (Vinet, Fukuda et al. 2009). Integration of LPG into phagosome membrane leads to extrusion of synaptotagmin V, which helps in acidification of pagosome by recruiting vesicular portion of ATPase. Thus, LPG-deficient parasites die rapidly before they fully adapted to an intracellular lifestyle.

Size of the parasite containing phagosomes also helps in parasite survival. Larger the size more is the dilutional effect on lesihmanicidal factors like nitric oxide. Lysosomal size is regulated by a Beige protein; also known as lysosomal trafficking regulator (LYST). Mutations in LYST gene (Chediak-Higashi syndrome) leads to increase in size of lysosomes whereas induction of this gene (Leishmaniasis) leads to decrease in size of lysosomes. Thus, LYST behaves as an inducible innate response gene during Leishmaniasis, leading to increased susceptible to killing by nitric oxide (Wilson, Huynh et al. 2008).

Iron has an important role in survival of *Leishmania* parasite as it is used by amastigotes (Huynh and Andrews 2008). There is an efflux pump present in phagosomal membrane which translocates Fe^{2+} and Mn^{2+} ions into the cytosol and thus limits iron availability to the parasite (Blackwell, Goswami et al. 2001). To overcome this decrease in iron availability, there occurs an upregulation of iron transporters, after its entry into macrophages. Thus intra-phagosomal competition for iron leads to activation of cytosolic iron sensors which helps in increased production of iron-binding protein transferrin and transferrin-mediated iron uptake (Das, Biswas et al. 2009).

Lipid microdomains present on macrophage surface helps the promastigotes of *Leishmania* to enter into macrophages (Fig 3). It also directs the entry of various virulence factors such as major surface protein also known as GP63 (Joshi, Rodriguez et al. 2009). These virulence factors can also be transferred to the macrophages by parasite-produced exosomes (Silverman and Reiner 2010). When promastigote enters into the phagosome, LPG inserts itself into lipid rafts and inhibits phagosome-lysosome fusion (Winberg, Holm et al. 2009). The inhibition of fusion is accompanied by accumulation of periphagosomal filamentous actin (F-actin) near lipid microdomains. Various virulence factors also use lipid microdomains to channel themselves into cytoplasm of macrophages. Altered lipid rafts may also be responsible for defective antigen presentation and CD40 signalling, MHC class II, major histocompatibility complex class II.

Leishmania is known to activate various inhibitor molecules that inhibit intracellular signaling spathways such as a negative regulatory molecule is the PTP SHP-1 (Src homology 2 domain containing tyrosine phosphatase)(Yi, Cleveland et al. 1992). SHP-1 is responsible for the negative regulation of many signaling pathways (Gregory and Olivier 2005). The majority of documented SHP-1effects are the result of the inhibition by

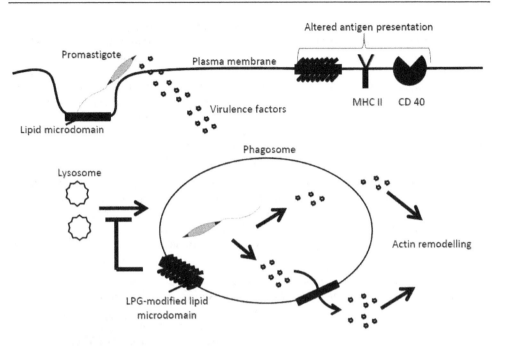

Fig. 3. Lipid microdomains, Leishmania parasite and macrophages. Role of lipid microdomains in transporting parasite and its virulence factors inside macrophages. Altered lipid domains by lipophosphoglycan (LPG) inhibits phagosome-lysosome fusion and also responsible for defective antigen presentation and CD40 signalling, MHC class II. Adapted from (Kaye and Scott 2011).

dephosphorylation of various kinases and their signaling pathways (Frearson and Alexander 1997). SHP-1 plays a vital role in limiting the activation of the JAK/STAT pathways following cytokine receptor stimulation. SHP-1 is known to be activated by MSP (major surface protein, GP63). *Leishmania spp.* contains multiple MSPs and can be found on the promastigote surface as well as in the parasite cytoplasm. Surface MSP is involved in parasite development within sandfly and the cytoplasmic MSP which is in preformed form is ready to use by the mammalian host (Yao, Donelson et al. 2007). This action is analogous to various effectors that are used by type III secretion system in bacteria which behaves like syringe and needle to inject various factors into cells (Winnen, Schlumberger et al. 2008). SHP-2 also known as PTPN 11 also shares many downstream targets with SHP-1 and provides anti-leishmanial immunity. The first line anti-leishmanial drug (sodium stibogluconate) also targets SHP-1 at concentrations that are used for chemotherapy in humans (Pathak and Yi 2001).

Another mechanism used by *Leishmania* parasite when inside the macrophages is by interference with host cell signalling at the level of macrophage protein C (PKC)(Olivier, Baimbridge et al. 1992). After initial contact with the target cells *Leishmania* parasite leads to leads to transient activation of MAPK and NF-kB. These signalling pathways lead to stimulation of cytokines and chemokines required for the efficient control of invading pathogen. Thus, amplitude and duration of this immune response must be maintained under strict control to avoid harmful effects on host itself. Important mechanism by which cells protect themselves is by developing refractoriness state to repeated stimulation. It is well known that prolonged stimulation of toll like receptors and macropahges by microbial components such as LPS (lipopolysaccharide), lead these cells to hyporesponsiveness to the same stimulus (Ben-Othman, Guizani-Tabbane et al. 2008). This phenomenon is termed as LPS tolerance similar phenomenon of and similar hyporesponsiveness is seen in macrophages infected by *L. major* promastigotes. *Leishmania* parasite is able to induce a state of tolerance which correlates with a blockade of intracellular MAPK and/or NF-kB signalling pathway (Ben-Othman, Guizani-Tabbane et al. 2008).

Type 1 interferon response is usually associated with viral infections but their role in leishmaniasis is increasingly becoming important. Such response has been seen in infection with *Leishmaniasis*, which induces the expression in macrophages of PKR, a protein kinase that is activated by double stranded RNA. PKR appears to promote parasite survival through induction of the macrophage-deactivating cytokine IL-10 (Pereira, Teixeira et al. 2010).

CD4+T$_H$1 cells are important for the control of *Leishmania* infections, owing their ability to make IFNγ, which activates macrophages and DCs, leading to parasite death (Fig 4). CD8+ T cells are known to provide immunity in visceral leishmaniasis and play an important role in resistance to reinfection (Muller, Kropf et al. 1993). CD8+ T cells are not always associated with disease resolution as seen in patients infected with *L. braziliensis*. These cells are correlated with disease progression when they express the granule-associated serine protease granzyme B. The factors that determine when CD8+ T cells are protective and when they promote disease remain puzzle to the investigators. Chronicity of infection with *L. donovani* appears to be caused by depletion of CD8+ T cells (Joshi, Rodriguez et al. 2009). Activation of CD8+ T cells depend upon dermal DCs and CD8+ T cells activated during Leishmaniasis infections can provide increased resistance to previously encountered pathogens.

Inspite of robust immune response, small number of parasites persist following disease resolution. The production of IL-10 dampens the immune response and allows the some parasites to escape destruction. The IL-10 is produced by a variety of cells following Leishmanial infection, such as regulatory T cells, T helper 1 cells, CD 8+ T cells, B cells, natural killer cells, DCs, macrophages and neutrophils. CD8+CD40+ T cells may act against regulatory T cells, limiting the production of IL-10 during the early phase of infection, but themselves become susceptible to IL-10 as the infection progresses (Belkaid, Piccirillo et al. 2002; Charmoy, Megnekou et al. 2007; Maroof, Beattie et al. 2008). Exactly how these immune mechanisms operate still remains unanswered and is an active area of research.

Dramatic remodelling occurs when leishmaniasis involve infection of lymphoid tissues like spleen and lymph nodes. Immune suppression occurs due to loss of architectural integrity. Interventions which can restore tissue microarchitecture can have important immune restorative functions.

A concept of concomitant immunity has been proposed in Leishmaniasis. It is a situation in which immunological resistance to reinfection co-exists at the same time as persistence of the original infection. The T cells which contribute to such immunity include CD4+T cells

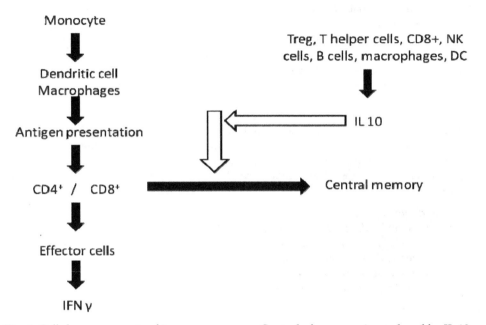

Fig. 4. Cellular components of immune response. Control of response is produced by IL 10, produced by different cell types. Effector cells produce interferon-γ which mediate parasite killing.

with a phenotype of central memory T cells, effector T helper type 1 cells, and resting effector T helper type 1 cells. CD8+ T cells are important in providing resistance to reinfection. Till date no successful vaccine has been developed but recent studies have shown that most protective CD4+ T cells are those which are multifunctional, capable of producing IFNγ, IL-2 and TNF. IL-10 appears to limit the generation of these protective T cells during vaccination (Kedzierski 2010). In future, the application of genomic approaches and study of host factors will lead to a better understanding of pathogenesis and immunology related to leishmaniasis. Further studies are required to investigate unanswered questions related to innate and T cell response in leishmaniasis.

4. *Leishmania* vaccines

WHO has classified Leishmaniasis is an emerging disease. The available treatment options are various chemotherapeutic drugs which are not only costly but also have many adverse side effects. Safe and cost effective vaccine is a need of an hour. Various vaccine strategies have been tried but these are of a little hope. The classical vaccinology or first generation vaccines have been tried in the past which includes infectious material for inoculation, live attenuated parasites and killed parasites for vaccination. Leishmanization, was based on the fact that individual is refractory to reinfection after the lesions of primary illness heals. Initially, infectious lesion material was used but later it was replaced by culture of parasites to inoculate uninfected individuals. This method was abandoned due to poor quality control, parasite persistence, emergence of HIV and ethical issues. Killed parasites replaced leishmanization, but they showed poor efficacy in clinical trials (Noazin, Modabber et al. 2008). Second generation vaccines (modern vaccinology) using subunit vaccines, DNA vaccines and recombinant vaccines are being tried but their efficacy in field trials have not been reported. The major hurdle in vaccine designing is the translation of data from animal models to human disease, and the transition of laboratory experiments to field trials. Table 3 summarizes the important vaccine candidates tested for the cure of leishmaniasis.

Killed vaccines

Vaccination trials in Brazil and Ecuador with killed *Leishmania* stocks have shown to provide immunity from natural infection. Killed vaccination induced Th1 type of immune response and delayed type of hypersensitivity skin test conversion can be used as a surrogate marker for protective immune response (Olivier, Baimbridge et al. 1992; Mendonca, De Luca et al.1995).

Convit and colleagues used a combination of killed *L. mexicana* or *L. braziliensis* promastigotes and *M. bovis* BCG to induce the immunity against South American leishmaniasis. High cure rate have been documented with the induction of Th1 type of immune response (Castes, Moros et al. 1989; Convit and Ulrich 1993). Recombinant IL-12 has been tried as an adjuvant in monkeys to provide the immunity against cutaneous leishmaniasis using killed *L. amazonensis* (Kenney, Sacks et al. 1999)

Live attenuated

Live attenuated vaccines are well known for their better immunogenicity but there are chances of reverting back to virulent forms. However, recent advances in genomics have provided an opportunity to manipulate the *Leishmania* genome by eliminating the virulent genes to produce the attenuated forms. Genes required for long term survival have been manipulated to produce the short lived forms in humans. In a mouse model, *L. major* parasites lacking the gene encoding for enzyme dihydrofolate reductase-thymidylate synthetase DHFR-TS have been produced to induce the protection against infection with either *L. major* or *L. amazonensis*. Mutant lacking genes encoding for cysteine proteases cpa and cpb have also been studied. Thus, the use of attenuated organisms is very useful as it closely mimics to natural infection and can lead to similar immune responses (Titus, Gueiros-Filho et al. 1995).

Synthetic recombinant vaccines:

These newer vaccines include recombinant DNA-derived antigens and peptides. The targets used as antigens may be species or life cycle stage specific. Recombinant antigens can be delivered as purified proteins, as the naked DNA encoding them, or as bacteria manufacturing the proteins of interest. These can be used as a potential vaccine candidate. Bioinformatics can be used to predict the immunogenic peptides which can be synthetically constructed. Though this approach sounds better but it suffers from many disadvantages such as the magnitude of the T-cell memory induced, the inability of all individuals in the population to respond to the peptide, and the high cost of production on large scale. Despite these limitations gp63 peptides have been successfully tested in animals (Campbell et.al 201; Carrión J. 2011).

Immunogens expressing Bacteria and Viruses as vaccines

Leishmaniolysin or gp63 is the first recombinant antigen to be used against as a vaccine candidate against leishmaniasis (Chang, Chaudhuri et al. 1990). The surface expressed glycoprotein leishmaniolysin (gp63) is one of the parasite receptors for host macrophages and mutants lacking this protein are avirulent. However, the T-cell responses to gp63 have been variable in animals and human studies (Olobo, Anjili et al. 1995). Parasite surface antigen have also been tested as a vaccine candidate. gp46/M2 or parasite surface antigen 2 (PSA-2) is expressed in all *Leishmania* species except *L. braziliensis*. Thus, providing an opportunity for developing pan-*Leishmania* vaccine (Handman, Symons et al. 1995). The leishmanial eukaryotic ribosomal protein (LeIF), a homologue of the ribosomal protein cIF4A, is an another important vaccine candidate as it can induce Th1-type cytokines in humans (Skeiky, Coler et al. 2002). This protein is highly conserved in evolution, but parasite specific epitopes can be used for vaccination, so that autoimmune responses can be avoided. Other vaccine candidates are amastigote specific proteins, such as A2, P4, and P8 of *L. mexicana pifanoi* (Soong, Duboise et al. 1995). Another vaccine candidate is a flagellar antigen, lcr1, from *L. donovani chagasi* (Streit, Recker et al. 2000) but its role in humans is debatable as asmastigote forms have a rudimentary flagellum.

Candidate vaccine	Advantages	Disadvantages
Whole killed	Cost effective Good safety profile in South America and Sudan	Quality control, difficult to standardize, variable potency
Surface expressed glycoprotein leishmaniolysin (gp63)	Good results in animals	Poor T cell response in humans
GPI-anchored membrane protein gp46 or Parasite Surface Antigen 2 (PSA-2)	Native polypeptides derived from promastigotes provide protection in mice	Recombinant protein derived from either promastigotes or amastigotes protein showed poor efficacy
Leishmania homologue for receptors of activated C kinase (LACK)	Promote IL-4 secreting T cells (Th2 responses)	Fails to provide protection against visceral leishmaniasis.
Leish-111f: Single molecule constructed by fusion of three molecules: *L. major* homologue of eukaryotic thiol-specific antioxidant (TSA *L. major* stress-inducible protein-1 (LmSTI1) *L. braziliensis* elongation and initiation factor (LeIF) Leish-110f: improved version of Leish-111f	Provides protection in mice against *L. major* and *L. amazonensis* infection Provides partial protection against visceral leishmaniasis in animal models Phase I and II clinical trials done	Failed to protect dogs against infection
Sandfly saliva components: maxadilan, 15 kDa protein, SP15, LJM19	LJM 19: protection in hamsters Dogs: IgG2 and IFN-γ	Experimental stage

Table 3. Summary of important vaccine candidates for leishmaniasis.

DNA vaccine

Vaccinations with DNA encoding gp63and PSA-2 have been tried. It has shown a good protection in animal models which is accompanied by Th1 immune responses (Gurunathan, Sacks et al. 1997; Walker, Scharton-Kersten et al. 1998). The genes encoding the vaccine candidate is cloned into mammalian expression vector, and the DNA is injected directly into muscle or skin. The plasmid DNA is taken up by cells and translocated to the nucleus, where it is transcribed into RNA and then translated in the cytoplasm. It has shown to induce both CD4+ and CD8+ T cell responses and they also ensure proper folding of proteins. Another advantage is that production on large scale is cheap and DNA is highly stable, so does not require cold chain. Research is still going on for developing a vaccine which can provide life long immunity without any side effects. Newer adjuvants are also being tried. Till date no successful vaccine has been developed but recent studies have shown that most protective CD4+ T cells are those which are multifunctional, capable of producing IFNγ, IL-2 and TNF. IL-10 appears to limit the generation of these protective T cells during vaccination (Kedzierski 2010). In future, the application of genomic approaches and study of host factors will lead to a better understanding of pathogenesis and immunology related to leishmaniasis. Further studies are required to investigate unanswered questions related to innate and T cell response in leishmaniasis.

5. Conclusions

Recent studies have provided new and important information on the biology of *Leishmania*. The *Leishmania* genome sequence is now available as well as new methods for its manipulation. We have learned that *Leishmania* can exchange genetic material during its journey in the sand fly, and we understand better the molecular mechanisms that allow *Leishmania* promastigotes and amastigotes to survive in their respective environments. Recent investigation have provided new insight into the role of cells of the innate immunity, such as neutrophils, monocytes, NK, and DCs, as well as 'non-immune' cells such as keratinocytes. Now we have better understand how *Leishmania* evade the mammalian immune response and avoid the development of sterilizing immunity, therefore increasing its chances to secure transmission to a new host. The identification of a greater range of antigen candidates with broad species coverage, and a greater understanding of the immunology of protective immunity, these arguments should be balanced by the need to develop a stronger base in clinical vaccinology. This end is only likely to be accomplished by an accelerated programme of well-defined clinical trials, and in this context the use of therapeutic vaccine trials as a first step has much to offer. New generation vaccines hold promises to control leishmaniasis and data suggest that prophylactic vaccination in humans and dogs could generate protection and may able to interrupt transmission, ultimately reducing disease incidence. These new generation vaccines in a therapeutic setting as an adjunct with various chemotherapies have demonstrated safety and efficacy against various manifestations of *Leishmania* infection. New generation's refined antigens and adjuvants for vaccines may provide the best range of vaccines aimed at controlling disease incidence and severity to *Leishmania* infection.

6. References

Belkaid, Y., C. A. Piccirillo, et al. (2002). "CD4+CD25+ regulatory T cells control Leishmania major persistence and immunity." Nature 420(6915): 502-507.

Ben-Othman, R., L. Guizani-Tabbane, et al. (2008). "Leishmania initially activates but subsequently down-regulates intracellular mitogen-activated protein kinases and nuclear factor-kappaB signaling in macrophages." Mol Immunol 45(11): 3222-3229.

Blackwell, J. M., T. Goswami, et al. (2001). "SLC11A1 (formerly NRAMP1) and disease resistance." Cell Microbiol 3(12): 773-784.

Castes, M., Z. Moros, et al. (1989). "Cell-mediated immunity in localized cutaneous leishmaniasis patients before and after treatment with immunotherapy or chemotherapy." Parasite Immunol 11(3): 211-222.

CFSPH (2009). "The Center for Food Security and Public Health, I.S.U., Leishmaniasis (cutaneous & visceral). Animal Disease Resource Index. Fact Sheet."

Chang, K. P., G. Chaudhuri, et al. (1990). "Molecular determinants of Leishmania virulence." Annu Rev Microbiol 44: 499-529.

Charmoy, M., S. Brunner-Agten, et al. (2010). "Neutrophil-derived CCL3 is essential for the rapid recruitment of dendritic cells to the site of Leishmania major inoculation in resistant mice." PLoS Pathog 6(2): e1000755.

Charmoy, M., R. Megnekou, et al. (2007). "Leishmania major induces distinct neutrophil phenotypes in mice that are resistant or susceptible to infection." J Leukoc Biol 82(2): 288-299.

Convit, J. and M. Ulrich (1993). "Antigen-specific immunodeficiency and its relation to the spectrum of American cutaneous leishmaniasis." Biol Res 26(1-2): 159-166.

Das, N. K., S. Biswas, et al. (2009). "Leishmania donovani depletes labile iron pool to exploit iron uptake capacity of macrophage for its intracellular growth." Cell Microbiol 11(1): 83-94.

Frearson, J. A. and D. R. Alexander (1997). "The role of phosphotyrosine phosphatases in haematopoietic cell signal transduction." Bioessays 19(5): 417-427.

Gabriel, C., W. R. McMaster, et al. (2010). "Leishmania donovani promastigotes evade the antimicrobial activity of neutrophil extracellular traps." J Immunol 185(7): 4319-4327.

Gelanew, T., K. Kuhls, et al. (2010). "Inference of population structure of Leishmania donovani strains isolated from different Ethiopian visceral leishmaniasis endemic areas." PLoS Negl Trop Dis 4(11): e889.

Gomez, M. A., I. Contreras, et al. (2009). "Leishmania GP63 alters host signaling through cleavage-activated protein tyrosine phosphatases." Sci Signal 2(90): ra58.

Gregory, D. J. and M. Olivier (2005). "Subversion of host cell signalling by the protozoan parasite Leishmania." Parasitology 130 Suppl: S27-35.

Gurunathan, S., D. L. Sacks, et al. (1997). "Vaccination with DNA encoding the immunodominant LACK parasite antigen confers protective immunity to mice infected with Leishmania major." J Exp Med 186(7): 1137-1147.

Handman, E., F. M. Symons, et al. (1995). "Protective vaccination with promastigote surface antigen 2 from Leishmania major is mediated by a TH1 type of immune response." Infect Immun 63(11): 4261-4267.

Haraldsen, G., J. Balogh, et al. (2009). "Interleukin-33 - cytokine of dual function or novel alarmin?" Trends Immunol 30(5): 227-233.

Huynh, C. and N. W. Andrews (2008). "Iron acquisition within host cells and the pathogenicity of Leishmania." Cell Microbiol 10(2): 293-300.

Joshi, T., S. Rodriguez, et al. (2009). "B7-H1 blockade increases survival of dysfunctional CD8(+) T cells and confers protection against Leishmania donovani infections." PLoS Pathog 5(5): e1000431.

Kaye, P. and P. Scott (2011). "Leishmaniasis: complexity at the host-pathogen interface." Nat Rev Microbiol 9(8): 604-615.

Kedzierski, L. (2010). "Leishmaniasis Vaccine: Where are We Today?" J Glob Infect Dis 2(2): 177-185.

Kenney, R. T., D. L. Sacks, et al. (1999). "Protective immunity using recombinant human IL-12 and alum as adjuvants in a primate model of cutaneous leishmaniasis." J Immunol 163(8): 4481-4488.

Lippuner, C., D. Paape, et al. (2009). "Real-time imaging of Leishmania mexicana-infected early phagosomes: a study using primary macrophages generated from green fluorescent protein-Rab5 transgenic mice." Faseb J 23(2): 483-491.

Lopez Kostka, S., S. Dinges, et al. (2009). "IL-17 promotes progression of cutaneous leishmaniasis in susceptible mice." J Immunol 182(5): 3039-3046.

Maroof, A., L. Beattie, et al. (2008). "Posttranscriptional regulation of Il10 gene expression allows natural killer cells to express immunoregulatory function." Immunity 29(2): 295-305.

Mendonca, S. C., P. M. De Luca, et al. (1995). "Characterization of human T lymphocyte-mediated immune responses induced by a vaccine against American tegumentary leishmaniasis." Am J Trop Med Hyg 53(2): 195-201.

Muller, I., P. Kropf, et al. (1993). "Gamma interferon response in secondary Leishmania major infection: role of CD8+ T cells." Infect Immun 61(9): 3730-3738.

Ng, L. G., A. Hsu, et al. (2008). "Migratory dermal dendritic cells act as rapid sensors of protozoan parasites." PLoS Pathog 4(11): e1000222.

Noazin, S., F. Modabber, et al. (2008). "First generation leishmaniasis vaccines: a review of field efficacy trials." Vaccine 26(52): 6759-6767.

Olivier, M., K. G. Baimbridge, et al. (1992). "Stimulus-response coupling in monocytes infected with Leishmania. Attenuation of calcium transients is related to defective agonist-induced accumulation of inositol phosphates." J Immunol 148(4): 1188-1196.

Olobo, J. O., C. O. Anjili, et al. (1995). "Vaccination of vervet monkeys against cutaneous leishmaniosis using recombinant Leishmania 'major surface glycoprotein' (gp63)." Vet Parasitol 60(3-4): 199-212.

Pathak, M. K. and T. Yi (2001). "Sodium stibogluconate is a potent inhibitor of protein tyrosine phosphatases and augments cytokine responses in hemopoietic cell lines." J Immunol 167(6): 3391-3397.

Pereira, R. M., K. L. Teixeira, et al. (2010). "Novel role for the double-stranded RNA-activated protein kinase PKR: modulation of macrophage infection by the protozoan parasite Leishmania." Faseb J 24(2): 617-626.

Ravichandran, K. S. and U. Lorenz (2007). "Engulfment of apoptotic cells: signals for a good meal." Nat Rev Immunol 7(12): 964-974.

Silverman, J. M. and N. E. Reiner (2010). "Exosomes and other microvesicles in infection biology: organelles with unanticipated phenotypes." Cell Microbiol 13(1): 1-9.

Skeiky, Y. A., R. N. Coler, et al. (2002). "Protective efficacy of a tandemly linked, multi-subunit recombinant leishmanial vaccine (Leish-111f) formulated in MPL adjuvant." Vaccine 20(27-28): 3292-3303.

Soong, L., S. M. Duboise, et al. (1995). "Leishmania pifanoi amastigote antigens protect mice against cutaneous leishmaniasis." Infect Immun 63(9): 3559-3566.

Streit, J. A., T. J. Recker, et al. (2000). "BCG expressing LCR1 of Leishmania chagasi induces protective immunity in susceptible mice." Exp Parasitol 94(1): 33-41.

Titus, R. G., F. J. Gueiros-Filho, et al. (1995). "Development of a safe live Leishmania vaccine line by gene replacement." Proc Natl Acad Sci U S A 92(22): 10267-10271.

Vinet, A. F., M. Fukuda, et al. (2009). "The Leishmania donovani lipophosphoglycan excludes the vesicular proton-ATPase from phagosomes by impairing the recruitment of synaptotagmin V." PLoS Pathog 5(10): e1000628.

Walker, P. S., T. Scharton-Kersten, et al. (1998). "Genetic immunization with glycoprotein 63 cDNA results in a helper T cell type 1 immune response and protection in a murine model of leishmaniasis." Hum Gene Ther 9(13): 1899-1907.

WHO (2004). "Scientific working group on Leishmaniasis. Meeting report. 2–4 February 2004, Geneva, Switzerland. http://apps.who.int/tdr/publications/tdr-research-publications/swg-report-leishmaniasis/pdf/swg_leish.pdf.".

WHO (2010). "WHO, Control of the Leishmanises, in WHO Technical Report Series 2010, World Health Organization: Geneva. ."

Wilson, J., C. Huynh, et al. (2008). "Control of parasitophorous vacuole expansion by LYST/Beige restricts the intracellular growth of Leishmania amazonensis." PLoS Pathog 4(10): e1000179.

Winberg, M. E., A. Holm, et al. (2009). "Leishmania donovani lipophosphoglycan inhibits phagosomal maturation via action on membrane rafts." Microbes Infect 11(2): 215-222.

Winnen, B., M. C. Schlumberger, et al. (2008). "Hierarchical effector protein transport by the Salmonella Typhimurium SPI-1 type III secretion system." PLoS One 3(5): e2178.

Xin, L., D. A. Vargas-Inchaustegui, et al. (2010). "Type I IFN receptor regulates neutrophil functions and innate immunity to Leishmania parasites." J Immunol 184(12): 7047-7056.

Yao, C., J. E. Donelson, et al. (2007). "Internal and surface-localized major surface proteases of Leishmania spp. and their differential release from promastigotes." Eukaryot Cell 6(10): 1905-1912.

Yi, T. L., J. L. Cleveland, et al. (1992). "Protein tyrosine phosphatase containing SH2
    domains: characterization, preferential expression in hematopoietic cells, and
    localization to human chromosome 12p12-p13." Mol Cell Biol 12(2): 836-
    846.

8

Adaptive Immunity from Prokaryotes to Eukaryotes: Broader Inclusions Due to Less Exclusivity?

Edwin L. Cooper
Laboratory of Comparative Neuroimmunology
Department of Neurobiology, David Geffen School of Medicine at UCLA
University of California, Los Angeles
USA

1. Introduction

1.1 The prevailing view: blurring, innate and adaptive

The currently held view of the immune system proposes generally acceptable descriptions supported by strong evidence. There are two primary systems: innate and adaptive but distributed "unequally" among the two major animal groups (ignoring mostly all plants). Animal groups include the multitudinous invertebrates and vertebrates with vertebrates being the greatest beneficiaries of a fully functional complex immune apparatus that combines the two systems. Despite this super armamentarium, the overwhelming problems of possessing this dual system, as the vertebrates i.e. the innate and adaptive does not seem to guard or even prevent the development of one internal threat to survival. This is the scourge: development of cancer. By contrast invertebrates whose immune system is primarily of the innate type manage to eat, reproduce and survive without developing cancer. Briefly the immune system consists of: Innate: natural, nonspecific, no memory, non-anticipatory, non-clonal, germ line; Adaptive: acquired, specific, memory, anticipatory, clonal, somatic. In general, both systems and in the simplest reductionist terms, each must possess a cell that recognizes an antigen and digests it. The second cell if appropriately stimulated must react to destroy a potentially detrimental antigen. During evolution more cells were added to this armamentarium giving rise to increasing functions associated with effector activity. Emerging information supports the view that overlap or blurring exists between these two sometimes rigidly defined systems. Clearly evidence suggests that lines of demarcation within and between innate and adaptive may not be so strictly delineated — there is immunologic flexibility designated as blurring, not "black and white".

1.2 Evolution of the immune systems

1.2.1 The agnathans (jawless fish)

We have been alerted to numerous analyses of the vertebrate and more specifically the mammalian immune system that reveal profound interrelationships and fundamental differences between the adaptive and innate systems of immune recognition (Fig.) [Du

Pasquier and Litman, 2000]. There is increasing experimental accessibility of non-mammalian jawed vertebrates (*gnathosomes*; *cartilaginous* and bony fish), jawless vertebrates (*agnathans*) (hagfish, lampreys), protochordates and invertebrates and an enthusiasm by comparative immunologists to explore. Thus we have intriguing new information that suggests likely patterns that reveal emergence of immune-related molecules during metazoan phylogeny. Moreover there is the promise that we may find evolution of alternative mechanisms that ensure receptor diversification. These such findings have already blurred traditional distinctions between adaptive and innate immunity. The adaptive must rely on the innate throughout evolution, the immune system has benefited by using a remarkably extensive variety of well-equipped mechanistic solutions to meet fundamentally similar requirements for host protection.

The range of such molecules, which includes the fibrinogen-related proteins (FREPs) in a mollusk, variable regioncontaining chitin-binding proteins (VCBPs) in a cephalochordate, variable lymphocyte receptors (VLRs) in jawless vertebrates, and novel immune-type receptors (NITRs) in bony fish, encompasses both the immunoglobulin gene superfamily (IgSF) and leucine-rich repeat (LRR) proteins. Although these molecules vary markedly in form and likely in function, growing evidence suggests that they participate in various types of host immune responses. These results represent significant alternatives to prevailing paradigms of innate and adaptive immune receptors. Thus unusual genetic mechanisms may support mechanisms for diversifying recognition proteins and it may be a ubiquitous characteristic of animal immunity (Fig. 2) (Theodor, 1970; Hildemann et al, 1977; Franc et al, 1996; Pancer, 2000; Watson et al, 2005; Sun et al, 1990; Flajnik and Pasquier, 2004; Zhang et al, 2004), not restricted rigidly to innate and adaptive.

Our immune system rarely acts alone but functions in association with the other two linked regulating systems (the nervous and endocrine systems; not to be examined in this review). Second, when we examine the immune systems close up, there are several generalizations that emerge. The immune system is ubiquitous, found in all creatures including plants and is therefore not restricted to humans. If carefully traced stepwise during evolution treating extremely limited fossil forms, reveals progressively more complex development after we critically examine various levels of plant and animal evolution. There is evidence for innate immunity in plants. According to Luke and O'Neill (2011), "Every organism has to contend with the risk of infection. To cope, organisms have evolved two types of immune responses: the more recent "adaptive" system, found only in vertebrates; and the more ancient "innate" system, which is present in both plants and animals. Researchers have uncovered remarkable evolutionary conservation of innate immune mechanisms between plants and animals. (Figure 3) They use similar receptor molecules to sense pathogens and for immune system signaling (Luke and O'Neill 2011).

This review will: 1) for the first time present an emerging view that "adaptive immunity" mechanisms need not be restricted to complex eukaryotic organisms. Although this may be revolutionary, we might ask: why not since microbes survive? In fact, there is compelling information that prokaryotes may possess adaptive immune mechanisms; 2) deemphasize the over reliance on embryologically defining the animal kingdom and forcing the immune system's evolution into two separate categories, i.e. the protostomes and deuterostomes; 3) support concepts that propelled the immune system into prominent discourse in the life sciences; 4) indicate that the concern for immunologic memory, development of cancer, autoimmunity, and clonal selection may not be essential for effective immunity to evolve; 5) consider analogous mechanisms in prokaryotes that concern CRISPR that are direct repeats found in the DNA of many bacteria and archaea; 6) to understand the mechanism of action of CRISPR systems reveals a prokaryotic analog of eukaryotic RNA supporting the view that bacteria possess a form of acquired immunity; 7) suggest a molecular mechanism by which the nervous system may sense inflammatory responses and respond by controlling stress response pathways at the organismal level; This supports the interconnectedness of two of the three monitoring systems: immune<>nervous<> endocrine to maintain a balanced internal milieu.

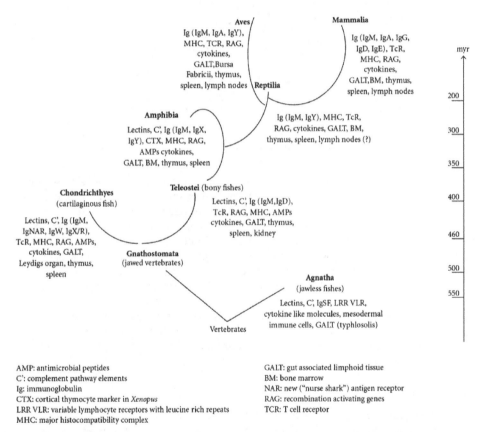

AMP: antimicrobial peptides
C': complement pathway elements
Ig: immunoglobulin
CTX: cortical thymocyte marker in *Xenopus*
LRR VLR: variable lymphocyte receptors with leucine rich repeats
MHC: major histocompatibility complex

GALT: gut associated limphoid tissue
BM: bone marrow
NAR: new ("nurse shark") antigen receptor
RAG: recombination activating genes
TCR: T cell receptor

Fig. 1. Evolution of molecular and histological structures of the vertebrate immune system. Regarding lymphatic tissues, the thymus, and spleen appeared early in fishes, while lymph filtering lymph nodes are observed only in birds and mammals. Among the development of various immunoglobulin isotypes, IgD is expressed in bony fishes, later only mammals are using this B-cell receptor. Reproduced by permission from (Kvell K, Cooper EL, Engelmann P, Bovari J, Nemeth P. Blurring borders: Innate immunity with adaptive features. Clin Dev Immunol (2007):836–71).

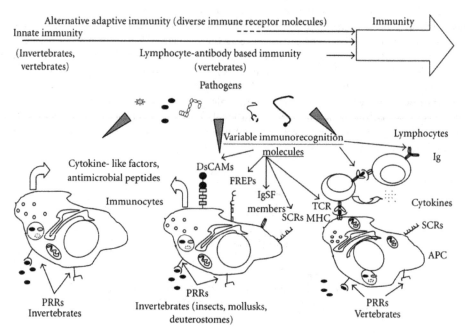

Fig. 2. Schematic representation of innate and adaptive immune feature development in animals. All immune cells express nonspecific receptors, for example, pattern recognition receptors that recognize pathogen associated molecular patterns (PAMPs). Several clusters of innate receptors are conserved from plants to humans and are essential components in the defense of self-integrity. Immune cells of invertebrates also express various scavenger receptor-like proteins (Croquemort, SCRs), immunoglobulin superfamily members (hemolin, DsCAM), and fibrinogen-related peptides (FREPs); all involved in immune functions (eliminating apoptotic cells, parasites, etc.). Invertebrate immune systems also exhibit receptors with high diversity involved in immune functions: FREPs, SCRs, and DsCAMs have extreme individual variability-like vertebrate adaptive immune recognition molecules (Ig, TcR). Reproduced by permission from (Kvell K, Cooper EL, Engelmann P, Bovari J, Nemeth P. Blurring borders: Innate immunity with adaptive features. Clin Dev Immunol (2007):836–71).

1.3 Self/ not-self

Now *Self/not self, adaptive immunity* and a fresh and renewed vision of a vigorous *innate immunity* are acceptable first for invertebrates and now essential for mammals. However, self/not self is now challenged by the controversial, alternative *danger hypothesis*. (Cooper, 2010; Cooper et al, 2002; Engelmann and Nemeth, 2010; Cossarizza, 2010; Parrinello 2010 Pradeu and Carosella 2004; 2006). Since Metchnikoff discovered phagocytosis, controversy persisted concerning two points. First, innate immunity was accorded minor significance to most of immunology while adaptive immunity emerged as predominant, perhaps due to anthropocentricity of 19th and early 20th century immunologists. Later adaptive immunity acquired a significant hypothetical base. Second, clonal selection and specific memory cast a shadow over Metchnikoff's leukocytes, perhaps bolstered by discovering them in invertebrates and not in mammals (Cooper, 2008; Cooper 2010)

Pradeu and Carosella criticize origins and legitimacy of self/non-self. They advocate a critical analysis both conceptually and experimentally to redefine self/non-self that reveals certain shortcomings; they even advocate possibly rejecting that model in favor of an alternative theoretical view for immunology: *continuity*. The '*continuity hypothesis*' attempts to support immunogenicity that avoids criticism of the self-model. Pradeu and Carosella assert that the main objective of immunology is to establish why (teleological?) and when an immune response occurs: to support immunogenicity. Is there an experimental model?

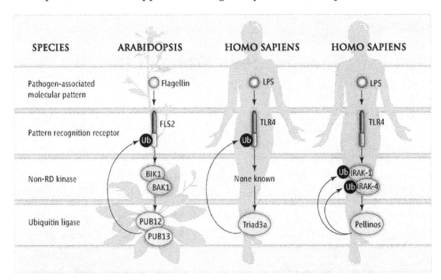

Fig. 3. Innate immunity, conserved.

Arabidopsis and humans have evolutionarily conserved innate immune signaling processes that involve a posttranslational modification process called ubiquitination. In Arabidopsis, bacterial flagellin is sensed by FLS2, which recruits the non-arginine/aspartate (Non-RD) kinases BAK1 and BIK1. BAK1 phosphorylates and activates PUB12/13, which ubiquitinates (Ub) FLS2 and leads to degradation. In humans, TLR4 senses lipopolysaccharide (LPS). This can activate Triad3a (third column), which ubiquitinates TLR4 and leads to its degradation. TLR4 can also activate IRAK-1 and IRAK-4 (fourth column), which activates nuclear factor kappa B (not shown), and also Pellino proteins (Pellinos), which ubiquitinate the IRAKs and lead to their degradation.

1.4 Clonal selection

Another view pertinent to prevailing immunologic concepts includes clonal selection which is a Darwinian corollary. In other words lymphocytes with appropriate receptors could be stimulated to divide leaving progenitor offspring lymphocytes. Now we may be able to deconstruct clonal selection since it may be not applicable to invertebrate mechanisms; all evidence indicates that clonal selection is purely a vertebrate strategy. Some views may insist that anthropocentric mammalian immunologists utilized a tool to propel: the universal innate immune system of ubiquitous and plentiful invertebrates as an essential system for vertebrates. Immunology benefited and innate immunity acquired an extended *raison d'être*. Innate immunity should help if there is a failure of the adaptive immune system. As an internal threat cancer would be subject to the immune system's efficiency. Still to be answered are questions concerning immunologic surveillance that includes clonal selection. According to the question does immunologic surveillance play a role in the survival of invertebrates that seem to not develop cancer as we identify metastasizing transplantable vertebrate type? As a possible explanation, perhaps invertebrate efficient innate immune systems and short life spans evolved certain "canceling devices" that maintain survival, thus precluding their demise by metastasis. (Cooper et al, 2002; Burnet, 1959; Burnet 1962)

Phylogenetic Tree of Life

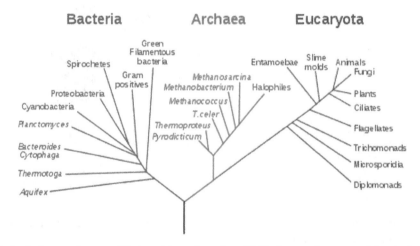

Fig. 4. A phylogenetic tree of living things, based on RNA data and proposed by Carl Woese, showing the separation of bacteria, archaea, and eukaryotes. Trees constructed with other genes are generally similar, although they may place some early-branching groups very differently, thanks to long branch attraction. The exact relationships of the three domains are still being debated, as is the position of the root of the tree. It has also been suggested that due to lateral gene transfer, a tree may not be the best representation of the genetic relationships of all organisms. For instance some genetic evidence suggests that eukaryotes evolved from the union of some bacteria and archaea (one becoming an organelle and the other the main cell). Author : Eric Gaba. Published : Sep. 2006. Nasa Astrobiology Institute. http://en.wikipedia.org/wiki/File:Phylogenetic_tree.svg

2. What are prokaryotes?

It is essential to define prokaryotes. The prokaryotes are a group of organisms that lack a cell nucleus (= karyon), or any other membrane-bound organelles. The organisms that have a cell nucleus are called eukaryotes. (Figure 4) Most prokaryotes are unicellular, but a few such as myxobacteria have multicellular stages in their life cycles. The word *prokaryote* comes from the Greek πρό- *(pro-)* "before" + καρυόν *(karyon)* "nut or kernel". Prokaryotes do not have a nucleus, mitochondria, or any other membrane-bound organelles. In other words, neither their DNA nor any of their other sites of metabolic activity are collected together in a discrete membrane-enclosed area. Instead, everything is openly accessible within the cell, some of which is free-floating. Prokaryotes belong to two taxonomic domains: the bacteria and the archaea. Archaea were recognized as a domain of life in 1990. These organisms were originally thought to live only in inhospitable conditions such as extremes of temperature, pH, and radiation but have since been found in all types of habitats."

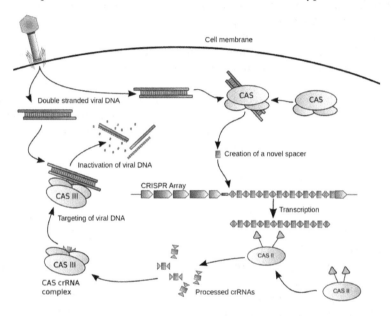

Fig. 5. Diagram of the possible mechanism for CRISPR. http://en.wikipedia.org/wiki/ File:Crispr.png Author: James Atmos 15 September 2009.

3. CRIPSR: Clustered, Regularly Interspaced Short Palindromic Repeat

3.1 CRIPSR (Clustered Regularly Interspaced Short Palindromic Repeats)

CRISPRs are loci containing multiple short direct repeats that are found in the genomes of approximately 40% of bacteria and 90% of archaea. CRISPR functions as a prokaryotic immune system, in that it confers resistance to exogenous genetic elements such as plasmids and phages. The CRISPR system provides a form of acquired immunity. Short segments of foreign DNA, called spacers, are incorporated into the genome between CRISPR repeats, and serve as a 'memory' of past exposures. CRISPR spacers are used to recognize and silence exogenous genetic elements in a way analogous to RNAi in eukaryotic organisms (Fig 5) (2, Grissa et al 2007; Barrangou et al 2007; Marraffini and Sontheimer 2010; Marraddini and Sontheimer 2010).

3.2 Self versus non-self discrimination during CRISPS RNA-directed immunity

All immune systems must distinguish self from non-self to repel invaders without inducing autoimmunity. Clustered, regularly interspaced, short palindromic repeat (CRISPR) loci protect bacteria and archaea from invasion by phage and plasmid DNA through a genetic interference pathway. CRISPR loci are present in ~ 40% and ~90% of sequenced bacterial and archaeal genomes respectively and evolve rapidly, acquiring new spacer sequences to adapt to highly dynamic viral populations. Immunity requires a sequence match between the invasive DNA and the spacers that lie between CRISPR repeats[1]. Each cluster is genetically linked to a subset of the *cas* (CRISPR-associated) genes that collectively encode >40 families of proteins involved in adaptation and interference. CRISPR loci encode small CRISPR RNAs (crRNAs) that contain a full spacer flanked by partial repeat sequences. CrRNA spacers are thought to identify targets by direct Watson-Crick pairing with invasive "protospacer" DNA, but how they avoid targeting the spacer DNA within the encoding CRISPR locus itself is unknown. Here we have defined the mechanism of CRISPR self/non-self discrimination. In *Staphylococcus epidermidis*, target/crRNA mismatches at specific positions outside of the spacer sequence license foreign DNA for interference, whereas extended pairing between crRNA and CRISPR DNA repeats prevents autoimmunity. Hence, this CRISPR system uses the base-pairing potential of crRNAs not only to specify a target but also to spare the bacterial chromosome from interference. Differential complementarity outside of the spacer sequence is a built-in feature of all CRISPR systems, suggesting that this mechanism is a broadly applicable solution to the self/non-self dilemma that confronts all immune pathways" (Marrafini & Sontheimer 2010).

3.3 CRISPR based adaptive and heritable immunity in prokaryotes

The recently discovered CRISPR (clustered regularly interspaced short palindromic repeat) defense system protects bacteria and archaea against mobile genetic elements. This immunity system has potential to continuously adjust its reach at the genomic level, implying that both gain and loss of information is inheritable. The CRISPR system consists of typical stretches of interspaced repetitive DNA (CRISPRs) and associated cas genes (van der Oost et al. 2009).

3.4 Hallmark of ingenious antiviral defense mechanisms

According to Al-Attar et al, many prokaryotes contain the recently discovered defense system against mobile genetic elements. (i) CRISPR-Adaptation, the invader DNA is encountered by the CRISPR/Cas machinery and an invader-derived short DNA fragment is incorporated in the CRISPR array. (ii) CRISPR-Expression, the CRISPR array is transcribed and the transcript is processed by Cas proteins. (iii) CRISPR-Interference, the invaders' nucleic acid is recognized by complementarity to the crRNA and neutralized (2011). An application of the CRISPR/Cas system is the immunization of industry-relevant prokaryotes (or eukaryotes) against mobile-genetic invasion. In addition, the high variability of the CRISPR spacer content can be exploited for phylogenetic and evolutionary studies. Despite impressive progress during the last couple of years, the elucidation of several fundamental details will be a major challenge in future research. (Fig 5)

3.5 Structural basis for CRIPSR RNA-guided DNA recognition by cascade and biology seahorse vs. pathogen

Here is the composition and low-resolution structure of casecade and how it recognizes double-stranded DNA (dsDNA) targets in a sequence-specific manner. Cascade is a 405-kDa complex comprising five functionally essential CRISPR-associated (Cas) proteins (CasA(1)B(2)C(6)D(1)E(1)) and a 61-nucleotide CRISPR RNA (crRNA) with 5'-hydroxyl and 2',3'-cyclic phosphate termini. Cascade recognizes target DNA without consuming ATP, which suggests that continuous invader DNA surveillance takes place without energy investment. The structure of Cascade shows an unusual seahorse shape that undergoes conformational changes when it binds target DNA (Jore et al. 2011). Jore et al. have analyzed the composition and low-resolution structure of the Cascade complex, which lies at the heart of the CRISPR Immune response. The snippets of invader sequence are transcribed and converted into CRISPR RNA (crRNA), which is bound by the Cascade complex. The overall structure of the Cascade complex surprisingly resembled the shape of the seahorse, with the spine and head consisting of a tight curved polymer of six CasC protein subunits, which might binf the crRNA- GR (Riddihough 2011).

3.6 Structures of the RNA-guided surveillance complex from a bacterial immune system

According to Wiedenheft et al (2011), bacteria and archaea acquire resistance to viruses and plasmids by integrating short fragments of foreign DNA into clustered regularly interspaced short palindromic repeats (CRISPRs). In *Escherichia coli*, crRNAs are incorporated into a multisubunit surveillance complex called Cascade (CRISPR-associated complex for antiviral defence), which is required for protection against bacteriophages. They used cryo-electron microscopy to determine the subnanometre structures of Cascade before and after binding to a target sequence. Cascade engages invading nucleic acids through high-affinity base-pairing interactions near the 5' end of the crRNA. Base pairing extends along the crRNA, resulting in a series of short helical segments that trigger a concerted conformational change. This conformational rearrangement may serve as a signal that recruits a trans acting nuclease (Cas3) for destruction of invading nucleic-acid sequences.

4. What are eukaryotes?

A eukaryote is an organism whose cells contain complex structures enclosed within membranes (Figure 4). Eukaryotes may more formally be referred to as the taxon Eukarya or Eukaryota. The defining membrane-bound structure that sets eukaryotic cells apart from prokaryotic cells is the nucleus, or nuclear envelope, within which the genetic material is carried. The presence of a nucleus gives eukaryotes their name, which comes from the Greek ευ (eu, "good") and κάρυον (karyon, "nut" or "kernel"). Most eukaryotic cells also contain other membrane-bound organelles such as mitochondria, chloroplasts and the Golgi apparatus. All species of large complex organisms are eukaryotes, including animals, plants and fungi, although most species of eukaryote are protist microorganisms.[Cell division in eukaryotes is different from that in organisms without a nucleus (prokaryotes). It involves separating the duplicated chromosomes, through movements directed by microtubules. There are two types of division processes. In mitosis, one cell divides to produce two genetically identical cells. In meiosis, which is required in sexual reproduction, one diploid

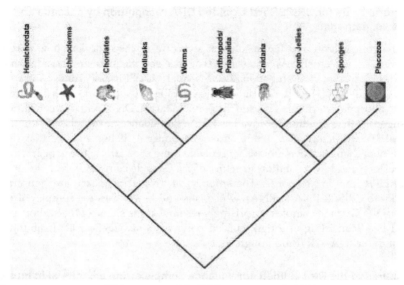

Fig. 6 New metazoan tree of life presented in Schierwater, et al. 2009
http://www.amnh.org/science/papers/metazoan.php Credit: AMNH

cell (having two instances of each chromosome, one from each parent) undergoes recombination of each pair of parental chromosomes, and then two stages of cell division, resulting in four haploid cells (gametes). Each gamete has just one complement of chromosomes, each a unique mix of the corresponding pair of parental chromosomes Eukaryotes appear to be monophyletic, and so make up one of the three domains of life. The two other domains, Bacteria and Archaea, are prokaryotes and have none of the above features. Eukaryotes represent a tiny minority of all living things; even in a human body there are 10 times more microbes than human cells.However, due to their much larger size their collective worldwide biomass is estimated at about equal to that of prokaryotes

5. Why was the 19th century crucial to the birth of immunology?

This provides an appropriate background for the analysis of eukaryotes. Darwin and Metchnikoff were laying the foundation for the "big bang" in immunology. It is not crystal clear when that occurred but surely whether directly or indirectly this revelation was the product of a coalescence of all the ferment that the 19th century inspired. In a sense, both were field biologists highly observant and meticulous – willing to take chances on the unexplored and to express their ideas. The inquisitiveness of Darwin and the consequence of Metchnikoff's single prescient observation by the sea both represent a *tour de force* in the annals of biology (Cooper et al 2002) The origin of species by natural selection underwent metamorphosis in its application to immunology and became the clonal selection theory with its inherent application to and explanation of adaptive immunity (Ribatti 2009] By contrast, Metchnikoff's phagocytosis in starfish larvae became the ancestor of innate immunity, even with the much later advent of T-cells (Silverstein 1989;, Tauber and Chernyak 1991, Besredka 1979). Darwin's well-known epic *The Origin of Species* was first published in 1859 when he was 50 years old and when Metchnikoff was only 14 years old.

The crossings and crisscrossing do continue. At 14 years Metchnikoff was already the budding zoologist imbued with an interest in animals, their lives and habitats quite the central thesis of Darwin's work as well that resulted from his now famous expeditions. Metcnikoff's observation split the monolithic field of immunology into two main camps, cellular and humoral giving cause to celebrate both investigations in 2008–2009.

6. From Darwin and Metchnikoff to Burnet and beyond

Phagocytosis in unicellular animals represents the most ancient and ubiquitous form of defense against foreign material. Unicellular invertebrates can phagocytose for food and defense. Multicellular invertebrates and vertebrates possess phagocytic cells and have evolved more complex functions attributed to immunodefense cells that specialized into sources of cellular and humoral immune responses. Thus all animals possess: innate, natural, nonspecific (no memory) nonanticipatory, nonclonal, germline (hard wired) host defense functions. In addition, all vertebrates possess: adaptive, induced, specific (memory), anticipatory, clonal, somatic (flexible) immune responses. A similar situation exists with respect to components of the signaling system, immunity and development. With multicellularity, clearly numerous immune response characteristics are not possible in unicellular forms or even those that straddle the divide between unicellularity and multicellularity, beginning with colonial/social protozoans. Still, it is instructive to elucidate a hierarchy of animals based upon immunologic characteristics and how they parallel other physiological traits. Evidence is presented that the most primitive of invertebrates prior to the evolution of multicellular organisms possess varying degrees of complexity at the molecular level of those hallmarks that now characterize the immune system.

According to Cooper (2008) we can now explore easily how potential external threats to life by continuously mutating microbes are first perceived, recognized, and the resulting signals interpreted and presumably survival from infection insured – or the blocking of cancer development an internal threat averted. This chapter will focus primarily on unicellular (Protozoa) and examples of multicellular animals (Sponges, Cnidarians); more complex invertebrates are excluded. Three reasons are presented. First, these two animal groups are situated at the nexus between single cell life and the emergence of multicellularity. Second, the unjustified thinking of immunologists would discredit these two groups with having evolved any semblance of an immune response other than phagocytosis. Third, the information that is included, i.e. the recent discovery of Toll-like receptors (TLRs) justified their inclusion. Finally, TLRs correlate with earlier information that substantiated the immunodefense capabilities as we knew them long ago and credit them today (Tables 1 and 2, Cooper 2008)

6.1 Emergence of modern immunology may be indebted to invertebrates?

This discovery of invertebrate phagocytosis dramatically changed the monolithic world of immunology. His careful and detailed observations of white cell motility toward and engulfment of foreign bodies in transparent larvae of starfish and in the water flea *Daphnia* provoked a major re-evaluation of the nature of immune systems, admittedly restricted to the human good. Before his prescient observations, immune systems were believed to be wholly humoral and there was little emphasis on the role of leukocytes or white cells. Metchnikoff's discovery, however, added cellular immunity to the known armory of

Genus & Species	Assessment of self and non- self activity	Results	Adhesion protein families and/or recognition system
Amoeba (*Amoeba preteus*) Amoeba discordes	Transplantation Allogeneic nuclei Xenogeneic nuclei	90% clones 0% clones 0% clones	-
Social amoebae (*Dictyostelium discoideum*) Slime molds	S cells Phagocytosis of bacteria	-	TIR domain proteins
Choanoflagellates (Unicellular colonial)	-	-	C-type lectins Tyrosine kinase signaling components
Ciliata Stentor Stenor coeruleus *Stentor polymorphus*	Lack of Chimera formation	Ejection of symbiotic *Chlorella*	-

Table 1. Recent evidence of signaling systems supported by early evidence of self and nonself recognition in unicellular species.

Genus & Species	Assessment of self and non- self activity	Results	Adhesion protein families and/or recognition system
Porifera Sponges *Microciona prolifera* *Cliona celata*	Mixing of red and yellow sponges	Disaggregated sponges to not reaggregate together	-
Demosponges *Suberites* *Domuncula*	Response to bacterial lipopeptides	-	TLR, IRAK-41, effector caspase sequence (SDCA, SL) Homologies in family-specific domains
Cnidaria Hydrozoa *Hydra* *Chlorphydra* *Pelmatohydra*	Allografts and xenografts	Incompatible transplant reactions	-
Anthozoa *Aborescent Cnidarians*	Autografts Allografts	Compatible Incompatible	-
Staghorn corals *Acropora*	Autografts Isografts Allografts	Compatible Incompatible Incompatible	-
Hydra magnipapillata *Nematostella vectensis*	- -		- -
Coral (*Acropora millepora*)			Canonical Toll/TLR Receptor C3, MAC/PF

Table 2. Evidence of signaling systems and early evidence of self and non-self recognition in multicellular animals (Porifera and Cnidaria).

humoral immunodefense mechanisms. Serendipity surely intervened and there was probably the impulse to shout Archimedes' *eureka* when the interpretation of why cells were moving toward a foreign body was easily visualized. Thus, the foundation for invoking the concept of self non-self recognition was laid (Cooper 1993).

Moreover, there is a much greater willingness to accept that invertebrate model systems have much more to contribute than was thought, even in the early 1960s when modern immunology was beginning to develop. Broadly interpreted, Darwin led us into the field and Metchnikoff into the laboratory at least with respect to comparative immunology (Cooper 1974; Cooper et al 1992). Evolutionary immunology reaped the benefits of Metchnikoff and modern immunology advanced conceptually when the clonal selection theory of Burnet was advanced – in essence a Darwinian corollary (Cooper 1974, Perlovsky 2010). According to Burnet (1962), 'The clonal-selection theory is a generalization about a wide range of biological phenomena but may suffer from the inherent weakness of all biological generalizations. The essence of the clonal-selection theory is that immunity and antibody production are functions of clones of mesenchymal cells. Each clone is characterized by the ability of its component cells to react immunologically with a very small number of antigenic determinants (Ribatti 2009).

Contact with the right antigenic configuration acts as a trigger to action and it is the essence of a clonal theory that such stimulation plays a major part in determining the observed changes in type and numbers of the mesenchymal cells of the body. The trigger of immunological contact is believed to provoke actions which, depending on many associated factors, may take one or other several forms. The cells may be killed or damaged, with release of cell-damaging or stimulating products; they may be stimulated to proliferate, with or without change of morphological type; or they may be converted to the plasma-cell form, with its capacity for active synthesis and liberation of antibody. Which particular reaction ensures will depend essentially on the physiological state of the cell and the nature of the internal environment to which it is exposed after stimulation.' (Burnet 1970) .

6.2 Origins of immune system components

6.2.1 Unicellular colonial protozoans

One approach to origin of animals is to determine which developmental proteins predated them and were subsequently co-opted for their development. Another strategy involves comparative genomics that can identify the minimal set of intact genes from the beginning of animal evolution that reveals those shared by all animals and their nearest relatives. Resolving the mystery of origins, these workers have sampled gene diversity expressed by choanoflagellates, unicellular and colonial protozoa that are closely related to metazoa, crucial for providing a possible clue into early animal evolution. Results revealed that choanoflagellates express representatives of a surprising number of cell-signaling and adhesion protein families not previously isolated from nonmetazoans; these include cadherins, C-type lectins, several tyrosine kinases and tyrosine kinase signaling pathway components. Choanoflagellates have a complex and dynamic tyrosine phosphoprotein profile, and tyrosine kinase inhibitors selectively affect cell proliferation. The expression in choanoflagellates of proteins involved in cell interaction in metazoa demonstrates that these proteins evolved before the origin of animals and were later co-opted for development. A similar situation exists with respect to components of the signaling system with respect to immunity and development. (Fig 6)

6.2.2 Emergence of multicellularity: social amoeba

Social amoebae feed on bacteria in the soil but aggregate when starved to form a migrating slug. Chen et al (2007) discovered an unknown cell type in social amoeba that is apparently involved in detoxification and immune-like functions; they call it the sentinel (S) cells. S cells engulf bacteria and sequester toxins while circulating within the slug, eventually being sloughed off. A Toll/interleukin-1 receptor (TIR) domain protein, TirA, is also required for certain S cell functions and for vegetative amoebae to feed on live bacteria. This apparent innate immune function in social amoebae, and the use of TirA for bacterial feeding, suggests an ancient cellular foraging mechanism that may have been adapted to defense functions well before the diversification of animals. Multicellularity likely increased the selective pressure on an organism's ability to avoid exploitation by pathogens. The role of TirA in *Dictyostelium's* response to bacteria provides t he first glimpse of an immune-related signaling system in amoeba and suggests that the use of TIR domain based signaling for defense represents an ancient function present in the progenitor of all crown group eukaryotes. If true, it would suggest that this system of pathogen recognition was advantageous to organisms before the evolution of multicellularity.

6.2.3 Sponges

Sponges (phylum Porifera) are filter feeders, therefore they are extremely exposed to microorganisms that represent a potential threat. Examining sponges, therefore moving to a higher taxonomic level, Wiens et al. 2007 have identified, cloned and deduced the protein sequence from 3 major elements of the poriferan innate response (to bacterial lipopeptides according to these definitions): the TLR, the interleukin-1 (IL-1) receptor-associated kinase-4-like protein (IRAK-4l), and a novel effector caspase from the demosponge *Suberites domuncula*. Each molecule shares significant sequence similarity with its homologues in higher metazoa. There are sequence homologies within the family-specific domains Toll/IL-1 receptor/resistance (TLR family), Ser/Thr/Tyr kinase domain (IRAK family), and CASc (caspase family).

6.2.4 Hydra and corals

Recently, whole genome sequences became available for two cnidarians, *Hydra magnipapillata* and *Nematostella vectensis*, and large expressed sequence tag datasets are available for them and for the coral *Acropora millepora*. (Powell 2007) A canonical Toll/TLR pathway in representatives of cnidarians of the class Anthozoa was observed. Neither a classic Toll/TLR receptor nor a conventional nuclear factor-β was identified in *Hydra* – an anthozoan. The detection of complement C3 and several membrane attack complex/perforin domain (MAC/PF) proteins suggests that a prototypic complement effector pathway may exist in anthozoans, but not in hydrozoans. Together with information for several other gene families, they suggest that *Hydra* may have undergone substantial secondary gene loss during evolution. Such patterns of gene distribution may underscore possible significance of gene loss during animal evolution but indicate ancient origins for components of vertebrate innate immune systems. (Miller et al 2007)

6.3 Toll-like receptors: innate sensing

Chen et al. (2007) review the earliest work in relation to current views. Phagocytes that engulf bacteria form part of the innate immune system of animals in the defense against pathogens. According to Beutler et al (2003), in humans innate immune sensing usually proceeds through the activation of 10TLRs, and these in turn lead to the production of cytokine mediators that create the inflammatory milieu and collaborate in developing an adaptive immune response. Each TLR senses a different molecular component of microbes that have invaded the host.

TLR4 senses bacterial endotoxins (lipopolysaccharide), TLR9 unmethylated DNA, and TLR3 double-stranded RNA. Each receptor has a conserved signaling element called the TIR (Toll/IL-1 receptor/resistance) motif that transduces a signal through five cytoplasmic adapter proteins, each of which has a homologous motif. (Hoffman 2004). With respect to TLRs, the integration of signals that receptors emit is a crucial mechanism that requires resolution. (Ferrandon et al 2004) By creating random germline mutations in mice and screening for individuals with differences in signaling potential, the complex biochemical circuitry of the innate immune response can be unraveled. Up to now, more than 35,000 germline mutants have been produced, and approximately 20,000 have been screened to predict innate immunodeficiency states (Medzhitov 2000).

6.3.1 Toll-like receptors in invertebrates and vertebrates: application to human diseases seems real

6.3.1.1 Annelids

Toll-like receptors (TLRs) are an important component of the innate immunity system and are found throughout the animal kingdom, but have not yet been fully analyzed in annelids. We searched shotgun reads of the genomes of the leech *Helobdella* and polychaete *Capitella* for TLR homologs. We found 10^5 TLR homologs in *Capitella* and 16 in *Helobdella* (Davidson et al 2011). The deduced phylogeny of these sequences, together with TLRs from other animal phyla, reveals three major clades (A clade is a group consisting of a species [extinct or extant] and all its descendants.). One clade consists of a mixture of both vertebrates and invertebrates, including sequences from *Capitella* and *Helobdella*, while the other two clades contain only invertebrate TLRs. Now these represent a beginning in need of further analysis especially with respect to p53 (TLR) and existence of cancer. This is needed since earthworm immune responses are well defined (Cooper et al 2002). Moreover early attempts to induce cancer were not successful (Cooper 1969); new trials are proposed combined with analyses of p53.

6.3.1.2 Molluscs

Toll-like receptor (TLR) signaling pathway is an important and evolutionarily conserved innate immune pathway. Phylogenetic lineage of this pathway in the Lophotrochozoans is still less understood. (The Lophotrochozoa comprise one of the major groups herein annelids and molluscs within the animal kingdom, In turn, the Lophotrochozoa belongs to a larger group within the Animalia called the Bilateria, because they are bilaterally symmetrical with a left and a right side to their bodies) is still less understood. Zhang and Zhang (2011) have cloned a novel TLR, a key component of TLR pathway, from the oyster, and named it CgToll-1. Real-time reverse transcription polymerase chain reaction analysis revealed that the highest CgToll-1 expression level was in hemolymph, and this pattern increased dramatically in the presence of bacteria *Vibrio anguillarum*. TLR pathway core genes of molluscs were searched and compared with model invertebrates revealing that their genes were closer to the fruit fly *Drosophila melanogaster* than to the purple sea urchin *Strongylocentrotus purpuratus*, while three upstream genes (MyD88, IRAK, TRAF6) were not closer. They also found that these two downstream genes were significantly more conserved than the three upstream genes based on amino acid sequence alignment. Results suggests that CgToll-1 is a constitutive and inducible protein that could play a role in immune responses against bacterial infection.

6.3.1.3 Ascidians

It is appropriate to present information on the ascidian since they are the nearest invertebrate relative of vertebrates (see Figs 1 and 2). According to Sasake et al (2009), key transmembrane proteins in the innate immune system, Toll-like receptors (TLRs), probably occur in the genome of non-mammalian organisms including invertebrates. However, authentic invertebrate TLRs have only been recently investigated structurally and functionally. Inflammatory cytokine production of the ascidian *Ciona intestinalis*, designated as Ci-TLR1 and Ci-TLR2 have been analyzed. The amino acid sequence of Ci-TLR1 and Ci-TLR2 possessed unique structural organization with moderate sequence similarity to functionally characterized vertebrate TLRs. *ci-tlr1* and *ci-tlr2* genes were mostly expressed in the stomach, and in hemocytes. Both Ci-TLR1 and Ci-TLR2 stimulate NF-κB induction in response to multiple pathogenic ligands such as double-stranded RNA, and bacterial cell wall components that are differentially recognized by respective vertebrate TLRs.This revealed that Ci-TLRs recognize broader pathogen-associated molecular patterns than vertebrate TLRs. The Ci-TLR-stimulating pathogenic ligands also induced expression of Ci-TNFα in intestine and stomach where Ci-TLRs are expressed. These results provide evidence that TLR-triggered innate immune systems are essentially conserved in ascidians, and that Ci-TLRs possess "hybrid" biological and immunological functions, compared with vertebrate TLRs. This is significant since ascidians are the nearest ancestor to vertebrates.

6.3.1.4 Birds

The Toll-Like receptor (TLR) pathway plays is crucial in innate immunity and is maintained with amazing consistency in all vertebrates. Considering this background of substantial conservation, any subtle differences in this pathway's composition may have important implications for species-specific defense against key pathogens. Cormican et al (2009) used a homology-based comparative method to characterize the TLR pathway the employed the recently sequenced chicken and zebra finch genomes from two distantly related bird species. Primary features of the TLR pathway are conserved in birds and mammals, despite some clear differences. TLR receptors show a pattern of gene duplication and gene loss in both birds when compared to mammals. They found avian specific duplication of both TLR1 and TLR2 and a duplication of the TLR7 gene in zebra finch. Both positive selection and gene conversion may shape evolution of avian specific TLR2 genes. Results contribute to characterization of differing immune responses that have evolved in individual vertebrates in response to their microbiological environment. Birds have been considered since they usually receive less coverage than mammals. Moreover without them we would have been slow to recognize the T and B system.

6.3.1.5 Disease and TLR

Now we consider an example of another disease related to the immune system, having presented cancer as the first example. It is well to remember however that cancer can now be considered to occur in invertebrates. This is a major resolution after many years of speculation concerning its absence. Ngoi et al (2001) have raised awareness of the incidence of allergic disorders and increased autoimmune diseases especially in developed nations. The hygiene hypothesis suggests that as a living environment becomes more sanitized, children are not exposed to microbial and parasitic stimulations that were once commonly acquired since early in life; this caused a lack of immune sensitization tending towards T helper 2 (Th2) dominance. Thus we can conclude that the immune system perhaps like the nervous system requires early learning experiences in order to respond to antigen stimulation. This view may explain allergic disorders, which mostly result from hyper Th2 responses, but inadequate in explaining Th1 or Th17-based autoimmunity increases.

With respect to signaling, recent advances in experimental mouse models revealed that stimulation of Toll-like receptors (TLRs) by pathogen-associated molecular patterns could reduce symptoms of allergic airway disease and prevent the onset of autoimmunity. For one explanation, the underlying mechanism for protective effects of TLR ligands is currently under investigation and there are indications that IL-10-producing B cells, regulatory T cells, and innate immune cells play an important role during this process. That early exposure to microbial byproducts probably contributes to modulation of immunological disorders may once again modify our interpretation of the hygiene hypothesis.

7. Cancer development in invertebrates may be linked to the presence of tumor suppressor genes independent of the innate immune system?

According to immunosurveillance, the adaptive immune system evolved to protect multicellular organisms against harmful invaders (bacteria, viruses, fungi — any disturbance of *non-self* material not acceptable to *self*) earlier thought of exclusively as threats from the external environment; however, internal threats may now include cancer cells growing out of control. These characteristics were restricted to vertebrates with adaptive immune responses. And invertebrates were not considered since it was assumed based mostly upon field observations that invertebrates with an innate system did not develop cancer. Some even assumed that the short life span of countless invertebrates precluded the development of any visible tumors. Thus the generalization: innate immunity either protects against cancer or it is so fast acting and efficient, more than the seemingly more complex vertebrate system that they do not develop cancer. Now it is becoming increasingly clear that invertebrates may also develop cancer. It seems safe to conclude that the influence may rest partially on **p53** or its family members: **p63, 73.**

p53 (also known as **protein 53** or **tumor protein 53**), is a tumor suppressor protein that in humans is encoded by the *TP53* gene. **p53** is crucial in multicellular organisms, where it regulates the cell cycle and, thus, functions as a tumor suppressor that is involved in preventing cancer. As such, **p53** has been described as "the guardian of the genome", the "guardian angel gene", and the "master watchman", referring to its role in conserving stability by preventing genome mutation. *p53* continues to be one of the most intensively studied genes in cancer biology. **p53** was initially identified >20 years ago as a binding partner for the SV40 T oncoprotein. Further studies revealed that **p53** is a tumor suppressor gene that is mutated or inactivated in >50% of human cancers. Furthermore, germ-line **p53** mutations cause hereditary cancer in both mice and humans. Molecular and biochemical assays revealed that the **p53** protein is a sequence-specific DNA-binding transcription factor. **p53** plays a central role in cellular responses to aberrant growth signals and certain cytotoxic stresses, such as DNA damage, by enhancing the transcription of genes that regulate a variety of cellular processes including cell cycle progression, apoptosis, genetic stability, and angiogenesis.

According to Walker et. al., (2011) the human **p53** tumor suppressor protein is inactivated in many cancers; it is also crucial in apoptotic responses to cellular stress. **p53** protein and the two other members (**p63, p73**) are encoded by distinct genes, whose functions have been extensively documented for humans and other vertebrates. The structure and relative expression levels for members of the **p53** superfamily have also been reported for most invertebrates. Using classical model organisms (nematodes, anemones and flies) reveal that the gene family originally evolved to mediate apoptosis of damaged germ cells or to protect germ cells from genotoxic stress. Analyses of **p53** signaling pathways in marine bivalve cancer and stress biology studies suggest that **p53** and **p63/73**-like proteins in soft shell clams (*Mya arenaria*), blue mussels (*Mytilus edulis*) and Northern European squid (*Loligo forbesi*) have identical core sequences. Still we know little about the molecular biology of marine invertebrates to address molecular mechanisms that characterize particular diseases. Understanding the molecular basis of naturally occurring diseases in marine bivalves is a virtually unexplored aspect of toxicoproteomics and genomics and related drug discovery. Marine bivalves could provide the most relevant and best understood models for experimental analyses by biomedical and marine environmental researchers.

The *Drosophila* tumor-suppressor gene lethal malignant brain tumor [l(3)mbt] (Bonasio et al., 2010) was first identified as a temperature-sensitive mutation that caused malignant growth in the larval brain (Gateff, et al 1993). These long awaited observations provided ample background for further analysis after discovery of tumor suppressors. According to Janic et al (2010), model organisms such as the fruit fly *Drosophila melanogaster* can help to elucidate the molecular basis of complex diseases such as cancer. Mutations in the *Drosophila* gene lethal malignant brain tumor (mbt) cause malignant growth in the larval brain. It has been shown that l(3)mbt tumors exhibited a soma-to-germline transformation through the ectopic expression of genes normally required for germline stemness, fitness, or longevity. Orthologs of these genes are also known to be expressed in human somatic tumors. Moreover, inactivation of any of the germline genes *nanos, vasa, piwi*, or *aubergine* suppressed l(3)mbt malignant growth. There was a consensus: results demonstrated that germline traits are necessary for tumor growth in this *Drosophila* model. Moreover inactivation of germline genes might have tumor-suppressing effects in other species which could inspire further investigations especially in those other invertebrates such as earthworms in which innate immune systems are well defined (Cooper et al 2002).

Receiving support for the work of Janic et al, Wu and Ruvkun (2010) suggest that cancer cells and germ cells share several characteristics. For instance, both have the ability to rapidly proliferate, typically do not lose the ability to divide as they age (lack senescence), and exist in undifferentiated states. Although some genes involved in cancer may initiate disease simply by activating cell division, others may promote tumors by activating early developmental pathways associated with programming for multipotency (the ability to differentiate into different cell types). Janic et al. (2010) have revealed that in fruit flies several genes typically involved in early programming of germline cells also play a role in the formation of malignant brain tumor. Moreover by inactivating these germ cell genes—some of which have related genes abnormally expressed in certain human cancers—can suppress tumor growth, suggesting new and future avenues for developing therapy.

If the expression of germline characteristics is common in tumors, for instance, it should be observable in gene expression analyses of human tumors. Indeed, the Piwil2 protein, a human Piwi family member, is widely expressed in several solid tumors. It should be feasible to examine more carefully the expression of germ cell genes, including *vasa* and *nanos*, in human tumors by microarray or deep RNA sequencing. The retinoblastoma tumor that stimulated analysis of this pathway provides a suitable candidate for studying germline gene activity in tumorigenesis. In addition, mutations in the human homologs of L(3)MBT, Rb, and its chromatin cofactors may be common in cancer genomes as they are sequenced. A query of the human homologs of these genes at the Cosmic web site (www.sanger.ac.uk/genetics/CGP/cosmic), for instance, revealed somatic mutations in L(3)MBT, Rb, and CHD3 (an Mi2 homolog) in a small fraction of tumors. Because there are so many mutations in these tumors, however, a more sophisticated statistical analysis is needed. The up-regulation of germline pathways in the l(3)mbt brain tumors and the required role for some of these genes in tumor growth also suggest new possibilities for tumor therapy. These genes are also conserved in mammals and could be potential targets for drugs that treat tumors similar to those analyzed by Janic et al. (2010)

Let us focus on new information that correlates with an animal model and cancer development. According to Read, (2011) glioblastomas (GBM), the most common primary brain tumors, infiltrate the brain, grow rapidly, and are refractory to current therapies. To analyze the genetic and cellular origins of this disease, a novel *Drosophila* GBM model is now available; Glial progenitor cells give rise to proliferative and invasive neoplastic cells that create transplantable tumors in response to constitutive co-activation of the EGFR-Ras and PI3K pathways. Since there is relevance of *Drosophila* to human cancer, neurological disease, and neurodevelopment, this fly model represents a neurological disease model wherein malignant cells are created by mutations in genetic pathways that may act in a homologous human disease. By using lineage analysis and cell-type specific markers, neoplastic glial cells presumably originated from committed glial progenitor cells, and not from multipotent neuroblasts. Genetic analyses demonstrated that EGFR-Ras and PI3K induce fly glial neoplasia through activation of a combinatorial genetic network that is partially comprised of other genetic pathways that are also mutated in human glioblastomas. Future research should focus on extensive genetic screens utilizing this model that could reveal new insights into origins and treatments of human glioblastoma.

8. Perspectives on parasitsm, cancer and immunity

For the past half-century, the dominant paradigm of oncogenesis has been mutational changes that disregulate cellular control of proliferation. The growing recognition of the molecular mechanisms of pathogen-induced oncogenesis and the difficulty of generating oncogenic mutations without first having large populations of dysregulated cells, however, suggests that pathogens, particularly viruses, are major initiators of oncogenesis for many if not most cancers, and that the traditional mutation-driven process becomes the dominant process after this initiation. Molecular phylogenies of individual cancers should facilitate testing of this idea and the identification of causal pathogens (Ewald 2009).

9. Pathogen survival in the external enviornment and the evolution of virulence

Recent studies have provided evolutionary explanations for much of the variation in mortality among human infectious diseases. Walther and Ewald's findings bear on several areas of active research and public health policy: (1) many pathogens used in the biological control of insects are potential sit-and-wait pathogens as they combine three attributes that are advantageous for pest control: high virulence, long durability after application, and host specificity; (2) emerging pathogens such as the 'hospital superbug' methicillin-resistant *Staphylococcus aureus* (MRSA) and potential bio-weapons pathogens such as smallpox virus and anthrax that are particularly dangerous can be discerned by quantifying their durability; (3) hospital settings and the AIDS pandemic may provide footholds for emerging sit-and-wait pathogens; and (4) studies on food-borne and insect pathogens point to future research considering the potential evolutionary trade-offs and genetic linkages between virulence and durability (2004).

All evidence indicates that clonal selection is purely a vertebrate strategy and therefore irrelevant to invertebrates. Some views may insist that anthropocentric mammalian immunologists utilized a tool to propel: the universal innate immune system of ubiquitous and plentiful invertebrates as an essential system for vertebrates. Innate immunity should help if there is a failure of the adaptive immune system. Still to be answered are questions concerning immunologic surveillance that includes clonal selection. We can then ask does immunologic surveillance play a role in the survival of invertebrates that most universally seem to not develop cancer at least of the vertebrate type. Perhaps invertebrates with their efficient innate immune system evolved certain "canceling devices" that maintain survival with short life spans, thus precluding their demise by metastasis.

10. Ancient neurons regulate immunity: innate innervation

According to Tracy (2011), the most evolutionarily ancient type of immunity, called "innate," exists in all living multicellular species. When exposed to pathogens or cellular damage, cells of an organism's innate immune system activate responses that coordinate defense against the insult, and enhance the repair of tissue injury. There is a modern-day cost associated with these processes, however, because innate mechanisms can damage normal tissue and organs, potentially killing the host. Human life is a balance between dual threats of insufficient innate immune responses – which would allow pathogens to prevail – and overabundant innate immune responses – which would kill or impair directly. What has been the key to maintaining this balance throughout years of mammalian evolution?

In this study, the nervous system controlled the activity of a noncanonical UPR pathway required for innate immunity in *Caenorhabditis elegans*. OCTR-1, a putative octopamine G protein–coupled catecholamine receptor (GPCR, G protein–coupled receptor), functioned in sensory neurons designated ASH and ASI to actively suppress innate immune responses by down-regulating the expression of noncanonical UPR genes*pqn/abu* in nonneuronal tissues. Findings suggest a molecular mechanism by which the nervous system may sense inflammatory responses and respond by controlling stress-response pathways at the organismal level.

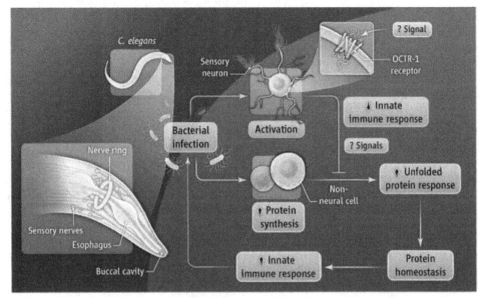

Fig. 7. Infection of *C. elegans* with a pathogen stimulates the innate immune response and activates the synthesis of new proteins, potentially causing the accumulation of unfolded proteins in host cells. (Tracey, 2011) The OCTR-1 receptor in the sensory neurons is required for this effect (figure 5). http://designmatrix.wordpress.com/ 2009/02/03/front-loading-neurons-more-supporting-evidence.

11. Perspectives

Clearly engaging TLRs activates various inflammatory and innate immune responses throughout the animal and plant kingdoms. This is associated with the innate immune system and must depend therefore on the presence, at least for now, of a multicellular system. Thus we would not expect as far as we have current information that prokaryotes would have evolved such a system. At the moment it is even with great difficulty to imagine such. Of course the thrust of this chapter refutes common dogma for it reports the existence of adaptive immunity in prokaryotes! But this impasse has been due to restricted definitions and these in turn due to restricted information based primarily on the dearth of molecular data. Ongoing efforts in many laboratories have led to the identification of TLR-specific signaling components and cellular responses within every major group –setting aside a wealth of new taxonomic data based on TLR. Perhaps this is a turning point in that the existence of TLR is so very basic, it seems inconceivable that investigations will reveal significant departures from what we know already. TLRs function in combination with additional pattern-recognition receptors and co-receptors to add further diversity to their role *in vivo*. How hosts integrate information that is signaled through TLRs and any co-receptors will ultimately control progression of the immune response to pathogens. Understanding this process will surely lead to newer fields that seek to develop novel therapeutics and immune boosting products.

Toll-like receptors (TLRs) are pattern-recognition receptors related to the *Drosophila* Toll protein (Adams 2009). TLR activation alerts the immune system to microbial products and initiates innate and adaptive immune responses. The naturally powerful immunostimulatory property of TLR agonists can be exploited for active immunotherapy against cancer. Antitumor activity has been demonstrated in several cancers, and TLR agonists are now undergoing extensive clinical investigation. Once there is more information, field and will focus on opportunities for clinical development of TLR agonists as single agent immunomodulators, vaccine adjuvants and in combination with conventional cancer therapies.

12. Conclusion

Perlovsky (2010) poses a pervasive and difficult question that challenges the utility of the immune system in relation to survival "Why deadly diseases exist from an evolutionary viewpoint? Some diseases, e.g. Influenza are clear; the disease agents are multiplying inside the host. But why cancer exists? According to surveillance, cancer poses an internal threat, in which cells no longer become recognizable as *self* (self/not self model) and therefore become cancerous and out of control. In this instance, the driving force for evolution of the immune system could be to effectively keep potentially cancerous cells in check, not allowing their uncontrolled metastases.

This review has covered enormous ground with respect to the immune system beginning with the view that microbes possess a form of adaptive immunity for protection against invading viruses. This is an interesting view and renders the immune system more encompassing than previous conceptions. By including the prokaryotes and eukaryotes and analyzing their responses to survival the immune system embraces a newer and broader scope than before when it was restricted to the higher eukaryotes. Gradually we have come to accept the innate immune system that characterizes the armamentarium of plants, invertebrates and vertebrates, it is only the vertebrates which at the moment whose immune system is associated with the appearance of cancer. Now two other points are worthy to raise and may bring us to another level of understanding of the immune system and in this light, I present at least two views concerning living systems in general and the immune system in particular.

In a recent review, the existence of artificial immune systems (AIS) has been presented (Cooper, 2010). Although not clearly defined, it is assumed that the field of AIS concerns an analysis of and development of computationally interesting abstractions of the immune system. Relevant to the current review there is the suggestion that to understand AIS could be inspired from organisms that possess only innate immune system. Moreover there is the suggestion that AISs should employ systemic models of the immune system in order to construct their overall design. For precision AIS should include plant and invertebrate immune systems.

Now we approach a new view presented recently by Bruce Alberts, Editor in Chief of Science (2011). He suggests recently: "A Grand Challenge in Biology" posing several questions and solutions aimed at advancing the field of synthetic biology. He emphasizes the need for basic research aimed at attaining a deep understanding of the chemistry of life. He further urges that a complete catalog of the tens of thousands of different molecules present in a human or mouse cell, along with a map of their myriad mutual interactions, is likely to be obtained with the wide variety of different techniques that are now available. Now, we are even closer to the present chapter and certainly suggestive of relevance to prokaryote immune systems. Albert's suggests: "Because all living things on earth are related through evolution, one can bootstrap one's way to understanding human cells by discovering how simpler cells and organisms work". A detailed study of *Mycoplasma genitalium*, a tiny bacterium that causes human disease, suggests that it can grow and divide with a minimal set of only about 430 genes. This suggests that we may be largely ignorant of some critical functions of proteins, such as their roles in the exquisite spatial organization of the molecules inside cells. (Alberts 2011). Of particular relevance is an article in the news section devoted to virus immunity by George Church, written by Bohannon, J. (2011)

13. Acknowledgements

Acknowledgement: I acknowledge with pleasure the superb assistance of Jesus Heredia and Kyle Hirabayashi.

14. References

Adams S. (2009). Toll-like receptor agonists in cancer therapy. *Immunotherapy*. 2009 , 6, pp.(949-64), 101485158

Janic A, Mendizabal L, Llamazares S, Rossell D & Gonzalez C. (2010). Ectopic expression of germline genes drives malignant brain tumor growth in *Drosophila*. *Science*. 2010 Dec, pp.(1824-1827)

Al-Attar S., Westra E.R., van der Oost J., Brouns S.J. (2011) Clustered regularly interspaced short palindromic repeats (CRISPRs) the hallmark of an ingenious antiviral defense mechanism in prokaryotes. *Biol Chem*, 392, 4, pp. (277-89), 9700112

Alberts B. (2011). A grand challenge in biology. *Science* 333, 2011, pp.(120), 0404511

Barrangou R, Fremaux C, Deveau H, Richards M, Boyaval P, Moineau S, Romero DA & Horvath P. (2007). *CRISPR* provides acquired resistance against viruses in prokaryotes. *Science*. 2007 Mar. pp.(1709-1712)

Besredka A. (1979). *The story of an idea*. Rivenson A, Oestreicher R, Trans.]. Bend, OR: Maverick; 1979

Beutler B, Hoebe K, Du X, Ulevitch RJ: How we detect microbes and respond to them: the Toll-like receptors and their transducers. *J Leukoc Biol*, 74, 4 2003, October, 74 pp.(479–485), 0741-5400

Bonasio R, Lecona E, & Reinberg D. (2010). MBT domain proteins in development and disease.*Semin Cell Dev Biol*. 2010, 2, pp(221-30), 9607332

Bohannon, J. (2011). The Life Hacker. *Science* 333, pp.(1236-1237), 0404511 [

Burnett FM. (1959). The clonal selection theory of acquired immunity. Nasville, Vanderbilt University Press; 1959

Burnet, M. Role of the thymus and related organs in immunity. Br Med J. 1962 Sep 29;2(5308):807-11.

Burnet FM. (1970). *Immunological surveillance*. Oxford: Pergamon; 1970.

Chen G, Zhuchenko O, Kuspa A. (2007). Immune-like phagocyte activity in the social amoeba. *Science*. 2007, 317. pp.(678–81), 0404511

Cooper, E. L. 1969. Neoplasia and transplantation immunity in annelids. J. Nat. Cancer Inst. 31: 655-669.

Cooper EL, Rinkevich B, Uhlenbruck G, Valembois P. (1992). Invertebrate immunity: Another viewpoint. *Scand J Immunol* 1992;35, pp.(247–66), 0323767

Cooper EL. In: Cooper EL, Nisbet-Brown E, editors. *Developmental immunology.* New York: Oxford University Press; 1993. pp. (3–30),

Cooper EL, Kauschke E, Cossarizza A. (2002). Digging for innate immunity since Darwin and Metchnikoff. (2002). *Bioessays.* 2002 Apr;24(4) pp.(319-333) 8510851

Cooper EL, Kvell K, Engelmann P, Nemeth. Still waiting for the toll? P.*Immunol Lett.* 2006, Apr 15, 104, 1 pp,(18-28) , 7910006

Cooper, EL. From Darwin and Metchnikoff to Burnet and beyond. (2008). Contrib Microbiol. 2008, 15. pp(1-11), 1662-291X, 9815689

Cooper, E.L. Evolution of immune systems from self/not self to danger to artificial immune systems (AIS). *Phys Life Rev.* 2010 Mar;7(1):55-78 2009, 101229718

Cooper, E.L. Self/not self, innate immunity, danger, cancer potential. *Phys Life Rev.* 2010. Feb, pp.(85-86) 101229718

Cooper, EL. (2010). Evolution of immune systems from self/not self to danger to artificial immune systems (AIS). *Phys Life Rev. 2010 Mar, pp.(55-78),* 101229718

Cooper, EL. (2010). Self/not self, innate immunity, danger, cancer potential. *Phys Life Rev.* 2010 Feb 1. pp.(55-78) ,101229718

Cossarizza, A. (2010). Know thyself and recognize dangers: An evolutionistic view. Phys Life Rev. 2010 Mar. pp.(81-82), 1873-1457, 101229718

Davidson CR, Best NM, Francis JW, Cooper EL, & Wood TC. (2011). Toll-like receptor genes (TLRs) from *Capitella capitata* and *Helobdella robusta* (Annelida). *Jourl of Biol Chem.* 2011, 284, pp.(608-612), 7708205

Du Pasquier L, & Litman GW. (2000) Origin and evolution of he vertebrate immune system, current topics in microbiology and immunology.2000, Heidelberg, Germany, Springer, 3540664149

Engelmann P. and Nemeth. (2010). Immune evolution and autoimmunity. *Phys life Rev,* 2010. 7, 1, pp.(79-80), 101229718

Ewald PW. (2009). An evolutionary perspective on parasitism as a cause of cancer. *Adv Parasitol.* 2009, 68, pp.(21-43), 0370435

Ferrandon D, Imler JL, Hoffmann JA. Sensing infection in Drosophila: Toll and beyond. *Semi. Immunol.* 2004, 16,. pp.(43-53), 9009458

Franc NC, Dimarcq J-L, Lagueux M, Hoffmann J, & Ezekowitz RAB. (1996). Croquemort, a novel *Drosophila* hemocyte/macrophage receptor that recognizes apoptotic cells. *Immunity.* 1996, 4.5, pp.(431–43), 9432918

Gateff et al 1993. A temperature-sensitive brain tumor suppressor mutation of Drosophila melanogaster: developmental studies and molecular localization of the gene. Mech Dev. 1993 Apr, pp.(15-31),

Grissa I, Bouchon P, Pourcel C & Vergnaud G. (2008). On-line resources for bacterial micro-evolution studies using MLVA or CRISPR typing. *Biochimi.* 2008, April, pp.(660-668)

Hildemann WH, Raison RL, Cheung G, Hull CJ, Akaka L, & Okamoto J.(1977). Immunological specificity and memory in a scleractinian coral. *Nature.* 1977, 270, pp.(219–2230), 0410462

Hoffmann JA. (2004). Primitive Immune Systems., *Immunological Reviews* 2004, 198, pp.(5-9), 1600-065X

Jore, M.M., Lundgren, M., van Duijn, E., Bultema, J.B., Westra, E.R., Waghmare, S.P., Wiedenheft, B., Pul, U., Wurm, R., Wagner, R., Beijer, M.R., Barendregt, A., Zhou, K., Snijders, A.P., Dickman, M.J., Doudna, J.A., Boekema, E.J., Heck, A.J., van der Oost, J., Brouns, S.J. (2011) Structural basis for CRISPR RNA-guided DNA recognition by Cascade. *Nat Struct Mol Biol.* 2011 May, 18, 5, pp.(529-36), 101186374

Kvell K, Cooper EL, Engelmann P, Bovari J, Nemeth. (2007). Blurring borders: innate immunity with adaptive features. (2007). *P.Clin Dev Immunol.* 2007, pp.(1-10), 101183692

Luke A.J. O'Neill. (2011) Innate Immunity in Plants Goes to the PUB. (2011). *Science* 332, 2011, June, pp.(1386-1387), 0404511

Marraffini LA & Sontheimer EJ. (2010). CRISPR interference: RNA-directed adaptive immunity in bacteria and archaea. *Nat Rev Genet.* 2010 Mar, pp.(181-190)

Marraffini LA & Sontheimer EJ. (2010). Self versus non-self discrimination during CRISPR RNA-directed immunity. *Nature* 2010, pp.(568-571)

Medzhitov R, Janeway Jr.C. (2000). The toll receptor family and microbial recognition. *Trends Microbiol* 2000, 10, pp.(452–456), 9310916

Mendizabal JL, LLamazares S, Rossell D, & Gonzalez C. (2010). Ectopic Expression of Germline Genes Drives Malignant Brain Tumor Growth in Drosophila. *Science.* 2010, 330, pp.(1824-1827), 0404511

Miller DJ, Hemmrich G, Ball EE, Hayward DC, Khalturin K, Funayama N, Agata K, Bosch TC. (2007). The innate immune repertoire in cnidaria—ancestral complexity and stochastic gene loss. *Genome Biol* 2007;8. pp.(1–13), 100960660

Ngoi SM, Sylvester FA, & Vella AT. (2011). The role of microbial byproducts in protection against immunological disorders and the hygiene hypothesis. *Discov Med.* 2011, 12.66, pp.(405-12), 101250006

Pancer Z. (2000). Dynamic expression of multiple scavenger receptor cysteine-rich genes in coelomocytes of the purple sea urchin. *Proc Natl Acad Sci.* 2000, 97, pp.(13156–61), 7505876

Parrinello. (2010). "Has innate immunity evolved through different routes?" 85-7. *Phys Life Rev* 2010, 7, pp.(83-84), 101229718

Perlovsky L. 2010; Cooper, E.L. Self/not self, innate immunity, danger, cancer potential. Phys Life Rev, 2010 pp.(55-78), 101229718

Powell AE, Nicotra ML, Moreno MA, Lakkis FG, Dellaporta SL, Buss LW. (2007). Differential effect of allorecognition loci on phenotype in *Hydractinia symbiolongicarpus* (Cnidaria: Hydrozoa). *Genetics.* 2007, 177, pp.(2101-2107) 0374636

Pradeu T. and E.D. Carosella. (2004). Critical analysis of the immunological self/non-self model and of its implicit metaphysical foundations. 2004, 325, 5, pp.(481–492), 101140040

Pradeu T. and E.D. Carosella. (2006). On the definition of a criterion of immunogenicity. *Proc Natl Acad Sci USA*, 2006, 103, 47, pp. (17858–1786), 7505876

Read RD. (2011). Drosophila melanogaster as a model system for human brain cancers. *Glia.* 2011, 59., pp.(1364-76), 8806785

Ribatti D. (2009). Sir Frank Macfarlane Burnet and the clonal selection theory of antibody formation, Clin Exp Med 2009, December, 4, pp.(253-258), 100973405

Riddihough, G. (2011). Structural biology Seahorse Versus Pathogen. *Nat. Struct. Mol. Biol,* 2011, pp.(10), 18, 10.1038/nsmb.2019 (2011).

Sasake Ni, Ogasawara M, Sekiguchi, T, Kusumoto S, & Satake H. (2011). Prototypes with Hybrid Functionalities of Vertebrate Toll-Like Receptors. *Fish Shellfish Immunol.* 2011, 30, pp.(653-660), 2985121R

Silverstein AM. *A history of immunology.* San Diego: Academic Press; 1989.

Sun S-C, Lindstrom I, Boman HG, Faye I, & Schmidt O. (1990). Hemolin: An insect-immune protein belonging to the immunoglobulin superfamily. *Science.* 1990, 250, pp.(1729-32), 0404511

Tauber AI, Chernyak L. (1991). *Metchnikoff and the origins of immunology: From metaphor to theory.* New York: Oxford University Press; 1991.

Theodor JL. (1970). Distinction between "self" and "not-self" in lower invertebrates. *Nature* 1970,227, pp.(690-692), 0410462

Tracey KJ. (2011). Ancient Neurons Regulate Immunity. *Science.* 2011, May, 332, 6030 pp.(673-674), 0404511

Van der Oost J, Jore MM, Westra ER, Lundgren M, Brouns SJ. CRISPR-based adaptive and heritable immunity in prokaryotes. *Trends Biochem Sci.* 2009, Aug, 34, 8, pp.(401-407), 7610674

Walther BA, Ewald PW. Pathogen survival in the external environment and the evolution of virulence. *Biol Rev Camb Philos Soc.* 2004, Nov, 79, 4, pp.(849-869), 0414576

Walker CW, Van Beneden RJ, Muttray AF, Böttger SA, Kelley ML, Tucker AE, & Thomas WK. (2011). Superfamily proteins in marine bivalve cancer and stress biology. *Adv Mar Biol.* 2011, 59, pp.(1-36), 0370431

Watson FL, Püttmann-Holgado R, & Thomas F. (2005). Immunology: Extensive diversity of Ig-superfamily proteins in the immune system of insects. *Science.* 2005, 309. pp.(1874-8), 0404511

Wiedenheft, B., Lander, G.C., Zhou, K., Jore, M.M., Brouns, S.J.J., van der Oost, J., Doudna, J.A., & Nogales E., Structures of the RNA-guided surveillance complex from a bacterial immune system. *Nature* 477, pp.(486–489), 0410462

Wiens M, Korzhev M, Perovic-Ottstadt S, Luthringer B, Brandt D, Klein S, Müller WE: Toll-like receptors are part of the innate immune defense system of sponges (demospongiae: Porifera). *Mol Biol Evol.* 2007, 24. pp.(792–804), 8501455

Wikipedia CRISPR. http://en.wikipedia.org/wiki/CRISPR

Wikipedia Prokaryotes. http://en.wikipedia.org/wiki/Eukaryote

Wu X & Ruykun G. (2010). Cancer. Germ cell genes and cancer..Science. 2010, 330 pp.(1761-1762), 0404511

Zhang S-M, Adema CM, Kepler TB, & Loker ES. (2004). Diversification of Ig superfamily genes in an invertebrate. *Science.* 2004, 305, pp.(251–4). 0404511

Zhang L., Li L., & Zhang G (2011). *Crassostrea gigas* Toll-like receptor and comparative analysis of TLR pathway in invertebrates. *Fish Shellfish Immunol.* 2011, 2, pp.(653-60), 9505220

Permissions

The contributors of this book come from diverse backgrounds, making this book a truly international effort. This book will bring forth new frontiers with its revolutionizing research information and detailed analysis of the nascent developments around the world.

We would like to thank Dr. Jagat R. Kanwar, for lending his expertise to make the book truly unique. He has played a crucial role in the development of this book. Without his invaluable contribution this book wouldn't have been possible. He has made vital efforts to compile up to date information on the varied aspects of this subject to make this book a valuable addition to the collection of many professionals and students.

This book was conceptualized with the vision of imparting up-to-date information and advanced data in this field. To ensure the same, a matchless editorial board was set up. Every individual on the board went through rigorous rounds of assessment to prove their worth. After which they invested a large part of their time researching and compiling the most relevant data for our readers. Conferences and sessions were held from time to time between the editorial board and the contributing authors to present the data in the most comprehensible form. The editorial team has worked tirelessly to provide valuable and valid information to help people across the globe.

Every chapter published in this book has been scrutinized by our experts. Their significance has been extensively debated. The topics covered herein carry significant findings which will fuel the growth of the discipline. They may even be implemented as practical applications or may be referred to as a beginning point for another development. Chapters in this book were first published by InTech; hereby published with permission under the Creative Commons Attribution License or equivalent.

The editorial board has been involved in producing this book since its inception. They have spent rigorous hours researching and exploring the diverse topics which have resulted in the successful publishing of this book. They have passed on their knowledge of decades through this book. To expedite this challenging task, the publisher supported the team at every step. A small team of assistant editors was also appointed to further simplify the editing procedure and attain best results for the readers.

Our editorial team has been hand-picked from every corner of the world. Their multi-ethnicity adds dynamic inputs to the discussions which result in innovative outcomes. These outcomes are then further discussed with the researchers and contributors who give their valuable feedback and opinion regarding the same. The feedback is then collaborated with the researches and they are edited in a comprehensive manner to aid the understanding of the subject.

Apart from the editorial board, the designing team has also invested a significant amount of their time in understanding the subject and creating the most relevant covers. They scrutinized every image to scout for the most suitable representation of the subject and create an appropriate cover for the book.

The publishing team has been involved in this book since its early stages. They were actively engaged in every process, be it collecting the data, connecting with the contributors or procuring relevant information. The team has been an ardent support to the editorial, designing and production team. Their endless efforts to recruit the best for this project, has resulted in the accomplishment of this book. They are a veteran in the field of academics and their pool of knowledge is as vast as their experience in printing. Their expertise and guidance has proved useful at every step. Their uncompromising quality standards have made this book an exceptional effort. Their encouragement from time to time has been an inspiration for everyone.

The publisher and the editorial board hope that this book will prove to be a valuable piece of knowledge for researchers, students, practitioners and scholars across the globe.

List of Contributors

Nathalie Compté and Stanislas Goriely
Institute for Medical Immunology, Université Libre de Bruxelles, Belgium

Miroslava Kuricova, Jana Tulinska, Aurelia Liskova, Mira Horvathova, Silvia Ilavska, Zuzana Kovacikova, Marta Hurbankova, Silvia Cerna, Eva Jahnova, Eva Neubauerova, Ladislava Wsolova and Sona Wimmerova
Slovak Medical University, Bratislava, Slovak Republic

Maria Dusinska
Slovak Medical University, Bratislava, Slovak Republic
NILU Norwegian Institute for Air Research, Kjeller, Norway

Elizabeth Tatrai
Department of Pathology, National Institute of Occupational Health, Budapest, Hungary

Laurence Fuortes
University of Iowa, College of Public Health, Iowa City, Iowa, USA

Soterios A. Kyrtopoulos
National Hellenic Research Foundation, Institute of Biological Research and Biotechnology, Athens, Greece

Johan Garssen and Léon M.J. Knippels
Pharmacology, Utrecht Institute for Pharmaceutical Sciences (UIPS), University of Utrecht, The Netherlands
Danone Research – Centre for Specialised Nutrition, Wageningen, The Netherlands and Friedrichsdorf, The Netherlands

Bastiaan Schouten
Danone Research – Centre for Specialised Nutrition, Wageningen, The Netherlands and Friedrichsdorf, The Netherlands

JoAnn Kerperien and Linette E.M. Willemsen
Pharmacology, Utrecht Institute for Pharmaceutical Sciences (UIPS), University of Utrecht, The Netherlands

Günther Boehm
Danone Research – Centre for Specialised Nutrition, Wageningen, The Netherlands and Friedrichsdorf, The Netherlands
Sophia Children's Hospital, Erasmus University Rotterdam, The Netherlands

Belinda van't Land
Danone Research – Centre for Specialised Nutrition, Wageningen, The Netherlands and Friedrichsdorf, The Netherlands
Wilhelmina Children's Hospital, University Medical Center, Utrecht, The Netherlands

Saba Tufail, Ravikant Rajpoot and Mohammad Owais
Aligarh Muslim University, India

Jalil Mehrzad
Sections Immunology and Biotechnology, Department of Pathobiology, Faculty of Veterinary Medicine, Iran
Institute of Biotechnology, Ferdowsi University of Mashhad, Mashhad, Iran

Alexandre de Castro
Laboratory of Computational Mathematics, National Center of Technological Research on Informatics for Agriculture (Embrapa Agriculture Informatics), Brazilian Agricultural Research Corporation (Embrapa), Campinas, Brazil

Rupinder Kanwar and Jagat R. Kanwar
Nanomedicine-Laboratory of Immunology and Molecular Biomedical Research (LIMBR), Centre for Biotechnology and Interdisciplinary Biosciences (BioDeakin), Institute for Technology & Research Innovation (ITRI), Deakin University, Geelong, Technology Precinct (GTP), Waurn Ponds, Geelong, Victoria, Australia

Rakesh Sehgal and Kapil Goyal
Department of Parasitology, Postgraduate Institute of Medical Education & Research, Chandigarh, India

Alka Sehgal
Government Medical College & Hospital, Sector 32, Chandigarh, India

Edwin L. Cooper
Laboratory of Comparative Neuroimmunology, Department of Neurobiology, David Geffen School of Medicine at UCLA, University of California, Los Angeles, USA